Aids to Radiological Differential Diagnosis

Aids to Radiological Differential Diagnosis

2nd Edition

Stephen Chapman

MB, BS, MRCP, FRCR

Consultant Radiologist
The Children's Hospital, Birmingham;
Honorary Senior Clinical Lecturer
University of Birmingham;
Senior Lecturer in Radiological Anatomy
University of Birmingham.

Richard Nakielny

MA, BM, BCh, FRCR

Consultant Radiologist
CT Body Scan Department
Royal Hallamshire Hospital, Sheffield;
Honorary Clinical Lecturer
University of Sheffield.

Baillière Tindall
London Philadelphia Toronto Sydney Tokyo

<u>Baillière Tindall</u>   24–28 Oval Road
W.B. Saunders   London NW1 7DX

The Curtis Center
Independence Square West
Philadelphia, PA 19106–3399, USA

55 Horner Avenue
Toronto, Ontario M8Z 4X6, Canada

Harcourt Brace Jovanovich Group (Australia) Pty Ltd
30–52 Smidmore Street
Marrickville
NSW 2204, Australia

Harcourt Brace Jovanovich Japan Inc
Ichibancho Central Building, 22–1 Ichibancho
Chiyoda-ku, Tokyo 102, Japan

©1990 Baillière Tindall

This book is printed on acid-free paper ∞

First published 1984
Second Edition 1990

Typeset by Photo·graphics, Honiton, Devon
Printed and bound in Great Britain by Richard Clay Ltd, Bungay, Sulfolk

---

British Library Cataloguing in Publication Data

Chapman, Stephen, *1953–*
Aids to radiological differential diagnosis. 2nd Edn.
I. Diagnosis, Radioscopic
I. Title II. Nakielny, Richard
616.07'57   RC78

ISBN 0-7020-1440-0

Contributors

Michael Collins
FRCR

Consultant Radiologist Royal Hallamshire Hospital, Sheffield; Honorary Clinical Lecturer University of Sheffield.

Keith Harding
BSc, MB, FRCP

Consultant in Nuclear Medicine Dudley Road Hospital, Birmingham; Senior Clinical Lecturer in Medicine University of Birmingham.

Josephine McHugo
MB BS, MRCP, FRCR

Consultant Radiologist Birmingham Maternity Hospital; Honorary Senior Clinical Lecturer University of Birmingham.

Contents

Foreword   xix

Preface to the First Edition   xx

Preface to the Second Edition   xxii

Explanatory Notes   xxiii

Abbreviations   xxiv

PART 1

1   Bones   3

1.1   Retarded skeletal maturation   3
1.2   Generalized accelerated skeletal maturation   4
1.3   Premature closure of a growth plate   4
1.4   Asymmetrical maturation   5
1.5   Dwarfing skeletal dysplasias   5
1.6   Lethal neonatal dysplasias   6
1.7   Conditions exhibiting dysostosis multiplex   7
1.8   Generalized increased bone density — children   8
1.9   Generalized increased bone density — adults   9
1.10   Solitary sclerotic bone lesion   10
1.11   Multiple sclerotic bone lesions   11
1.12   Bone sclerosis with a periosteal reaction   12
1.13   Solitary sclerotic bone lesion with a lucent centre   12
1.14   Coarse trabecular pattern   13
1.15   Excessive callus formation   13
1.16   Skeletal metastases — most common radiological
         appearances   13
1.17   Sites of origin of primary bone neoplasms   15
1.18   Peak age incidence of primary bone neoplasms   16
1.19   Lucent bone lesion in the medulla — well-defined,
         marginal sclerosis, no expansion   17
1.20   Lucent bone lesion in the medulla — well-defined,
         no marginal sclerosis, no expansion   17
1.21   Lucent bone lesion in the medulla — ill-defined   18
1.22   Lucent bone lesion in the medulla — well-defined,
         eccentric expansion   19
1.23   Lucent bone lesion — grossly expansile   20
1.24   Subarticular lucent bone lesion   21

1.25	Lucent bone lesion — containing calcium or bone	22
1.26	'Moth-eaten bone'	22
1.27	Regional osteopenia	23
1.28	Generalized osteopenia	23
1.29	Osteoporosis	24
1.30	Osteomalacia and rickets	26
1.31	Periosteal reactions — types	27
1.32	Periosteal reaction — solitary and localized	29
1.33	Periosteal reactions — bilaterally symmetrical in adults	30
1.34	Hypertrophic osteoarthropathy	31
1.35	Periosteal reactions — bilaterally symmetrical in children	32
1.36	Periosteal reactions — bilaterally asymmetrical	33
1.37	Differential diagnosis of skeletal lesions in non-accidental injury	34
1.38	Pseudarthrosis	35
1.39	Irregular or stippled epiphyses	36
1.40	Avascular necrosis	37
1.41	Solitary radiolucent metaphyseal band	38
1.42	Alternating radiolucent and dense metaphyseal bands	38
1.43	Solitary dense metaphyseal band	39
1.44	Dense vertical metaphyseal lines	39
1.45	Fraying of metaphyses	39
1.46	Cupping of metaphyses	40
1.47	Erlenmeyer flask deformity	40
1.48	Erosions of the medial metaphysis of the proximal humerus	40
1.49	Erosion or absence of the outer end of the clavicle	41
1.50	Focal rib lesion (solitary or multiple)	41
1.51	Rib notching — inferior surface	42
1.52	Rib notching — superior surface	43
1.53	Arachnodactyly	43
1.54	Distal phalangeal destruction	44
1.55	Short metacarpal(s) or metatarsal(s)	46
1.56	Carpal fusion	46
1.57	Madelung deformity	47
2	**Spine**	**52**
2.1	Scoliosis	52
2.2	Solitary collapsed vertebra	55
2.3	Multiple collapsed vertebrae	56
2.4	Platyspondyly in childhood	57
2.5	Erosion, destruction or absence of a pedicle	58
2.6	Solitary dense pedicle	58
2.7	Enlarged vertebral body	59
2.8	Squaring of one or more vertebral bodies	59

2.9	Block vertebrae	60
2.10	Ivory vertebral body	61
2.11	Atlanto-axial subluxation	62
2.12	Intervertebral disc calcification	63
2.13	Bony outgrowths of the spine	64
2.14	Coronal cleft vertebral bodies	65
2.15	Anterior vertebral body beaks	66
2.16	Posterior scalloping of vertebral bodies	66
2.17	Anterior scalloping of vertebral bodies	67
2.18	Anterior scalloping of the sacrum	68
2.19	Syndromes with a narrow spinal canal	68
2.20	Widened interpedicular distance	69
2.21	Spinal block	70
2.22	Extradural spinal masses	71
2.23	Intradural, extramedullary spinal masses	72
2.24	Intradural, intramedullary spinal masses	73

3	**Joints**	**77**
3.1	Monoarthritis	77
3.2	The major polyarthritides	78
3.3	Arthritis with osteoporosis	79
3.4	Arthritis with preservation of bone density	79
3.5	Arthritis with a periosteal reaction	79
3.6	Arthritis with preserved or widened joint space	79
3.7	Arthritis mutilans	80
3.8	Diffuse terminal phalangeal sclerosis	80
3.9	Erosion (enlargement) of the intercondylar notch of the distal femur	80
3.10	Calcified loose body (single or multiple) in a joint	81
3.11	Calcification of articular (hyaline) cartilage (chondrocalcinosis)	81
3.12	Sacroiliitis	82
3.13	Protrusio acetabuli	83
3.14	Widening of the symphysis pubis	83
3.15	Fusion or bridging of the symphysis pubis	84

4	**Respiratory Tract**	**87**
4.1	Acute upper airway obstruction	87
4.2	Chronic upper airway obstruction in a child	88
4.3	Chronic upper airway obstruction in an adult	90
4.4	Unequal lung size, lucency and vascularity. Which is the abnormal side?	91
4.5	Unilateral hypertransradiant hemithorax	92
4.6	Bilateral hypertransradiant hemithoraces	94
4.7	Bronchial stenosis or occlusion	95

x *Contents*

4.8	Increased density of a hemithorax	96
4.9	Pneumatocoeles	97
4.10	Slowly resolving or recurrent pneumonia	97
4.11	Pneumonia with an enlarged hilum	98
4.12	Lobar pneumonia	99
4.13	Consolidation with bulging of fissures	99
4.14	Bronchiectasis	100
4.15	Widespread air-space (acinar) disease	100
4.16	Localized air-space disease	102
4.17	Pulmonary oedema	103
4.18	Unilateral pulmonary oedema	104
4.19	Septal lines (Kerley B lines)	105
4.20	'Honeycomb lung'	106
4.21	Pneumoconioses	107
4.22	Multiple pin-point opacities	108
4.23	Multiple opacities (0.5–2 mm)	108
4.24	Multiple opacities (2–5 mm)	109
4.25	Solitary pulmonary nodule	110
4.26	Multiple pulmonary nodules (> 5 mm)	112
4.27	Lung cavities	113
4.28	Opacity with an air bronchogram	116
4.29	Pulmonary calcification or ossification	116
4.30	Unilateral hilar enlargement	118
4.31	Bilateral hilar enlargement	119
4.32	'Eggshell' calcification of lymph nodes	120
4.33	Upper zone fibrosis	121
4.34	Pleural effusion	122
4.35	Pleural effusion due to extrathoracic disease	123
4.36	Pleural effusion with an otherwise normal chest X-ray	124
4.37	Pneumothorax	125
4.38	Pneumomediastinum	126
4.39	Right-sided diaphragmatic humps	127
4.40	Unilateral elevated hemidiaphragm	128
4.41	Bilateral elevated hemidiaphragms	129
4.42	Pleural calcification	129
4.43	Local pleural masses	130
4.44	Rib lesion with an adjacent soft tissue mass	131
4.45	The chest radiograph following chest trauma	132
4.46	Neonatal respiratory distress	134
4.47	Ring shadows in a child	136
4.48	Drug-induced lung disease	136
4.49	Anterior mediastinal masses	138
4.50	Middle mediastinal masses	141
4.51	Posterior mediastinal masses	142
4.52	CT mediastinal mass containing fat	144
4.53	CT mediastinal cysts	145
4.54	CT thymic mass	146

5	**Cardiovascular System**	**151**
5.1	Gross cardiac enlargement	151
5.2	Small heart	151
5.3	Enlarged right atrium	152
5.4	Enlarged right ventricle	153
5.5	Enlarged left atrium	154
5.6	Enlarged left ventricle	155
5.7	Bulge on the left heart border	156
5.8	Cardiac calcification	156
5.9	Valve calcification	157
5.10	Large aortic arch	158
5.11	Small aortic arch	158
5.12	Right-sided aortic arch	159
5.13	Enlarged superior vena cava	159
5.14	Enlarged azygos vein	160
5.15	Enlarged pulmonary arteries	160
5.16	Enlarged pulmonary veins	161
5.17	Neonatal pulmonary venous congestion	161
5.18	Neonatal cyanosis	162
5.19	Cardiovascular involvement in syndromes	163
5.20	Complications of subclavian vein catheterization	164
6	**Abdomen and Gastrointestinal Tract**	**168**
6.1	Extraluminal intra-abdominal gas	168
6.2	Pneumoperitoneum	169
6.3	Gasless abdomen	170
6.4	Ascites	170
6.5	Abdominal mass in a neonate	171
6.6	Abdominal mass in a child	172
6.7	Intestinal obstruction in a neonate	174
6.8	Abnormalities of bowel rotation	175
6.9	Haematemesis	177
6.10	Dysphagia — adult	178
6.11	Dysphagia — neonate	180
6.12	Pharyngeal/oesophageal 'diverticula'	181
6.13	Oesophageal ulceration	182
6.14	Oesophageal strictures — smooth	184
6.15	Oesophageal strictures — irregular	185
6.16	Tertiary contractions in the oesophagus	186
6.17	Stomach masses and filling defects	186
6.18	Thick stomach folds	188
6.19	Linitis plastica	190
6.20	Gastrocolic fistula	190
6.21	Gastric dilatation	191
6.22	'Bull's eye' (target) lesion in the stomach	192
6.23	Gas in the stomach wall	193
6.24	Cobblestone duodenal cap	194

6.25	Decreased/absent duodenal folds	194
6.26	Thickened duodenal folds	195
6.27	Dilated duodenum	196
6.28	Dilated small bowel	197
6.29	Strictures in the small bowel	198
6.30	Thickened folds in non-dilated small bowel — smooth and regular	199
6.31	Thickened folds in non-dilated small bowel — irregular and distorted	201
6.32	Multiple nodules in the small bowel	202
6.33	Malabsorption	204
6.34	Protein-losing enteropathy	206
6.35	Lesions in the terminal ileum	207
6.36	Colonic polyps	208
6.37	Colonic strictures	211
6.38	Gas in the wall of the colon	212
6.39	Megacolon in an adult	213
6.40	Megacolon in a child	214
6.41	'Thumbprinting' in the colon	214
6.42	Aphthoid ulcers	215
6.43	Anterior indentation of the rectosigmoid junction	216
6.44	Widening of the retrorectal space	217
6.45	CT retroperitoneal cystic mass	218
6.46	CT mesenteric cystic lesion	218
7	**Gallbladder, Liver, Spleen, Pancreas and Adrenals**	**223**
7.1	Non-visualization of the gall bladder	223
7.2	Filling defect in the gall bladder	224
7.3	Gas in the biliary tract	225
7.4	Gas in the portal veins	226
7.5	Hepatomegaly	227
7.6	Hepatic calcification	228
7.7	Fetal or neonatal liver calcification	230
7.8	Ultrasound liver — generalized hypoechoic	230
7.9	Ultrasound liver — generalized hyperechoic ('bright' liver)	231
7.10	Ultrasound liver — focal hyperechoic	231
7.11	Ultrasound liver — focal hypoechoic	231
7.12	Ultrasound liver — periportal hyperechoic	232
7.13	CT liver — focal hypodense lesion pre intravenous contrast	232
7.14	CT liver — focal hyperdense lesion	235
7.15	CT liver — generalized low density pre intravenous contrast	236
7.16	CT liver — generalized increase in density pre intravenous contrast	237

7.17	CT liver — patchy areas of low density post intravenous contrast	237
7.18	Splenomegaly	238
7.19	Splenic calcification	239
7.20	Pancreatic calcification	240
7.21	CT focal pancreatic mass	242
7.22	Adrenal calcification	244
7.23	CT adrenal masses	245

8	**Urinary Tract**	**250**
8.1	Loss of renal outline on the plain film	250
8.2	Renal calcification	251
8.3	Renal calculi	253
8.4	Gas in the urinary tract	254
8.5	Non-visualization of one kidney during excretion urography	255
8.6	Unilateral scarred kidney	256
8.7	Unilateral small smooth kidney	258
8.8	Bilateral small smooth kidneys	259
8.9	Unilateral large smooth kidney	260
8.10	Bilateral large smooth kidneys	261
8.11	Localized bulge of the renal outline	263
8.12	Renal neoplasms	265
8.13	CT kidney — focal hypodense lesion	266
8.14	Classification of renal cysts	268
8.15	CT renal cysts	270
8.16	Renal mass in the newborn and young infant	271
8.17	Hydronephrosis in a child	271
8.18	Nephrogenic patterns	272
8.19	Renal papillary necrosis	273
8.20	Renal induced hypertension	274
8.21	Renal vein thrombosis	276
8.22	Non-visualization of a calyx	277
8.23	Radiolucent filling defect in the renal pelvis or a calyx	278
8.24	Dilated calyx	279
8.25	Dilated ureter	280
8.26	Retroperitoneal fibrosis	281
8.27	Filling defect in the bladder (in the wall or in the lumen)	282
8.28	Bladder calcification	283
8.29	Bladder fistula	284
8.30	Bladder outflow obstruction in a child	285
8.31	Calcification of the seminal vesicles or vas deferens	286

9	**Soft Tissues**	**290**
9.1	Gynaecomastia	290

9.2   Linear and curvilinear calcification in soft tissues   291
9.3   Conglomerate calcification in soft tissues   292
9.4   Sheets of calcification/ossification in soft tissues   293
9.5   Periarticular soft-tissue calcification   293
9.6   Soft-tissue ossification   294
9.7   Increased heel pad thickness   294

10   Mammography/*Michael Collins*   **297**

10.1   Benign *vs* malignant   297
10.2   Calcification   300
10.3   Benign conditions that mimic malignancy   302
10.4   Benign lesions with typical appearances   302
10.5   Single, well-defined soft tissue opacity   303
10.6   Multiple, well-defined soft tissue opacities   303
10.7   Large (> 5 cm) well-defined opacity   303
10.8   Mixed density, well-defined single opacity   304
10.9   Causes of disappearance of calcification   304
10.10   Oedematous breast   304
10.11   Ultrasound in breast disease   305
10.12   Breast cancer screening — Forrest report   305
10.13   Radiation risk from mammography   306

11   Face and neck   **309**

11.1   Unilateral exophthalmos   309
11.2   CT characteristics of orbital masses in children   310
11.3   Optic nerve enlargement   312
11.4   Optic nerve glioma *vs* orbital meningioma clinical
           and CT differentiation   313
11.5   Enlarged orbit   314
11.6   'Bare' orbit   314
11.7   Enlarged optic foramen   315
11.8   Enlarged superior orbital fissure   316
11.9   Intraorbital calcification   316
11.10   Hyperostosis in the orbit   317
11.11   Small or absent sinuses   317
11.12   Opaque maxillary antrum   317
11.13   Mass in the maxillary antrum   318
11.14   Cystic lesion in the mandible   319
11.15   'Floating' teeth   319
11.16   Loss of lamina dura of teeth   320
11.17   Mass in the nasopharynx   320
11.18   Prevertebral soft-tissue mass in the cervical region   321

12   Skull and Brain   **324**

12.1   Lucency in the skull vault, with no surrounding
           sclerosis — adult   324

12.2	Lucency in the skull vault, with no surrounding sclerosis — child	326
12.3	Lucency in the skull vault, with surrounding sclerosis	327
12.4	Multiple lucent lesions in the skull vault	328
12.5	Generalized thickening of the skull vault in children	328
12.6	Bone dysplasias with increased density of the skull	329
12.7	Generalized increase in density of the skull vault	330
12.8	Localized increase in density of the skull vault	331
12.9	Increase in density of the skull base	331
12.10	Destruction of the petrous bone — apex	332
12.11	Destruction of the petrous bone — middle ear	332
12.12	Metastases in the skull base	333
12.13	Basilar invagination	334
12.14	'Hair-on-end' skull vault	335
12.15	Craniostenosis	336
12.16	Wormian bones	337
12.17	Defective ossification of skull vault	338
12.18	Raised intracranial pressure	338
12.19	Large head in infancy	339
12.20	Wide sutures	340
12.21	Pneumocephalus	341
12.22	Small pituitary fossa	341
12.23	Expanded pituitary fossa	342
12.24	J-shaped sella	343
12.25	Erosion and osteoporosis of the sella, with no expansion	344
12.26	Unifocal intracranial calcification	345
12.27	Multifocal intracranial calcification	347
12.28	Parasellar calcification	348
12.29	Basal ganglia calcification	348
12.30	Curvilinear calcification	349
12.31	Surface enhancement of the brain	350
12.32	Posterior fossa neoplasms in childhood	351
12.33	CT attenuation of cerebral masses	353
12.34	CT appearances of cerebral masses	355
13	**Nuclear Medicine**/*Keith Harding*	**360**
13.1	Increased uptake on bone scans	360
13.2	Increased uptake on bone scans not due to skeletal abnormality	361
13.3	Photopenic areas (defects) on bone scans	362
13.4	Abnormal bone scan with normal or minimal radiographic changes	363
13.5	Positive radiograph with normal bone scan	363
13.6	Localization of infection	364
13.7	Gallium uptake	365

13.8	Whole body iodine scan for localizing metastases	366
13.9	Photopenic (cold) areas in thyroid imaging	366
13.10	Parathyroid imaging	367
13.11	Brain isotope angiogram	368
13.12	Ventilation perfusion mismatch	369
13.13	Myocardial perfusion imaging	370
13.14	Gated blood pool imaging	370
13.15	Photopenic (cold) areas in colloid liver scans	371
13.16	Non visualization of the gall bladder with HIDA	372
13.17	Spleen imaging	373
13.18	Meta iodo benzyl guanidine (MIBG) imaging	374
13.19	Unilateral adrenal visualization	374
13.20	Cortical defects in renal images	375
13.21	Localization of gastrointestinal bleeding	376
13.22	Meckel's diverticulum	377

14   Obstetric and Gynaecological Ultrasonography/*Josephine McHugo*   380

14.1	Measurements for dating (in weeks post LMP)	380
14.2	Ultrasound features of a normal intrauterine pregnancy (using abdominal scanning)	381
14.3	Indications for ultrasound scanning in the first trimester	382
14.4	Threatened abortion	382
14.5	Blighted ovum (anembryonic pregnancy)	383
14.6	Ectopic pregnancy	383
14.7	Absent intrauterine pregnancy with positive pregnancy test	384
14.8	Liquor volume	384
14.9	Fetal hydrops	385
14.10	Raised serum alphafeto protein (AFP)	386
14.11	Ultrasound signs suggesting chromosomal abnormality	387
14.12	Cystic structures seen in the fetal abdomen	387
14.13	Major structural abnormalities diagnosable antenatally	388
14.14	Fetal growth	390
14.15	Normal placental development	392
14.16	Placental grading	393
14.17	Placenta and membranes in twin pregnancy	394
14.18	Abnormalities of the placenta	395
14.19	Placental haemorrhage	396
14.20	Causes of a thickened placenta (>4cm)	397
14.21	Causes of a thin placenta	397
14.22	Gestational trophoblastic disease	397
14.23	The normal uterus	398
14.24	Endometrial thickness	399

14.25	Enlarged uterus	399
14.26	The normal ovary	399
14.27	Ovarian masses	400
15	**Evaluating Statistics**	**404**

PART 2

Achondroplasia	411
Acquired Immune Deficiency Syndrome (AIDS) in Adults	412
Acquired Immune Deficiency Syndrome (AIDS) in Children	414
Acromegaly	416
Alkaptonuria	417
Aneurysmal Bone Cyst	418
Ankylosing Spondylitis	418
Asbestos Inhalation	420
Calcium Pyrophosphate Dihydrate Deposition Disease	421
Chondroblastoma	422
Chondromyxoid Fibroma	422
Chondrosarcoma	423
Cleidocranial Dysplasia	424
Coal Miner's Pneumoconiosis	425
Cretinism (Congenital Hypothyroidism)	426
Crohn's Disease	427
Cushing's Syndrome	429
Cystic Fibrosis	430
Down's Syndrome (Trisomy 21)	431
Enchondroma	432
Eosinophilic Granuloma	432
Ewing's Tumour	432
Extrinsic Allergic Alveolitis	433
Fibrous Dysplasia	434
Giant Cell Tumour	435
Gout	435
Haemangioma	437
Haemochromatosis	437
Haemophilia	438
Histiocytosis X	439
Homocystinuria	440
Hurler's Syndrome	440
Hyperparathyroidism, Primary	441
Hypoparathyroidism	443
Hypophosphatasia	443
Hypothyroidism	444
Juvenile Chronic Arthritis	444

Lymphoma	446
Marfan's Syndrome	449
Morquio's Syndrome	450
Multiple Endocrine Neoplasia (MEN) Syndromes	450
Multiple Myeloma/Plasmacytoma	451
Neurofibromatosis	453
Neuropathic Arthropathy	455
Non-Accidental Injury	456
Non-ossifying Fibroma (Fibrous Cortical Defect)	458
Ochronosis	458
Osteoblastoma	459
Osteochondroma (Exostosis)	459
Osteogenesis Imperfecta	460
Osteogenic Sarcoma	461
Osteoid Osteoma	462
Osteomalacia	462
Osteopetrosis	463
Paget's Disease	464
Plasmacytoma	465
Polycystic Disease, Infantile	466
Polycystic Disease, Adult	467
Pseudohypoparathyroidism	467
Pseudopseudohypoparathyroidism	467
Psoriatic Arthropathy	468
Pulmonary Embolic Disease	469
Reiter's Syndrome	470
Renal Osteodystrophy	471
Rheumatoid Arthritis	472
Rickets	474
Sarcoidosis	475
Scleroderma (Progressive Systemic Sclerosis)	478
Scurvy	479
Sickle-cell Anaemia	480
Silicosis	481
Simple Bone Cyst	482
Steroids	482
Systemic Lupus Erythematosus	483
Thalassaemia	484
Tuberous Sclerosis	484
Turner's Syndrome	486
Ulcerative Colitis	487
Index	**489**

Foreword

The first edition of this book was aimed to help relatively inexperienced radiologists through that very taxing time after they have become familiar with the fundamental concepts of radiodiagnosis and need a logical guide to their application. By offering diagnostic lists in order of probability and commonness, the authors hoped to help both the rigorous preparation for the Fellowship examinations and the preparation for subsequent clinical practice of the highest standard. The immediate and sustained success of the book, which has now been translated into two additional languages, is an eloquent vindication of the authors' labours.

But radiology has not stood still during the past five years and in addition to a burgeoning international literature, there are refocused interests such as mammography, new interfaces such as ultrasound in obstetrics, and well established links with allied disciplines like nuclear medicine, that benefit from strengthening. The authors have attended to all of these facets by their own meticulous scrutiny, and by commissioning contributions from three new authors.

There is still no substitute for practical experience, but it can be hastened and broadened by absorbing the distilled experiences of Doctors Chapman, Nakielny and colleagues, presented in this book. I have no doubt that the efforts of the authors will be rewarded by a successful contribution to radiological education.

E. Rhys Davies
Professor of Radiodiagnosis
University of Bristol

Preface to the First Edition

During the period of study prior to taking the final Fellowship of the Royal College of Radiologists, or other similar radiological examinations, many specialist textbooks and the wealth of radiological papers are carefully scoured for lists of differential diagnoses of radiological signs. These will supplement the information already learned and enable that information to be used logically when analysing a radiograph. All this takes precious time when effort is best spent trying to memorize these lists rather than trying to find them within the massive texts or, even worse, trying to construct them oneself.

Consequently we decided to write a book which contains as many useful lists as one might reasonably be expected to know for a postgraduate examination. To make it manageable, we have omitted those lists and conditions which have limited relevance to routine radiological practice. In addition, many of the lists are constructed in terms of a 'surgical sieve' and by using this method we would hope that the lists are easier to remember. We have tried to present the conditions in some order of importance, although we realize that local patient selection and the geographical distribution of diseases will have a great influence in modifying the lists. The lists will, almost certainly, not be acceptable to all radiologists. However, the basic lists are supplemented with useful facts and discriminating features about each condition and these should enable the trainee to give a considered opinion of the radiograph. So that this added information can be kept concise and to avoid unnecessary repetition we have summarized the radiological signs of many important conditions separately in Part 2 of the book.

The book has no radiographs. We have assumed a basic knowledge of radiology in the reader and expect him or her to already be able to recognize the abnormal signs. A limited number of line drawings have been used to emphasize radiographic abnormalities.

The aim of the book is to assist with logical interpretation of the radiograph. It is not intended for use on its own because it is not a complete radiological textbook. Recourse will need to be made to the larger general and specialist texts and journals and the reading of them is still a prerequisite to passing the postgraduate examinations.

More exhaustive lists are to be found in Felson & Reeder's *Gamuts in Radiology* (Pergamon Press, Oxford, 1975) and Kreel's *Outline of Radiology* (Heinemann, London, 1971) and these books are to be commended.

Stephen Chapman
Richard Nakielny

Preface to the Second Edition

In the five years since the publication of the first edition we have seen it accepted not only by radiologists in training but also by those who are more experienced. However, in preparing a second edition we have tried to keep to our premise to produce a book with relatively short lists, aimed primarily at those taking postgraduate examinations. The lists have been revised since the first edition by adding in information from the last five years of radiological literature.

Now that a knowledge of other methods of imaging is necessary for postgraduate examinations we decided that the scope of the book should be broadened. Further lists of CT differential diagnoses have been included and we are grateful for the co-operation of three of our specialist colleagues who have written new chapters on topics which are outside our own fields of expertise. Michael Collins, Keith Harding and Josephine McHugo have expertly accomplished the production of chapters on mammography, nuclear medicine and obstetric and gynaecological ultrasonography, respectively. The few general ultrasonography lists are, we admit, little more than a token gesture but to have included an extensive input in this field would have increased the size of the book beyond what will fit comfortably in a white coat pocket.

It is inevitable that our knowledgeable readers will not agree with the arrangement of all of our lists. We hope that such differences of opinion will be made known to us so that we can make any appropriate changes to future editions.

Stephen Chapman
Richard Nakielny

Explanatory Notes

The 'surgical sieve' classification used in the longer lists is presented in order of commonness, e.g. when 'neoplastic' is listed first then this is the commonest cause as a group. Within the group of neoplastic conditions, number 1 is more common or as common as number 2. However, it does not necessarily follow that all the conditions in the first group are more common than those in subsequent groups, e.g. infective, metabolic, etc.

The groups entitled 'idiopathic' or 'others' are usually listed last even though the disease or diseases within them may be common. This has been done for the sake of neatness only.

In order that the supplementary notes are not unnecessarily repeated in several lists, those conditions which appear in several lists are denoted by an asterisk (*) and a summary of their radiological signs is to be found in Part 2 of the book. In this section conditions are listed alphabetically.

Abbreviations

ACTH	Adrenocorticotrophic hormone
AD	Autosomal dominant
AFP	Alphafeto protein
AP	Anteroposterior
AR	Autosomal recessive
ASD	Atrial septal defect
AV	Atrioventricular
CMCJ	Carpometacarpal joint
CMV	Cytomegalovirus
CNS	Central nervous system
CSF	Cerebrospinal fluid
CT	Computerized tomography
CXR	Chest X-ray
DIC	Disseminated intravascular coagulopathy
DIPJ	Distal interphalangeal joint
HCG	Human chorionic gonadotrophin
HOA	Hypertrophic osteoarthropathy
HOCM	Hypertrophic obstructive cardiomyopathy
IAM	Internal auditory meatus
IUCD	Intrauterine contraceptive device
IVU	Intravenous urogram
LAT	Lateral
MCPJ	Metacarpophalangeal joint
PA	Postero-anterior
PAS	Periodic acid-Schiff (stain)
PDA	Patent ductus arteriosus
PIPJ	Proximal interphalangeal joint
PMF	Progressive massive fibrosis
PPH	Post-partum haemorrhage
SIJ	Sacroiliac joint
SLE	Systemic lupus erythematosus
SOL	Space occupying lesion
SXR	Skull X-ray
TAPVD	Total anomalous pulmonary venous drainage
TB	Tuberculosis
TOF	Tracheo-oesophageal fistula
VSD	Ventricular septal defect

PART 1

Chapter 1
Bones

1.1 Retarded Skeletal Maturation

Chronic Ill Health
1. Congenital heart disease — particularly cyanotic.
2. Renal failure.
3. Inflammatory bowel disease.
4. Malnutrition.
5. Rickets*.
6. Maternal deprivation.
7. Any other chronic illness.

Endocrine Disorders
1. Hypothyroidism* — with granular, fragmented epiphyses. This causes severe retardation (five or more standard deviations below the mean).
2. Steroid therapy and Cushing's disease — see Cushing's syndrome*.
3. Hypogonadism — including older patients with Turner's syndrome.
4. Hypopituitarism — panhypopituitarism, growth hormone deficiency and Laron dwarfism.

Chromosome Disorders
1. Trisomy 21.
2. Most other chromosome disorders — severely depressed in trisomy 18.

Other Congenital Disorders
1. Most bone dysplasias.
2. Most malformation syndromes.

Further Reading
Poznanski A.K. (1984) *The Hand in Radiological Diagnosis*. Chapter 3, pp. 67–96. Philadelphia: Saunders.

1.2 Generalized Accelerated Skeletal Maturation

Endocrine Disorders
1. Idiopathic sexual precocity.
2. Intracranial masses in the region of the hypothalamus (hamartoma, astrocytoma and optic chiasm glioma), hydrocephalus and encephalitis.
3. Adrenal and gonadal tumours.
4. Hyperthyroidism.

Congenital Disorders
1. McCune–Albright syndrome — polyostotic fibrous dysplasia with precocious puberty.
2. Cerebral gigantism (Soto's syndrome).
3. Lipodystrophy.
4. Pseudohypoparathyroidism.
5. Acrodysostosis.
6. Weaver syndrome.
7. Marshall syndrome.

Others
1. Large or obese children.

Further Reading
Poznanski A.K. (1984) *The Hand in Radiological Diagnosis*. Chapter 3, pp. 67–96. Philadelphia: Saunders.
Rieth K.G., Comite F., Dwyer A.J., Nelson M.J., Pescovitz O., Shawker T.H., Cutler G.B & Loriaux D.L. (1987) CT of cerebral abnormalities in precocious puberty. *Am. J. Roentgenol.*, 148: 1231–8.

1.3 Premature Closure of a Growth Plate

1. Local hyperaemia — juvenile chronic arthritides, infection, haemophilia or arteriovenous malformation.
2. Trauma.
3. Vascular occlusion — infarcts and sickle cell anaemia*.
4. Thermal injury — burns, frostbite.
5. Multiple exostoses.

1.4 Asymmetrical Maturation

1. **Normal children** — minor differences only.
2. **Paralysis** — with osteopenia and overtubulation of long bones.
3. **Hemihypertrophy.**
4. **Russell–Silver dwarfism** — evident from birth. Triangular face with down-turned corners of the mouth, frontal bossing, hemihypertrophy and altered skeletal maturation.
5. **Klippel–Trenaunay–Weber syndrome** — hypertrophy of the skeleton and soft tissues of one limb or one side of the body is associated with angiomatous malformations.
6. **Increased or decreased blood supply.**

1.5 Dwarfing Skeletal Dysplasias

Without Significant Spinal Involvement
1. **Achondroplasia*** — rhizomelic (proximal) limb shortening.
2. **Hypochondroplasia** — resembles a mild form of achondroplasia.
3. **Asphyxiating thoracic dysplasia of Jeune** — narrow thorax with short ribs leading to respiratory distress. Spur-like projections of the acetabular roof. Premature ossification of the femoral capital epiphyses. Occasionally post-axial hexadactyly. Cone-shaped epiphyses in childhood. Acromelic (distal) limb shortening.
4. **Chondroectodermal dysplasia (Ellis–van Creveld syndrome)** — similar to asphyxiating throracic dysplasia but (a) hexadactyly is a constant finding, (b) there is severe hypoplasia of the fingers and nails, (c) congenital heart disease is common and (d) hypoplastic lateral tibial plateau is characteristic in childhood.
5. **Multiple epiphyseal dysplasia** — small, irregular epiphyses. Premature osteoarthritis.
6. **Chondrodysplasia punctata** — see 1.39.
7. **Metaphyseal chondrodysplasias.**

With Significant Spinal Involvement
1. Pseudoachondroplasia.
2. Spondyloepiphyseal dysplasia — retarded development of the symphysis pubis and femoral heads. Coxa vara, which may be severe. +/− odontoid hypoplasia.
3. Spondylometaphyseal dysplasia.
4. Metatropic dwarfism — dumb-bell shaped long bones.
5. Diastrophic dwarfism — progressive kyphoscoliosis, hitch-hiker thumb, delta-shaped epiphyses, interpedicular narrowing of the lumbar spine.
6. Kniest syndrome.

1.6 Lethal Neonatal Dysplasias

1. Osteogenesis imperfecta* — type II.
2. Thanatophoric dwarfism — small thorax, severe platyspondyly and 'telephone handle shaped' long bones.
3. Chondrodysplasia punctata — rhizomelic form — see 1.39.
4. Asphyxiating thoracic dysplasia of Jeune — see 1.5.
5. Campomelic dwarfism — bowed long bones.
6. Achondrogenesis — types I and II.
7. Short rib syndrome, type Saldino–Noonan.
8. Short rib syndrome, type Majewski.
9. Homozygous achondroplasia*.
10. Hypophosphatasia* — lethal type.

1.7 Conditions Exhibiting Dysostosis Multiplex

Dysostosis multiplex is a constellation of radiological signs which are exhibited, in total or in part by a number of conditions due to defects of complex carbohydrate metabolism. These signs include (a) abnormal bone texture, (b) widening of diaphyses, (c) tilting of distal radius and ulna towards each other, (d) pointing of the proximal ends of the metacarpals, (e) large skull vault with calvarial thickening, (f) anterior beak of upper lumbar vertebrae and (g) 'J–shaped' sella.

Mucopolysaccharidoses
1. MPS I–H (Hurler)*.
2. MPS I–S (Scheie).
3. MPS II (Hunter).
4. MPS III (Sanfilippo).
5. MPS IV (Morquio)*.
6. MPS VI (Maroteaux–Lamy).
7. MPS VII (Sly).

Mucolipidoses
1. MLS I (neuraminidase deficiency).
2. MLS II (I–Cell Disease).
3. MLS III (Pseudopolydystrophy of Maroteaux).

Oligosaccharidoses
1. Fucosidosis I.
2. Fucosidosis II.
3. GM_1 Gangliosidosis.
4. Mannosidosis.
5. Aspartylglucosaminuria.

1.8   Generalized Increased Bone Density — Children

N.B. Infants in the first few months of life can exhibit 'physiological' bone sclerosis which regresses spontaneously.

Dysplasias
1. **Osteopetrosis***.
2. **Pycnodysostosis** — short stature, hypoplastic lateral ends of clavicles, hypoplastic terminal phalanges, bulging cranium and delayed closure of the anterior fontanelle. AR.
3. **The craniotubular dysplasias** — abnormal skeletal modelling +/− increased bone density.
   (a) Metaphyseal dysplasia (Pyle).
   (b) Craniometaphyseal dysplasia.
   (c) Craniodiaphyseal dysplasia.
   (d) Frontometaphyseal dysplasia.
   (e) Osteodysplasty (Melnick–Needles).
4. **The craniotubular hyperostoses** — overgrowth of bone with alteration of contours and increased bone density.
   (a) Endosteal hyperostosis, Van Buchem type.
   (b) Endosteal hyperostosis, Worth type.
   (c) Sclerosteosis.
   (d) Diaphyseal dysplasia (Camurati–Engelmann).

Metabolic
1. **Renal osteodystrophy*** — rickets + osteosclerosis.

Poisoning
1. **Lead** — dense metaphyseal bands. Cortex and flat bones may also be slightly dense. Modelling deformities later, e.g. flask-shaped femora.
2. **Fluorosis** — more common in adults. Usually asymptomatic but may present in children with crippling stiffness and pain. Thickened cortex at the expense of the medulla. Periosteal reaction. Ossification of ligaments, tendons and interosseous membranes.
3. **Hypervitaminosis D** — slightly increased density of skull and vertebrae early, followed later by osteoporosis. Soft-tissue calcification. Dense metaphyseal bands and widened zone of provisional calcification.

4. **Chronic hypervitaminosis A** — not before 1 yr of age. Failure to thrive, hepatosplenomegaly, jaundice, alopecia and haemoptysis. Cortical thickening of long and tubular bones, especially in the feet. Subperiosteal new bone. Normal epiphyses and reduced metaphyseal density. The mandible is not affected (cf. Caffey's disease).

Idiopathic
1. **Caffey's disease (infantile cortical hyperostosis)** — see section 1.12.
2. **Idiopathic hypercalcaemia of infancy** — probably a manifestation of hypervitaminosis D. Elfin facies, failure to thrive and mental retardation. Generalized increased density or transverse dense metaphyseal bands. Increased density of the skull base.

Further Reading
Beighton P. & Cremin B.J. (1980) *Sclerosing Bone Dysplasias*. Berlin: Springer-Verlag.

1.9 Generalized Increased Bone Density — Adults

Myeloproliferative
1. **Myelosclerosis** — marrow cavity is narrowed by endosteal new bone. Patchy lucencies due to persistence of fibrous tissue. (Generalized osteopenia in the early stages due to myelofibrosis.) Hepatosplenomegaly.

Metabolic
1. **Renal osteodystrophy***.

Poisoning
1. **Fluorosis** — with periosteal reaction, prominent muscle attachments and calcification of ligaments and interosseous membranes. Changes are most marked in the innominate bones and lumbar spine.

Neoplastic (more commonly multifocal than generalized)
1. **Osteoblastic metastases** — most commonly prostate and breast. See section 1.16.
2. **Lymphoma***.
3. **Mastocytosis** — sclerosis of marrow containing skeleton with patchy areas of radiolucency. Urticaria pigmentosa. Can have symptoms and signs of carcinoid syndrome.

Idiopathic (more commonly multifocal than generalized)
1. **Paget's disease*** — coarsened trabeculae, bony expansion and thickened cortex.

Those Conditions with Onset in the Paediatric Age Group (q.v.)

1.10   Solitary Sclerotic Bone Lesion

Developmental
1. **Bone island.**
2. **Fibrous dysplasia***.

Neoplastic
1. **Metastasis** (q.v.) — most commonly prostate or breast.
2. **Lymphoma***.
3. **Osteoma/osteoid osteoma/osteoblastoma***.
4. **Healed or healing benign or malignant bone lesion** — e.g. lytic metastasis following radiotherapy or chemotherapy, bone cyst, fibrous cortical defect, eosinophilic granuloma or brown tumour.
5. **Primary bone sarcoma.**

Vascular
1. **Bone infarct** (q.v.).

Traumatic
1. **Callus** — especially a transverse density around a healing stress fracture.

Infective
1. **Sclerosing osteomyelitis of Garré.**

Idiopathic
1. **Paget's disease***.

1.11 Multiple Sclerotic Bone Lesions

Developmental
1. Bone islands.
2. Fibrous dysplasia*.
3. Osteopoikilosis — asymptomatic. 1–10 mm, round or oval densities in the appendicular skeleton and pelvis. Ribs, skull and spine are usually exempt. Tend to be parallel to the long axis of the affected bones and are especially numerous near the ends of bones.
4. Osteopathia striata (Voorhoeve's disease) — asymptomatic. Linear bands of dense bone parallel with the long axis of the bone. The appendicular skeleton and pelvis are most frequently affected; skull and clavicles are spared.
5. Tuberous sclerosis*.

Neoplastic
1. Metastases (q.v.) — most commonly prostate or breast.
2. Lymphoma*.
3. Mastocytosis.
4. Multiple healed or healing benign or malignant bone lesions — e.g. lytic metastases following radiotherapy or chemotherapy, eosinophilic granuloma and brown tumours.
5. Multiple myeloma* — sclerosis in up to 3% of cases.
6. Osteomata — e.g. Gardner's syndrome.

Idiopathic
1. Paget's disease*.

Vascular
1. Bone infarcts (q.v.).

Traumatic
1. Callus — around numerous fractures.

1.12   Bone Sclerosis with a Periosteal Reaction

Traumatic
1. Healing fracture with callus.

Neoplastic
1. Metastasis.
2. Lymphoma*.
3. Osteoid osteoma/osteoblastoma*.
4. Osteogenic sarcoma*.
5. Ewing's tumour*.
6. Chondrosarcoma*.

Infective
1. Osteomyelitis — including Garré's sclerosing osteomyelitis and Brodie's abscess.
2. Syphilis — congenital or acquired.

Idiopathic
1. **Infantile cortical hyperostosis (Caffey's disease)** — in infants up to 6 months of age. Multiple bones involved at different times, most frequently mandible, ribs and clavicles; long bones less commonly; spine, hands and feet are spared. Increased density of bones is due to massive periosteal new bone. In the long bones the epiphyses and metaphyses are spared.
2. **Melorheostosis** — cortical and periosteal new bone giving the appearance of molten wax flowing down a burning candle. The hyperostosis tends to extend from one bone to the next. Usually affects one limb but both limbs on one side may be affected. Sometimes it is bilateral but asymmetrical. Skull, spine and ribs are seldom affected.

1.13   Solitary Sclerotic Bone Lesion with a Lucent Centre

Neoplastic
1. Osteoid osteoma*.
2. Osteoblastoma*.

Infective
1. Brodie's abcess.

1.14 Coarse Trabecular Pattern

1. **Paget's disease*** — an enlarged bone with a thickened cortex. If only part of the bone is affected the demarcation between normal and pagetoid bone is clear cut.
2. **Osteoporosis** (see section 1.29) ⎱ resorption of secondary trabeculae accentuates the remaining
3. **Osteomalacia*** ⎰ primary trabeculae.
4. **Haemoglobinopathies** — especially thalassaemia*.
5. **Haemangioma** — especially in a vertebral body.
6. **Gaucher's disease.**

1.15 Excessive Callus Formation

1. Steroid therapy and Cushing's syndrome*.
2. Neuropathic arthropathy*.
3. Osteogenesis imperfecta*.
4. Non-accidental injury*.
5. Paralytic states.
6. Renal osteodystrophy*.
7. Multiple myeloma*.

1.16 Skeletal Metastases — Most Common Radiological Appearances

Lung
1. Carcinoma	lytic
2. Carcinoid	sclerotic

Breast
	lytic or mixed

Genito-urinary
1. Renal cell carcinoma	lytic, expansile
2. Wilms' tumour	lytic
3. Bladder (transitional cell)	lytic, occasionally sclerotic
4. Prostate	sclerotic

Reproductive Organs
1. Cervix	lytic or mixed
2. Uterus	lytic
3. Ovary	lytic
4. Testis	lytic; occasionally sclerotic

Thyroid
	lytic, expansile

Gastrointestinal Tract

1. Stomach	sclerotic or mixed
2. Colon	lytic; occasionally sclerotic
3. Rectum	lytic

Adrenal

1. Phaeochromocytoma	lytic, expansile
2. Carcinoma	lytic
3. Neuroblastoma	lytic; occasionally sclerotic

Skin

1. Squamous cell carcinoma	lytic
2. Melanoma	lytic, expansile

Further Reading

Kagan R.A., Steckel R.J., Bassett L.W. & Gold R.H. (1986) Radiologic contributions to cancer management. Bone metastases. *Am. J. Roentgenol.*, 147: 305–12.

Pagani J.J. & Libshitz H.I. (1982) Imaging bone metastases. *Radiol. Clin. North Am.*, 20(3): 545–60.

Thrall J.H. & Ellis B.I. (1987) Skeletal metastases. *Radiol. Clin. North Am.*, 25(6): 1155–70.

1.17 Sites of Origin of Primary Bone Neoplasms

(A composite diagram modified from Madewell et al., 1981.)

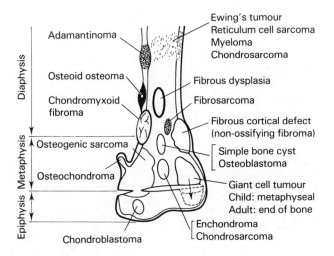

Diaphysis

Adamantinoma

Ewing's tumour
Reticulum cell sarcoma
Myeloma
Chondrosarcoma

Osteoid osteoma

Fibrous dysplasia

Chondromyxoid
fibroma

Fibrosarcoma

Fibrous cortical defect
(non-ossifying fibroma)

Metaphysis

Osteogenic sarcoma

Simple bone cyst
Osteoblastoma

Osteochondroma

Giant cell tumour
Child: metaphyseal
Adult: end of bone

Epiphysis

Enchondroma
Chondrosarcoma

Chondroblastoma

Further Reading

Madewell J.E., Ragsdale B.D. & Sweet D.E. (1981) Radiologica and pathologic analysis of solitary bone lesions. *Radiol. Clin. North Am.*, 19: 715–48.

1.18 Peak Age Incidence of Primary Bone Neoplasms

Decades	1st	2nd	3rd	4th	5th	6th	7th
Simple bone cyst							
Ewing's tumour							
Chondroblastoma							
Non-ossifying fibroma							
Osteochondroma							
Osteoblastoma							
Osteogenic sarcoma							
Osteoid osteoma							
Aneurysmal bone cyst							
Chondromyxoid fibroma							
Giant cell tumour							
Reticulum cell sarcoma							
Fibrosarcoma							
Osteoma							
Parosteal sarcoma							
Chondroma							
Haemangioma							
Chondrosarcoma							
Myeloma							
Chordoma							

1.19 Lucent Bone Lesion in the Medulla — Well-defined, Marginal Sclerosis, No Expansion

Indicates a slowly progressing lesion.

1. **Geode** — a subarticular cyst. Other signs of an arthritis. See section 1.24.
2. **Healing benign or malignant bone lesion** — e.g. metastasis, eosinophilic granuloma or brown tumour.
3. **Brodie's abscess.**
4. **Benign bone neoplasms**
   (a) Simple bone cyst* — 75% arise in the proximal humerus and femur.
   (b) Enchondroma* — more than 50% are found in the tubular bones of the hands. ± internal calcification.
   (c) Chondroblastoma* — in an epiphysis. Most common sites are proximal humerus, distal femur and proximal tibia. Internal hazy calcification.
5. **Fibrous dysplasia*.**

1.20 Lucent Bone Lesion in the Medulla — Well-defined, No Marginal Sclerosis, No Expansion

The absence of reactive bone formation implies a fast growth rate.

1. **Metastasis** — especially from breast, bronchus, kidney or thyroid.
2. **Multiple myeloma*.**
3. **Eosinophilic granuloma*.**
4. **Brown tumour of hyperparathyroidism*.**
5. **Benign bone neoplasms**
   (a) Enchondroma*.
   (b) Chondroblastoma*.

1.21   Lucent Bone Lesion in the Medulla — Ill-defined

An aggressive pattern of destruction.

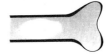

1. Metastatis.
2. Multiple myeloma*.
3. Osteomyelitis.
4. Lymphoma*.
5. Long-bone sarcomas
    (a) Osteogenic sarcoma*.
    (b) Ewing's tumour*.
    (c) Chondrosarcoma*.
    (d) Fibrosarcoma.
    (e) Reticulum cell sarcoma.

1.22 Lucent Bone Lesion in the Medulla — Well-defined, Eccentric Expansion

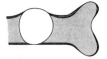

1. **Giant cell tumour*** — typically subarticular after epiphyseal fusion. (3% are metaphyseal prior to fusion). Ill-defined margins. Septa. ± soft-tissue extension and destroyed cortex. Mostly long bones.
2. **Aneurysmal bone cyst*** — in the unfused metaphysis or metaphysis and epiphysis following fusion of the growth plate. Intact but thin cortex. Well-defined endosteal margin. ± thin internal strands of bone. Fluid level on C.T.
3. **Enchondroma*** — diaphyseal. Over 50% occur in the tubular bones of the hands and feet. Internal ground glass appearance ± calcification within it. May be multilocular in long bones.
4. **Non-ossifying fibroma (fibrous cortical defect)*** — frequently in the distal tibia or femur and produces an eccentric expanded cortex. (In a thin bone such as the fibula central expansion is observed.) Metaphyseal. Smooth, sharp margins with a thin rim of surrounding sclerosis.
5. **Chondromyxoid fibroma*** — 75% in the lower limbs (50% in the proximal tibia). Metaphyseal and may extend into the epiphysis. Frequently has marginal sclerosis.

1.23 Lucent Bone Lesion — Grossly Expansile

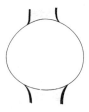

Malignant Bone Neoplasms
1. **Metastases** — renal cell carcinoma and thyroid; less commonly melanoma, bronchus, breast and phaeochromocytoma.
2. **Plasmacytoma*** — ± soft tissue extension. ± internal septa.
3. **Chondrosarcoma/reticulum cell sarcoma /fibrosarcoma** — when slow growing may have this appearance.

Benign Bone Neoplasms
1. **Aneurysmal bone cyst*** — in the unfused metaphysis or metaphysis and epiphysis following fusion of the growth plate. ± internal septa. Fluid level on C.T.
2. **Giant cell tumour*** — typically subarticular after epiphyseal fusion. Ill-defined endosteal margin. ± soft-tissue extension and destroyed cortex.
3. **Enchondroma*** — ground-glass appearance ± internal calcifications.

Non-neoplastic
1. **Fibrous dysplasia*** — ground-glass appearance ± internal calcification. Modelling deformities of affected bone.
2. **Haemophilic pseudotumour** (see Haemophilia*) — especially in the iliac wing and lower limb bones. Soft-tissue swelling. ± haemophilic arthropathy.
3. **Brown tumour of hyperparathyroidism*** — the solitary skeletal sign of hyperparathyroidism in 3% of patients. Most commonly in the mandible, followed by pelvis, ribs and femora. Usually unilocular.
4. **Hydatid.**

1.24 Subarticular Lucent Bone Lesion

Arthritides

1. **Osteoarthritis** — may be multiple 'cysts' in the load-bearing areas of multiple joints. Surrounding sclerotic margin. Joint-space narrowing, subchondral sclerosis and osteophytes.
2. **Rheumatoid arthritis*** — no sclerotic margin. Begin periarticularly near the insertion of the joint capsule. Joint-space narrowing and juxta-articular osteoporosis.
3. **Calcium pyrophosphate arthropathy** (see Calcium pyrophosphate dihydrate deposition disease*) — similar to osteoarthritis but frequently larger and with more collapse and fragmentation of the articular surface.
4. **Gout*** — ± erosions with overhanging edges and adjacent soft-tissue masses.
5. **Haemophilia***.

Neoplastic

1. **Metastases/multiple myeloma*** — single or multiple. Variable appearance.
2. **Aneurysmal bone cyst*** — solitary. Expansile. Narrow zone of transition.
3. **Giant cell tumour*** — solitary. Eccentric. Ill-defined endosteal margin.
4. **Chondroblastoma*** — solitary. Predilection for the proximal ends of the humerus, femur and tibia. Contains amorphous or spotty calcification in 50%.
5. **Pigmented villonodular synovitis** — mainly the lower limb, especially the knee. Soft-tissue mass. Cyst-like defects with sharp sclerotic margins. May progress to joint destruction.

Others

1. **Post-traumatic** — particularly in the carpal bones. Well defined.
2. **Osteonecrosis** (q.v.) — with bone sclerosis, collapse and fragmentation. Preservation of joint space.
3. **Tuberculosis** — wholly epiphyseal or partly metaphyseal. Well defined or ill-defined. No surrounding sclerosis.

Further Reading

Bullough P.G. & Bansal M. (1988) The differential diagnosis of geodes. *Radiol. Clin. North Am.*, 26: 1165–84.
Resnick D., Niwayama G. & Coutts R.D. (1977) Subchondral cysts (geodes) in arthritic disorders: Pathologic and radiographic appearance of the hip joint. *Am. J. Roentgenol.*, 128: 799–806.

1.25   Lucent Bone Lesion — Containing Calcium or Bone

Neoplastic

1. **Metastases** — especially from breast.
2. **Cartilage neoplasms**
   (a) Benign — enchondroma, chondroblastoma and chondromyxoid fibroma.
   (b) Malignant — chondrosarcoma.
3. **Bone (osteoid) neoplasms**
   (a) Benign — osteoid osteoma and osteoblastoma.
   (b) Malignant — osteogenic sarcoma.
4. **Fibrous-tissue neoplasms**
   (a) Malignant — fibrosarcoma.

Others

1. **Fibrous dysplasia***.
2. **Osteoporosis circumscripta***.
3. **Osteomyelitis** — with sequestrum.
4. **Eosinophilic granuloma***.

1.26   'Moth-eaten Bone'

Multiple scattered lucencies of variable size with no major central lesion. Coalescence may occur later. Cancellous and/or cortical bone is involved.

Neoplastic

1. **Metastases** — including neuroblastoma in a child.
2. **Multiple myeloma***.
3. **Leukaemia and lymphoma***.
4. **Long-bone sarcomas**
   (a) Ewing's tumour*.
   (b) Reticulum cell sarcoma.
   (c) Osteogenic sarcoma*.
   (d) Chondrosarcoma*.
   (e) Fibrosarcoma.
5. **Histiocytosis X*** — especially in older patients.

Infective

1. **Osteomyelitis.**

1.27 Regional Osteopenia

Decreased bone density confined to a region or segment of the appendicular skeleton.

1. **Disuse** — during the immobilization of fractures, in paralysed segments and in bone and joint infections. Usually appears after 8 weeks of immobilization. The patterns of bone loss may be uniform (commonest), spotty (mostly periarticular), band-like (subchondral or metaphyseal) or endosteal cortical scalloping and linear cortical lucencies.
2. **Sudeck's atrophy (reflex sympathetic dystrophy syndrome)** — is mediated via a neurovascular mechanism and associated with post-traumatic and post-infective states, myocardial infarction, calcific tendinitis and cervical spondylosis. It most commonly affects the shoulder and hand and develops rapidly. Pain and soft-tisse swelling are clinical findings. In addition to the radiological signs of disuse there may be subperiosteal bone resorption and small periarticular erosions.
3. **Transient osteoporosis of the hip** — a severe, progressive osteoporosis of the femoral head and, to a lesser degree, of the femoral neck and acetabulum. Full recovery is seen in 6 months.
4. **Regional migratory osteoporosis** — pain, swelling and osteoporosis affect the joints of the lower limbs in particular. The migratory nature differentiates it from other causes.

1.28 Generalized Osteopenia

1. **Osteoporosis** — diminished quantity of normal bone.
2. **Osteomalacia*** — normal quantity of bone but it has an excess of uncalcified osteoid.
3. **Hyperparathyroidism*** — increased bone resorption by osteoclasts.
4. **Diffuse infiltrative bone disease** — e.g. multiple myeloma and leukaemia.

1.29 Osteoporosis

1. Decreased bone density.
2. Cortical thinning with a relative increase in density of the cortex and vertebral end-plates. Skull sutures are relatively sclerotic.
3. Relative accentuation of trabecular stress lines because of resorption of secondary trabeculae.
4. Brittle bones with an increased incidence of fractures, especially compression fractures of vertebral bodies, femoral neck and wrist fractures.

Endocrine
1. **Hypogonadism**
    (a) Ovarian — menopausal, Turner's syndrome*.
    (b) Testicular — eunuchoidism.
2. **Cushing's syndrome***.
3. **Diabetes mellitus.**
4. **Acromegaly***.
5. **Addison's disease.**
6. **Hyperthyroidism.**
7. **Mastocytosis** — mast cells produce heparin.

Disuse

Iatrogenic
1. Steroids*.
2. Heparin.

Deficiency States
1. Vitamin C (scurvy*).
2. Protein.

Idiopathic
1. **In young people** — a rare self-limiting condition occurring in children of 8–12 years. Spontaneous improvement is seen.

Congenital
1. Osteogenesis imperfecta*.
2. Turner's syndrome*.
3. Homocystinuria*.
4. Neuromuscular diseases.
5. Mucopolysaccharidoses.
6. Trisomy 13 and 18.
7. Pseudo- and pseudopseudohypoparathyroidism*.
8. Glycogen storage diseases.
9. Progeria.

1.30   Osteomalacia and Rickets*

Vitamin-D Deficiency
1. Dietary.
2. Malabsorption.

Renal Disease
1. Glomerular disease (renal osteodystrophy*).
2. Renal tubular disease
   (a) Fanconi syndromes.
   (b) X-linked hypophosphataemia.
   (c) Renal tubular acidosis.

Hepatic Disease
1. Parenchymal failure.
2. Obstructive jaundice — especially congenital biliary atresia.

Anticonvulsants
1. Phenytoin and phenobarbitone.

Tumour Associated
1. Soft tissues — haemangiopericytoma.
2. Bone — non-ossifying fibroma, giant cell tumour, osteoblastoma (and fibrous dysplasia).

Not Related to Vitamin-D Metabolism
1. Hypophosphatasia* — low serum alkaline phosphatase.
2. Metaphyseal chondrodysplasia (type Schmid) — normal serum phosphate, calcium and alkaline phosphatase differentiate it from other rachitic syndromes.

If the patient is less than 6 months of age consider:
1. Biliary atresia.
2. Hypophosphatasia*.
3. Neonatal rickets — in premature infants because of combined dietary deficiency and impaired hepatic hydroxylation of vitamin D.
4. Vitamin D dependent rickets — rachitic changes are associated with a severe myopathy in spite of adequate dietary intake of vitamin D. Deformed tarsal and carpal bones and platyspondyly.

1.31 Periosteal Reactions — Types

(Modified from Ragsdale et al., 1981.)

Continuous		*Interrupted*
Cortex destroyed	Intact cortex	

Shell –
'expanded cortex'

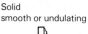

Solid
smooth or undulating

Buttress

Lobulated shell

Solid spiculated

Ridged shell –
'trabeculated'
'soap bubble'

Single lamina

Codman triangle
single lamina

Lamellated

Codman triangle
lamellated

Parallel spiculated –
'hair-on-end'

Spiculated

Divergent spiculated –
'sunray'

The different types are, in general, non-specific, having multiple aetiologies. However, the following comments can be made:

Continuous with Destroyed Cortex
This is the result of an expanding lesion. See sections 1.22 and 1.23.

Parallel Spiculated ('Hair-on-end')
1. Ewing's tumour*.
2. Syphilis.
3. Infantile cortical hyperostosis (Caffey's disease).

See section 12.14 for causes in the skull vault.

Divergent Spiculated ('Sunray')
1. Osteogenic sarcoma*.
2. Metastases — especially from sigmoid colon and rectum.
3. Ewing's tumour*.
4. Haemangioma*.
5. Meningioma.
6. Tuberculosis.
7. Tropical ulcer.

Codman Triangle (Single Lamina or Lamellated)
1. Aggressive malignant tissue extending into the soft tissues.
2. Infection — occasionally.

Further Reading
Ragsdale B.D., Madewell J.E. & Sweet D.E. (1981) Radiologic and pathologic analysis of solitary bone lesions. Part II: Periosteal reactions. *Radiol. Clin. North. Am.*, 19: 749–83.

1.32 Periosteal Reaction — Solitary and Localized

1. Traumatic.
2. Inflammatory.
3. Neoplastic
   (a) Malignant
      — primary.
      — secondary.
   (b) Benign — an expanding shell or complicated by a fracture.

1.33 Periosteal Reactions — Bilaterally Symmetrical in Adults

1. **Hypertrophic osteoarthropathy (HOA)** — clinically there is clubbing of the fingers and painful swelling of knees, ankles, wrists, elbows and metacarpophalangeal joints. The periosteal reaction occurs in the metaphysis and diaphysis of the radius, ulna, tibia, fibula and, less commonly, the humerus, femur and tubular bones of the hands and feet. It can be a single lamina, lamellated or solid and undulating. The thickness of the periosteal reaction correlates with the duration of disease activity. Periarticular osteoporosis, soft-tissue swelling and joint effusions are other features. The condition can be caused by the conditions in section 1.34 (q.v.).

2. **Pachydermoperiostosis** — a rare, self-limiting and familial condition, usually affecting boys at puberty and with a predilection for blacks. Clinically there is an insidious onset of thickening of the skin of the extremities (including the face), hyperhidrosis and clubbing. Compared with HOA it is relatively pain free. The bones most commonly affected are the tibia, fibula, radius and ulna (less commonly the carpus, tarsus and tubular bones of the hands and feet). The periosteal reaction is similar to HOA but is more solid and spiculated and also involves the epiphysis to produce outgrowths around joints. The concavity of the diaphysis may be filled in. ± ligamentous calcification.

3. **Vascular insufficiency (venous, lymphatic or arterial)** — the legs are almost exclusively affected with involvement of tibia, fibula, metatarsals and phalanges. There is a solid undulating periosteal reaction, which is, initially, separated from the cortex but later merges with it. No definite relationship to soft-tissue ulceration. Phleboliths may be associated with venous stasis. Soft-tissue swelling is a feature whatever the aetiology. Arterial insufficiency due to polyarteritis nodosa or other arteritides may also be associated with a mild periostitis and is also usually confined to the lower limbs.

4. **Thyroid acropachy** — in 0.5–10% of patients following thyroidectomy for thyrotoxicosis and who may now be euthyroid, hypothyroid or hyperthyroid. Clinically there is soft-tissue swelling, clubbing, exophthalmos and pretibial myxoedema. A solid, spiculated, almost lace-like periosteal reaction affects the diaphysis of the metacarpals and phalanges of the hands, especially the radial side of the thumbs and index fingers. Less commonly the feet, lower legs and forearms are involved.
5. **Fluorosis** — solid, undulating periosteal reaction with osteosclerosis. The long bones and tubular bones are most frequently affected. Ligamentous calcification.

Further Reading

Pineda C.J., Sartoris D.J., Clopton P. & Resnick D. (1987) Periostitis in hypertrophic osteoarthropathy: relationship to disease duration. *Am. J. Roentgenol.*, 148: 773–78.

1.34 Hypertrophic Osteoarthropathy

Pulmonary
1. **Carcinoma of bronchus.**
2. **Lymphoma***.
3. **Abscess.**
4. **Bronchiectasis** — frequently due to cystic fibrosis*.
5. **Metastases.**

Pleural
1. **Pleural fibroma** — has the highest incidence of accompanying HOA, although it is itself a rare cause.
2. **Mesothelioma.**

Cardiovascular
1. **Cyanotic congenital heart diease** — produces clubbing but only rarely a periosteal reaction.

Gastrointestinal
1. **Ulcerative colitis***.
2. **Crohn's disease***.
3. **Dysentery** — amoebic or bacillary.
4. **Lymphoma***.
5. **Whipple's disease.**
6. **Coeliac disease.**
7. **Cirrhosis** — especially primary biliary cirrhosis.
8. **Nasopharyngeal carcinomas** (Schmincke's tumour).
9. **Juvenile polyposis.**

1.35 Periosteal Reactions — Bilaterally Symmetrical in Children

1. **Normal infants** — diaphyseal, not extending to the growth plate.
2. **Juvenile chronic arthritis*** — in approx 25% of cases. Most common in the periarticular regions of the phalanges, metacarpals and metatarsals. When it extends into the diaphysis it will eventually result in enlarged, rectangular tubular bones.
3. **Acute leukaemia** — associated with prominent metaphyseal bone resorption ± a dense zone of provisional calcification. Osteopenia. Periosteal reaction is due to cortical involvement by tumour cells. Metastatic neuroblastoma can look identical.
4. **Rickets*** — the presence of uncalcified subperiosteal osteoid *mimics* a periosteal reaction because the periosteum and ossified cortex are separated.
5. **Scurvy*** — subperiosteal haemorrhage is most frequent in the femur, tibia and humerus. Periosteal reaction is particularly evident during the healing phase. Age 6 months or older.
6. **Congenital syphilis** — an exuberant periosteal reaction can be due to infiltration by syphilitic granulation tissue or the healing (with callus formation) of osteochondritis. The former is essentially diaphyseal and the latter around the metaphyseal/epiphyseal junction.
7. **Caffey's disease** — first evident before 5 months of age. Mandible, clavicles and ribs show cortical hyperostosis and a diffuse periosteal reaction. The scapulae and tubular bones are less often affected and tend to be involved asymmetrically.

1.36 Periosteal Reactions — Bilaterally Asymmetrical

1. **Metastases.**
2. **Osteomyelitis.**
3. **Arthritides** — especially Reiter's syndrome* and psoriatic arthropathy*.
4. **Osteoporosis** (q.v.) ⎱ because of the increased
5. **Osteomalacia** (q.v.) ⎰ liability to fractures.
6. **Non-accidental injury*.**
7. **Bleeding diatheses.**
8. **Hand–foot syndrome (sickle-cell dactylitis)** — see Sickle-cell anaemia*.

1.37   Differential Diagnosis of Skeletal Lesions in Non-accidental Injury*

Disease	Shaft fractures	Abnormal meta-physis	Osteo-penia	Periosteal reaction	Comments
Non-accidental injury*	+	+	−	+	
Accidental trauma	+	−	−	callus	
Birth trauma	+	+/−	−	+/−	Clavicle, humerus and femur are most frequent fractures
Osteogenesis imperfecta*	+	+/−	+	−	Highly unlikely in the absence of osteopenia, Wormian bones dentinogenesis imperfecta and a relevant family history
Osteomyelitis	−	+	localized	+	May be multifocal
Rickets*	+	+	+	+	↑ Alkaline phosphatase
Scurvy*	−	+	+	+	Not before 6 months age
Congenital syphilis	−	+	−	+	
Congenital insensitivity to pain	+	+	−	+	
Paraplegia	+	+	+	with fractures	Lower limb changes only
Prostaglandin E₁ therapy	−	−	−	+	
Menke's syndrome	−	+	+	+	Males only. Abnormal hair. Retardation. Wormian bones
Copper deficiency	+	+	+	+/−	See note 1

[1]   **Copper Deficiency**. Rare. Unlikely in the absence of at least one risk factor — prematurity, total parenteral nutrition, malabsorption or a low copper diet. Unlikely in full term infants less than 6 months age. Microcytic, hypochromic anaemia. Leukopenia. Normal serum copper and caeruloplasmin does not exclude the diagnosis.
Skull fracture never recorded in copper deficiency. Rib fractures only recorded in premature infants.

Further Reading
Kleinman P. (1987) *Diagnostic Imaging of Child Abuse*. Baltimore: Williams & Wilkins.
Shaw J.C.L. (1988) Copper deficiency and non-accidental injury. *Arch. Dis. Childhood*, 63: 448–55.

1.38   Pseudarthrosis

1. **Non-union of a fracture.**
2. **Congenital** — in the middle to lower third of the tibia ± fibula. 50% present in the first year. Later there may be cupping of the proximal bone end and pointing of the distal bone end.
3. **Neurofibromatosis***.
4. **Osteogenesis imperfecta***.
5. **Cleidocranial dysplasia*** — congenitally in the femur.
6. **Fibrous dysplasia***.
7. **Ankylosing spondylitis*** — in the fused bamboo spine.

Further Reading
Boyd H.B. & Sage F.P. (1958) Congenital pseudarthrosis of the tibia. *J. Bone Joint Surg.*, 40A: 1245–70.
Park W.M., Spencer D.G., McCall I.W., Ward D.J., Watson Buchanan W. & Stephens W.H. (1981) The detection of spinal pseudarthrosis in ankylosing spondylitis. *Br. J. Radiol.*, 54: 467–72.

1.39   Irregular or Stippled Epiphyses

1. **Avascular necrosis** (q.v.) — single, e.g. Perthes' disease (although 10% are bilateral), or multiple, e.g. sickle-cell anaemia.
2. **Cretinism*** — not present at birth. Delayed appearance and growth of ossification centres. Appearance varies from slightly granular to fragmentation. The femoral capital epiphysis may be divided into inner and outer halves.
3. **Morquio's syndrome*** — irregular ossification of the femoral capital epiphyses results in flattening.
4. **Multiple epiphyseal dysplasia** — onset 5–14 years. May be familial. Delayed appearance and growth of epiphyses but the time of fusion is normal. ± metaphyseal irregularity. Carpal and tarsal bones, hips, knees and ankles are most commonly affected. Tibio-talar slant. Short, stubby digits and metacarpals. Spine usually, but not always, normal. Early and severe osteoarthritis.
5. **Chondrodyslasia punctata** — autosomal dominant and (rarer) autosomal recessive types are recognized.
   (a) Autosomal dominant type (Conradi–Hünerman) — in the newborn stippling is evident in the long bone epiphyses, spine and larynx. +/− malsegmentation of vertebral bodies. Stippling disappears by 2 years of age. Asymmetrical shortening of limbs. Usually survive to adulthood.
   (b) Autosomal recessive (severe rhizomelic) type — marked symmetrical rhizomelia with humeri more severely affected than femora. Spinal stippling is mild. Stillborn or perinatal death.
6. **Trisomy 18 and 21.**
7. **Prenatal infections.**
8. **Warfarin embryopathy** — stippling of uncalcified epiphyses, particularly of the axial skeleton, proximal femura and calcanei. Disappears after 1st year.

1.40 Avascular Necrosis

Toxic
1. **Steroids*** — probably does not occur with less than 2 years of treatment.
2. **Anti-inflammatory drugs** — indomethacin and phenylbuta-zone.
3. **Alcohol** — possibly because of fat emboli in chronic alcoholic pancreatitis.
4. **Immunosuppressives.**

Traumatic
1. **Idiopathic** — e.g. Perthes' disease and other osteochondri-tides.
2. **Fractures** — especially femoral neck, talus and scaphoid.
3. **Radiotherapy.**
4. **Heat** — burns.
5. **Fat embolism.**

Inflammatory
1. **Rheumatoid arthritis*.** ⎱ in the absence of drugs
2. **Systemic lupus erythematosus*.** ⎰ probably due to a vasculitis.
3. **Scleroderma*.**
4. **Infection** — e.g. following a pyogenic arthritis.
5. **Pancreatitis.**

Metabolic and Endocrine
1. **Pregnancy.**
2. **Diabetes.**
3. **Cushing's syndrome*.**
4. **Hyperlipidaemias.**
5. **Gout*.**

Haemopoietic Disorders
1. **Haemoglobinopathies** — especially sickle-cell anaemia*.
2. **Polycythaemia rubra vera.**
3. **Gaucher's disease.**
4. **Haemophilia*.**

Thrombotic and Embolic
1. **Dysbaric osteonecrosis.**
2. **Arteritis.**

1.41   Solitary Radiolucent Metaphyseal Band

A non-specific sign which represents a period of poor endochondral bone formation.

1. **Normal neonate.**
2. **Any severe illness.**
3. **Metaphyseal fracture** — especially non-accidental injury*.
4. **Leukaemia and lymphoma***.
5. **Metastases.**
6. **Congenital infections** — especially syphilis.
7. **Intrauterine perforation.**
8. **Scurvy***.

Further Reading
Wolfson J.J. & Engel R.R. (1969) Anticipating meconium peritonitis from metaphyseal bands. *Radiology*, 92: 1055–60.

1.42   Alternating Radiolucent and Dense Metaphyseal Bands

1. **Growth arrest or Park's lines.**
2. **Rickets*** — especially those types that require prolonged treatment such as vitamin D dependent rickets.
3. **Osteopetrosis***.

Further Reading
Follis R.H. & Park E.A. (1952) Some observations on bone growth, with particular respect to zones and transverse lines of increased density in the metaphysis. *Am. J. Roentgenol.*, 68: 709–24.

1.43 Solitary Dense Metaphyseal Band

1. Normal infants.
2. Lead poisoning — dense line in the proximal fibula is said to differentiate from normal. Other poisons include bismuth, arsenic, phosphorus, mercury fluoride and radium
3. Radiation.
4. Cretinism*.
5. Osteopetrosis*.
6. Hypervitaminosis D.

1.44 Dense Vertical Metaphyseal Lines

1. Congenital rubella — celery stalk appearance. Less commonly in congenital CMV.
2. Osteopathia striata — +/− exostoses.
3. Hypophosphatasia*.

1.45 Fraying of Metaphyses

1. Rickets*.
2. Hypophosphatasia*.
3. Chronic stress (in the wrists of young gymnasts) — with wide, irregular, asymmetrical widening of the distal radial growth plate and metaphyseal sclerosis.
4. Copper deficiency.

Further Reading

Carter S.R., Aldridge M.J., Fitzgerald R. & Davies A.M. (1988) Stress changes of the wrist in adolescent gymnasts. *Br. J. Radiol.*, 61: 109–12.

Grünebaum M., Horodniceanu C. & Steinherz R. (1980) The radiographic manifestations of bone changes in copper deficiency. *Paed. Radiol.*, 9: 101–4.

1.46   Cupping of Metaphyses

Often associated with fraying.

1. **Normal** — especially of the distal ulna and proximal fibula of young children. No fraying.
2. **Rickets*** — with widening of the growth plate and fraying.
3. **Trauma** — to the growth plate and/or metaphysis. Asymmetrical and localized changes.
4. **Bone dysplasias** — a sign in a large number e.g. achondroplasia*, pseudoachondroplasia, metatropic dwarfism, diastrophic dwarfism, the metaphyseal chondrodysplasias and hypophosphatasia*.
5. **Scurvy*** — usually after fracture.

1.47   Erlenmeyer Flask Deformity

1. **Haemoglobinopathies** — especially thalassaemia*.
2. **Gaucher's disease.**
3. **Niemann–Pick disease.**
4. **Osteopetrosis*.**
5. **Craniometaphyseal dysplasias.**

1.48   Erosions of the Medial Metaphysis of the Proximal Humerus

1. **Normal variant.**
2. **Leukaemia.**
3. **Metastatic neuroblastoma.**
4. **Gaucher's disease.**
5. **Hurler's syndrome*.**
6. **Glycogen storage disease.**
7. **Niemen–Pick disease.**

Further Reading
Li J.K.W., Birch P.D. & Davies A.M. (1988) Proximal humerus defects in Gaucher's disease. *Br. J. Radiol.*, 61: 579–83.

1.49 Erosion or Absence of the Outer End of the Clavicle

1. Rheumatoid arthritis*.
2. Hyperparathyroidism*.
3. Multiple myeloma*.
4. Metastasis.
5. Post-traumatic osteolysis.
6. Cleidocranial dysplasia*.
7. Pyknodysostosis.

1.50 Focal Rib Lesion (Solitary or Multiple)

Neoplastic
Secondary more common than primary. Primary malignant more common than benign.
1. Metastases
   (a) **Adult male** — bronchus, kidney or prostate most commonly.
   (b) **Adult female** — breast.
   (c) **Child** — neuroblastoma.
2. Primary malignant
   (a) **Multiple myeloma/plasmacytoma***.
   (b) **Chondrosarcoma***.
   (c) **Ewing's tumour*** — in a child.
3. Benign
   (a) **Osteochondroma***.
   (b) **Enchondroma***.
   (c) **Histiocytosis X***.

Non-neoplastic
1. Healed rib fracture.
2. Fibrous dysplasia.
3. Paget's disease*.
4. Brown tumour of hyperparathyroidism*.
5. Osteomyelitis — bacterial, tuberculous or fungal.

Further Reading
Omell G.H., Anderson L.S. & Bramson R.T. (1973) Chest wall tumours. *Radiol. Clin. North Am.*, 11: 197–214.

1.51 Rib Notching — Inferior Surface

Arterial
1. **Coarctation of the aorta** — rib signs are unusual before 10 years of age. Affects 4–8th ribs bilaterally; not the upper two if conventional. Unilateral and right-sided if the coarctation is proximal to the left subclavian artery. Unilateral and left-sided if associated with an anomalous right subclavian artery distal to the coarctation. Other signs include a prominent ascending aorta and a small descending aorta with an intervening notch, left ventricular enlargement and possibly signs of heart failure.
2. **Aortic thrombosis** — usually the lower ribs bilaterally.
3. **Subclavian obstruction** — most commonly post Blalock operation (either subclavian-to-pulmonary artery anastomosis) for Fallot's tetralogy. Unilateral rib notching of the upper three or four ribs on the operation side.
4. **Pulmonary oligaemia** — any cause of decreased pulmonary blood supply.

Venous
1. Superior vena caval obstruction.

Arteriovenous
1. Pulmonary arteriovenous malformation.
2. Chest wall arteriovenous malformation.

Neurogenic
1. Neurofibromatosis* — 'ribbon ribs' may also be a feature.

Further Reading
Boone M.L., Swenson B.E. & Felson B. (1964) Rib notching: its many causes. *Am. J. Roentgenol.*, 91: 1075–88.

1.52 Rib Notching — Superior Surface

Connective Tissue Diseases
1. Rheumatoid arthritis*.
2. Systemic lupus erythematosus*.
3. Scleroderma*.
4. Sjögren's syndrome.

Metabolic
1. Hyperparathyroidism*.

Miscellaneous
1. Neurofibromatosis*.
2. Restrictive lung disease.
3. Poliomyelitis.
4. Marfan's syndrome*.
5. Osteogenesis imperfecta*.
6. Progeria.

Further Reading
Boone M.L., Swenson B.E. & Felson B. (1964) Rib notching: its many causes. *Am. J. Roentgenol.*, 91: 1075–88.

1.53 Arachnodactyly

Elongated and slender tubular bones of the hands and feet. The metacarpal index is an aid to diagnosis and is estimated by measuring the lengths of the 2nd, 3rd, 4th and 5th metacarpals and dividing by their breadths taken at the exact mid-points. These four figures are then added together and divided by 4.
Normal range 5.4–7.9.
Arachnodactyly range 8.4–10.4.
1. **Marfan's syndrome*** — although arachnodactyly is not necessary for the diagnosis.
2. **Homocystinuria*** — morphologically resembles Marfan's syndrome but 60% are mentally defective, they have a predisposition to arterial and venous thromboses and the lens of the eye dislocates downward rather than upward.

1.54   Distal Phalangeal Destruction

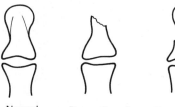

Normal   Resorption of   Resorption of   Periarticular
                the tuft   the mid portion

N.B. Because of reinforced Sharpey's fibres periosteal reaction is rare at this site.

Resorption of the Tuft
1. **Scleroderma***.
2. **Raynaud's disease.**
3. **Psoriatic arthropathy*** — can precede the skin changes.
4. **Neuropathic diseases** — diabetes mellitus, leprosy, myelomeningocoele, syringomyelia and congenital indifference to pain.
5. **Thermal injuries** — burns, frostbite and electrical.
6. **Trauma.**
7. **Hyperparathyroidism***.
8. **Epidermolysis bullosa.**
9. **Porphyria** — due to cutaneous photosensitivity leading to blistering and scarring.
10. **Phenytoin toxicity** — congenitally in infants of epileptic mothers.
11. **Subungual exostosis.**
12. **Snake and scorpion venom** — due to tissue breakdown by proteinases.

Resorption of the Mid Portion
1. **Polyvinyl chloride tank cleaners.**
2. **Acro-osteolysis of Hajdu and Cheney.**
3. **Hyperparathyroidism***.

Periarticular — i.e. erosion of the distal interphalangeal joints.
1. **Psoriatic arthropathy***.
2. **Erosive osteoarthritis.**
3. **Hyperparathyroidism***.
4. **Thermal injuries.**
5. **Scleroderma***.
6. **Multicentric reticulohistiocytosis.**

Poorly Defined Lytic Lesions
1. **Osteomyelitis** — mostly staphylococcal with diabetics at particular risk. Periosteal reaction is infrequent.
2. **Metastases** — bronchus is most common primary site. Bone metastases to the hand are commonest in the terminal phalanx and may be the only metastasis to bone. The subarticular cortex is usually the last to be destroyed.
3. **Multiple myeloma***.
4. **Aneurysmal bone cyst*** — rare at this site. Marked thinning and expansion of cortex.
5. **Giant cell tumour*** — usually involving the base of the phalanx.
6. **Leprosy** — at any age, but 30% present before 15 years of age.

Well defined Lytic Lesions
1. **Implantation dermoid/epidermoid cyst** — an expanding lesion, 1–20 mm, with minimal sclerosis ± soft tissue swelling.
2. **Enchondroma***.
3. **Sarcoidosis*** — associated 'lace-like' destruction of phalangeal shaft, subperiosteal erosion leading to resorption of terminal tufts and endosteal sclerosis.
4. **Glomus tumour** — soft tissue swelling with disuse osteoporosis because of pain. Bone involvement is uncommon but there may be pressure erosion or a well defined lytic lesion.
5. **Osteoid osteoma***.
6. **Fibrous dysplasia***.

Further Reading
Jones S.N. & Stoker D.J. (1988) Radiology at your fingertips; lesions of the terminal phalanx. *Clin. Radiol.*, 39: 478–85.
Qteishat W.A., Whitehouse G.H. & Hawass N-E-D. (1985) Acro-osteolysis following snake and scorpion envenomation. *Br. J. Radiol.*, 58: 1035–9.

1.55 Short Metacarpal(s) or Metatarsal(s)

1. **Idiopathic.**
2. **Post-traumatic** — iatrogenic, fracture, growth plate injury, thermal or electrical.
3. **Post-infarction** — e.g. sickle-cell anaemia*.
4. **Turner's syndrome*** — 4th ± 3rd & 5th metacarpals.
5. **Pseudo- and pseudopseudohypoparathyroidism*** — 4th & 5th metacarpals.

Further Reading

Bell J. (1951) On brachydactyly and symphalangism. In: Penrose L.S. (ed.) *The Treasury of Human Inheritance*, Vol. 5, Part 1, pp 1–31. Cambridge: University Press.

Poznanski A.K. (1984) *The Hand in Radiologic Diagnosis*. 2nd edn, Vol. 1, Chapter 9, pp. 209–62. Philadelphia: Saunders.

1.56 Carpal Fusion

Isolated

Tends to involve bones in the same carpal row (proximal or distal). More common in Negroes than Caucasians.

1. **Triquetral–lunate** — the most common site. Affects 1% of the population.
2. **Capitate–hamate.**
3. **Trapezium–trapezoid.**

Syndrome-related

Tends to exhibit massive carpal fusion affecting bones in different rows (proximal and distal).

1. **Acrocephalosyndactyly (Apert's syndrome).**
2. **Arthrogryposis multiplex congenita.**
3. **Ellis–van Creveld syndrome.**
4. **Holt–Oram syndrome.**
5. **Turner's syndrome*.**
6. **Symphalangism.**

Acquired
1. **Inflammatory arthritides** — especially juvenile chronic arthritis* and rheumatoid arthritis*.
2. **Pyogenic arthritis.**
3. **Post-traumatic.**
4. **Post-surgical.**

Further Reading
Cope J.R. (1974) Carpal coalition. *Clin. Radiol.*, 25: 261–6.

1.57 Madelung Deformity

1. **Dyschondrosteosis (Leri–Weil disease)** — consider if bilateral with mesomelic limb shortening. AD.
2. **Diaphyseal aclasis.**
3. **Turner syndrome***.
4. **Trauma.**
5. **Infection.**

Bibliography

General
Felson B. (ed.) (1970) *Semin. Roentgenol.*, 5(4).
Greenfield G.B. (1986) *Radiology of Bone Disease*, 4th edn. Philadelphia: Lippincott.
Murray R.O. & Jacobson H.G. (1977) *The Radiology of Skeletal Disorders*, 2nd edn. Edinburgh: Churchill Livingstone.
Poznanski A.K. (1984) *The Hand in Radiologic Diagnosis*, 2nd edn. Philadelphia: Saunders.
Reeder M. & Felson B. (1975) *Gamuts in Radiology*. Oxford: Pergamon Press.
Resnick D. & Niwayama G. (1988) *Diagnosis of Bone and Joint Disorders*, 2nd edn. Philadelphia: Saunders.
Sutton D. (1986) *Textbook of Radiology and Imaging*, 4th edn. Edinburgh: Churchill Livingstone.
Swischuk L.E. (1984) *Differential Diagnosis in Paediatric Radiology*. Baltimore: Williams & Wilkins.

Benign Neoplasms

Byers P.D. (1968) Solitary benign osteoblastic lesions of bone. *Cancer*, 22: 43–57.

Clough J.R. & Price C.H.G. (1968) Aneurysmal bone cysts. *J. Bone Joint Surg.*, 50B: 116–27.

Lodwick G.S. (1958) Juvenile unicameral bone cyst. *Am. J. Roentgenol.*, 83: 495–504.

McLeod R.A. & Beabout J.W. (1973) The roentgenographic features of chondroblastoma. *Am. J. Roentgenol.*, 118: 464–71.

Maudsley R.H. (1956) Non-osteogenic fibroma of bone (fibrous metaphyseal defect). *J. Bone Joint Surg.*, 38B: 714–33.

Murphy N.B. & Price C.H.G. (1971) The radiological aspects of chondromyxoid fibroma of bone. *Clin. Radiol.*, 22: 261–9.

Omojola M.F., Cockshott W.P. & Beatty E.G. (1981) Osteoid osteoma: an evaluation of diagnostic modalities. *Clin. Radiol.*, 32: 199–204.

Malignant Neoplasms

Barnes R. & Catto M. (1966) Chondrosarcoma of bone. *J. Bone Joint Surg.*, 48B: 729–64.

Dahlin D.C. (1967) Osteogenic sarcoma. A study of 600 cases. *J. Bone Joint Surg.*, 49A: 101–10.

Dahlin D.C., Coventry M.B. & Scanlon P.W. (1961) Ewing's sarcoma: a critical analysis of 165 cases. *J. Bone Joint Surg.*, 43A: 185–92.

Jacobs P. (1972) The diagnosis of osteoclastoma (giant cell tumour): a radiological and pathological correlation. *Br. J. Radiol.*, 45: 121–36.

Pagani J.J. & Libshitz H. I. (1982) Imaging bone metastases. *Radiol. Clin. North Am.*, 20(3): 545–60.

Infections

Chapman M., Murray R.O. & Stoker D.J. (1979) Tuberculosis of the bones and joints. *Semin. Roentgenol.*, 14: 266–82.

Cremin B.J. & Fisher R.M. (1970) The lesions of congenital syphilis. *Br. J. Radiol.*, 43: 333–41.

Enna C.D., Jacobson R.A. & Rausch R.O (1971) Bone changes in leprosy. *Radiology*, 100: 295–306.

Goldblatt M. & Cremin B.J. (1978) Osteoarticular tuberculosis: its presentation in coloured races. *Clin. Radiol.*, 29: 669–77.

Latham W.J. (1953) Hydatid disease. *J. Faculty Radiol.*, 5: 65–81 & 83–95.

Dysplasias
Beighton P. (1988) *Inherited Disorders of the Skeleton*, 2nd edn. Edinburgh: Churchill Livingstone.
Beighton P. & Cremin B.J. (1980) *Sclerosing Bone Dysplasias*. Berlin: Springer-Verlag.
Dorst J.P., Scott C.I. & Hall J.G. (1972) The radiological assessment of short-stature dwarfism. *Radiol. Clin. North Am.*, 10(3): 393–414.
Felson B. (ed.) (1973) Dwarfs and other little people. *Semin. Roentgenol.*, 8(2).
Koslowski K. & Beighton P. (1984) *Gamut Index of Skeletal Dysplasias*. Berlin: Springer-Verlag.
Spranger J.W., Langer L.O. & Wiedmann H.R. (1974) *Bone Dysplasias: An Atlas of Constitutional Disorders of Skeletal Development*. Philadelphia: Saunders.
Wynne-Davies R., Hall C.M. & Apley A.G. (1985) *Atlas of Skeletal Dysplasias*. Edinburgh: Churchill Livingstone.

Metabolic Bone Disease
Doyle F.H. (1975) Current concepts in metabolic bone disease. In: Lodge T. & Steiner R. (eds) *Recent Advances in Radiology*, No. 5. Edinburgh: Churchill Livingstone.
Grainger R.G. (1964) The radiology of metabolic bone disease. In: Lodge T. (ed.) *Recent Advances in Radiology*, No. 4, Edinburgh: Churchill Livingstone.

Ischaemia
Davidson J.K. (1979) Dysbaric osteonecrosis and pulmonary changes in divers. In: Lodge T. & Steiner R.E. (eds) *Recent Advances in Radiology and Medical Imaging* — 6, pp. 145–62. Edinburgh: Churchill Livingstone.
Edeiken J., Hodes P.J., Libshitz H.I. & Weller M.H. (1967) Bone ischaemia. *Radiol. Clin. North Am.*, 5(3): 515–29.

Notes

Notes

Chapter 2
The Spine

2.1 Scoliosis

Idiopathic

2% prevalence for curves >10°.

1. **Infantile** — diagnosed before the age of 4 years. 90% are thoracic and concave to the right. More common in boys. 90% resolve spontaneously.
2. **Juvenile** — diagnosed between 4 and 10 years. More common in girls. Almost always progressive.
3. **Adolescent** — diagnosed between 10 years and maturity. More common in females. Majority are concave to the left in the thoracic region.

Congenital

Prognosis is dependent on the anatomical abnormality and a classification (Figure 2.1) is, therefore, important.

Failure of Formation. A. Incarcerated hemivertebra. A straight spine with little tendency to progression. **B.** Free hemivertebra. May be progressive. **C.** Wedge vertebra. Better prognosis than a free hemivertebra. **D.** Multiple hemivertebrae. Failure of formation on the same side results in a severe curve. Hemivertebrae on opposite sides may compensate each other. **E.** Central defect. Butterfly vertebra.

Failure of Segmentation. A. Bilateral → block vertebra and a short spine, e.g. Klippel–Feil. **B.** Unilateral unsegmented bar. Severely progressive curve with varying degrees of kyphosis or lordosis depending on the position of the bar.

Mixed defects. A. Unilateral unsegmented bar and a hemivertebra. Severely progressive. **B.** Partially segmented incarcerated hemivertebra. **C.** Bilateral failure of segmentation incorporating a hemivertebra.

FAILURE OF FORMATION

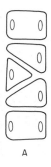
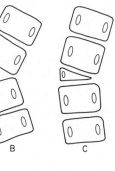
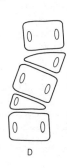
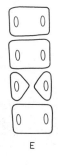

A   B   C   D   E

FAILURE OF SEGMENTATION

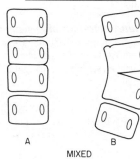

A   B

MIXED
e.g.

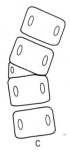

A   B   C

Fig 2.1

Indicators of serious progression are:
  (a) Deformity present at birth.
  (b) Severe deformity of the chest wall.
  (c) Unilateral unsegmented bars.
  (d) Thoracic abnormality.
Associated abnormalities may occur — urinary tract (18%), congenital heart disease (7%), undescended scapulae (6%) and diastematomyelia (5%).

Neuromuscular Diseases
1. Myelomeningocoele.
2. Spinal muscular atrophy.
3. Friedreich's ataxia.
4. Poliomyelitis.
5. Cerebral palsy.
6. Muscular dystrophy.

Mesodermal and Neuroectodermal Diseases
1. **Neurofibromatosis*** — in up to 40% of patients. Classically a sharply angled short segment scoliosis with a severe kyphosis. The apical vertebrae are irregular and wedged with adjacent dysplastic ribs. 25% have a congenital vertebral anomaly.
2. **Marfan's syndrome*** — scoliosis in 40–60%. Double structural curves are typical.
3. **Homocystinuria*** — similar to Marfan's syndrome.

Post Radiotherapy
Wedged and hypoplastic vertebrae ± unilateral pelvic or rib hypoplasia.

Leg Length Discrepancy
A flexible lumbar curve, convex to the side of the shorter leg. Disparity of iliac crest level.

Painful Scoliosis
1. **Osteoid osteoma*** — 10% occur in the spine. A lamina or pedicle at the apex of the curve will be sclerotic or overgrown.
2. **Osteoblastoma***.
3. **Intraspinal tumour** (q.v.).
4. Infection.

Further Reading
Winter R.B. (1983) *Congenital Deformities of the Spine.* New York: Thieme-Stratton.

2.2 Solitary Collapsed Vertebra

1. **Neoplastic disease**
   (a) Metastasis — breast, bronchus, prostate, kidney and thyroid account for the majority of patients with a solitary spinal metastasis. The disc spaces are preserved until late. The bone may be lytic, sclerotic or mixed. ± destruction of a pedicle.
   (b) Multiple myeloma/plasmacytoma* — a common site, especially for plasmacytoma. May mimic an osteolytic metastasis or be expansile and resemble an aneurysmal bone cyst.
   (c) Lymphoma*.
2. **Osteoporosis** (q.v.) — generalized osteopenia. Coarsened trabecular pattern in adjacent vertebrae due to resorption of secondary trabeculae.
3. **Trauma**.
4. **Infection** — with destruction of vertebral end-plates and adjacent disc spaces.
5. **Histiocytosis X*** — eosinophil granuloma is the most frequent cause of a solitary vertebra plana in childhood. The posterior elements are usually spared.
6. **Benign tumours** — haemangioma, giant cell tumour and aneurysmal bone cyst.

2.3 Multiple Collapsed Vertebrae

1. **Osteoporosis** (q.v.) — reduced bone density. Vertebral bodies may be wedged or biconcave (fish-shaped).
2. **Neoplastic disease** — wedge fractures are particularly related to osteolytic metastases and osteolytic marrow tumours, e.g. multiple myeloma, leukaemia and lymphoma. Altered or obliterated normal trabeculae. Disc spaces are usually preserved until late. Paravertebral soft-tissue mass is more common in myeloma than metastases.
3. **Trauma** — discontinuity of trabeculae, sclerosis of the fracture line due to compressed and overlapping trabeculae. Disc space usually preserved. The lower cervical, lower dorsal and upper lumbar spine are most commonly affected. Usually no soft-tissue mass.
4. **Scheuermann's disease** — irregular end plates and numerous Schmorl's nodes in the thoracic spine of children and young adults. Disc space narrowing. Often progresses to a severe kyphosis. Secondary degenerative changes later.
5. **Infection** — destruction of end plates adjacent to a destroyed disc. Although it is usually not possible to differentiate radiologically between pyogenic and tuberculous spondylitis in white patients the following signs are said to be helpful.

Pyogenic	Tuberculous
Rapidly progressive	Slower progression
Marked osteoblastic response	Less sclerosis
Less collapse	Marked collapse
Small or no paravertebral abscess	Large paravertebral abscess
Early bridging of affected vertebrae	

6. **Histiocytosis X*** — the spine is more frequently involved in eosinophilic granuloma and Hand–Schüller–Christian disease than in Letterer–Siwe disease. Most common in young people. The thoracic and lumbo-sacral spine are the usual sites of disease. Disc spaces are preserved.
7. **Sickle-cell anaemia*** — characteristic step-like depression in the central part of the end-plate.

Further Reading
Allen E.H., Cosgrove D. & Millard F.J.C. (1978) The radiological changes in infections of the spine and their diagnostic value. *Clin. Radiol.*, 29: 31–40.
Goldman A.B. & Freiberger R.H. (1978) Localised infections and neuropathic disease. *Semin. Roentgenol.*, 14: 19–32.

2.4 Platyspondyly in Childhood

This sign describes a decrease in the distance between the upper and lower vertebral end plates and should be differentiated from wedge shaped vertebrae. Platyspondyly may be *generalized*, affecting all the vertebral bodies, *multiple*, affecting some of the vertebral bodies or *localized*, involving one vertebral body (also termed vertebra plana).

Congenital Platyspondyly
1. **Thanatophoric dwarfism** — inverted 'U' or H-shaped vertebrae with a markedly increased disc space:body height ratio. Telephone handle shaped long bones.
2. **Metatropic dwarfism.**
3. **Osteogenesis imperfecta*** — type IIA.

Platyspondyly in Later Childhood
1. **Morquio's disease***.
2. **Spondyloepiphyseal dysplasia congenita.**
3. **Spondyloepiphyseal dysplasia tarda.**
4. **Kniest syndrome.**

Acquired Platyspondyly — see section 2.3.

Further Reading
Kozlowski K. (1974) Platyspondyly in childhood. *Paed. Radiol.*, 2: 81–8.

2.5   Erosion, Destruction or Absence of a Pedicle

1. **Metastasis** ⎫   metastatic carcinoma involves the
                   ⎪   pedicle relatively early and con-
                   ⎬   trasts with the late preservation of
                   ⎪   the pedicle in multiple myeloma.
2. **Multiple myeloma*** ⎭
3. **Intraspinal mass** (q.v.) — with widening of the interpedicular distance.
4. **Tuberculosis** — uncommonly. With a large paravertebral abscess.
5. **Benign bone tumour** — aneurysmal bone cyst or giant cell tumour.
6. **Congenital absence** — ± sclerosis of the contralateral pedicle.

Further Reading
Bell D. & Cockshott W.P. (1971) Tuberculosis of the vertebral pedicle. *Radiology*, 99: 43–8.

2.6   Solitary Dense Pedicle

1. **Osteoblastic metastasis** — no change in size.
2. **Osteoid osteoma*** — some enlargement of the pedicle ± radiolucent nidus.
3. **Osteoblastoma*** — larger than osteoid osteoma and more frequently a lucency with a sclerotic margin rather than a purely sclerotic pedicle.
4. **Secondary to spondylolysis** — ipsilateral or contralateral.
5. **Secondary to congenitally absent or hypoplastic contralateral posterior elements.**

Further Reading
Pettine K. & Klassen R. (1986) Osteoid osteoma and osteoblastoma of the spine. *J. Bone Joint Surg.*, 68A: 354–61.
Wilkinson R.H. & Hall J.E. (1974) The sclerotic pedicle: tumour or pseudotumour? *Radiology*, 111: 683–8.

2.7 Enlarged Vertebral Body

Generalized
1. Gigantism.
2. Acromegaly*.

Local (Single or Multiple)
1. Paget's disease*.
2. Benign bone tumour
   (a) Aneurysmal bone cyst* — typically purely lytic and expansile. Involves the anterior and posterior elements more commonly than the anterior or posterior elements alone. Rapid growth.
   (b) Haemangioma* — with a prominent vertical trabecular pattern.
   (c) Giant cell tumour* — involvement of the body alone is most common. Expansion is minimal.
3. **Hydatid** — over 40% of cases of hydatid disease in bone occur in vertebrae.

Further Reading
Beabout J.W., McLeod R.A. & Dahlin D.C. (1979) Benign tumours. *Semin. Roentgenol.*, 14: 33–43.
Dahlin D.C. (1977) Giant cell tumour of vertebrae above the sacrum. A review of 31 cases. *Cancer*, 39: 1350–6.
Mohan V., Gupta S.K., Tuli S.M. & Sanyal B. (1980) Symptomatic vertebral haemangiomas. *Clin. Radiol.*, 31: 575–9.

2.8 Squaring of One or More Vertebral Bodies

1. Ankylosing spondylitis*.
2. Paget's disease*.
3. Psoriatic arthropathy*.
4. Reiter's syndrome*.
5. Rheumatoid arthritis*.

2.9   Block Vertebrae

1. **Isolated congenital** — a failure of segmentation. Most common in the lumbar spine but also occurs in the cervical and thoracic regions. The ring epiphyses of adjacent vertebrae do not develop and thus the AP diameter of the vertebrae at the site of the segmentation defect is decreased. The articular facets, neural arches or spinous processes may also be involved. A faint lucency representing a vestigial disc may be observed.

2. **Klippel–Feil syndrome** — segmentation defects in the cervical spine, short neck, low hairline and limited cervical movement, especially rotation. The radiological appearance of the cervical spine resembles (1) above. C2–C3 and C5–C6 are most commonly affected. Other anomalies are frequently associated, the most important being
   (a) Scoliosis >20° in more than 50% of patients.
   (b) Sprengel's shoulder in 30%, ± an omovertebral body.
   (c) Cervical ribs.
   (d) Genito-urinary abnormalities in 66%; renal agenesis in 33%.
   (e) Deafness in 33%.

3. **Rheumatoid arthritis*** — especially juvenile onset rheumatoid arthritis and juvenile chronic arthritis with polyarticular onset. There may be angulation at the fusion site and this is not a feature of the congenital variety. The spinous processes do not fuse.

4. **Ankylosing spondylitis*** — squaring of anterior vertebral margins and calcification in the invertebral discs and anterior and posterior longitudinal ligaments.

5. **Tuberculosis** — vertebral body collapse and destruction of the disc space, ± paraspinal calcification. There may be angulation of the spine.

6. **Operative fusion.**

7. **Post-traumatic.**

2.10 Ivory Vertebral Body

Single or multiple very dense vertebrae. The list excludes
those causes where increased density is due to compaction
of bone following collapse. If there is generalized
involvement of the spine see section 1.9.

1. **Metastases** — sclerotic metastases or an initially lytic
   metastasis which, after treatment, has become sclerotic.
   Usually no alteration in vertebral body size. Disc spaces
   preserved until late.
2. **Paget's disease*** — usually a single vertebral body is
   affected. Expanded body with a thickened cortex and
   coarsened trabeculation. Disc space involvement is uncommon.
3. **Lymphoma*** — more frequent in Hodgkin's disease than
   the other reticuloses. Normal size vertebral body. Disc
   spaces intact.
4. **Low-grade infection** — with end-plate destruction, disc
   space narrowing and a paraspinal soft-tissue mass.

2.11 Atlanto-axial Subluxation

When the distance between the posterior aspect of the anterior arch of the atlas and the anterior aspect of the odontoid process exceeds 3 mm in adults and older children or 5 mm in younger children, or an interosseous distance that changes considerably between flexion and extension.

Trauma

Arthritides
1. **Rheumatoid arthritis*** — in 20–25% of patients with severe disease. Associated erosion of the odontoid may be severe enough to reduce it to a small spicule of bone.
2. **Psoriatic arthropathy*** — in 45% of patients with spondylitis.
3. **Juvenile chronic arthritis*** — most commonly in seropositive juvenile onset adult rheumatoid arthritis.
4. **Systemic lupus erythematosus***.
5. **Ankylosing spondylitis*** — in 2% of cases. Usually a late feature.

Congenital
1. **Down's syndrome*** — in 20% of cases. ± odontoid hypoplasia. May, rarely, have atlanto-occipital instability.
2. **Morquio's syndrome***.
3. **Spondylo–epiphyseal dysplasia.**
4. **Congenital absence/hypoplasia of the odontoid process** — many have a history of previous trauma. N.B. in children <9 years it is normal for the tip of the odontoid to fall well below the top of the anterior arch of the atlas.

Infection
1. **Retropharyngeal abscess in a child.**

Further Reading
Elliott S. (1988) The odontoid process in children — is it hypoplastic? *Clin. Radiol.*, 39: 391–3.
Martel W. (1961) the occipito-atlanto-axial joints in rheumatoid arthritis and ankylosing spondylitis. *Am. J. Roentgenol.*, 86: 223–40.
Rosenbaum D.M., Blumhagen J.D. & King H.A. (1986) Atlanto-occipital instability in Down syndrome. *Am. J. Roentgenol.*, 146: 1269–72.

2.12 Intervertebral Disc Calcification

1. **Degenerative spondylosis** — in the nucleus pulposus. Usually confined to the dorsal region. With other signs of degenerative spondylosis — disc-space narrowing, osteophytosis and vacuum sign in the disc. A frequent finding in the elderly.

2. **Alkaptonuria*** — symptoms of arthropathy first appear in the 4th decade. Widespread disc calcification, osteoporosis, disc-space narrowing and osteophytosis. The disc calcification is predominantly in the inner fibres of the annulus fibrosus but may be diffusely throughout the disc. Severe changes progress to ankylosis and may mimic ankylosing spondylitis.

3. **Calcium pyrophosphate dihydrate deposition disease*** — predominantly in the outer fibres of the annulus fibrous.

4. **Ankylosing spondylitis*** — in the nucleus pulposus. Ankylosis, square vertebral bodies and syndesmophytes.

5. **Juvenile chronic arthritis*** — may mimic ankylosing spondylitis.

6. **Haemochromatosis*** — in the outer fibres of the annulus fibrosus.

7. **Diffuse idiopathic skeletal hyperostosis (DISH)** — may mimic ankylosing spondylitis.

8. **Gout***.

9. **Idiopathic** — a transient phenomenon in children. The cervical spine is most often affected. Clinically associated with neck pain and fever but may be asymptomatic. Persistent in adults.

10. **Following spinal fusion.**

Further Reading

Weinberger A. & Myers A.R. (1978) Intervertebral disc calcification in adults: a review. *Semin. Arthritis Rheum.*, 18: 69–75.

2.13 Bony Outgrowths of the Spine

Syndesmophytes
Ossification of the annulus fibrosus. Thin, vertical and symmetrical. When extreme results in the 'bamboo spine'.

1. **Ankylosing spondylitis***.
2. **Alkaptonuria.**

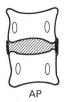

AP

Paravertebral Ossification
Ossification of paravertebral connective tissue which is separated from the edge of the vertebral body and disc. Large, coarse and asymmetrical.

1. **Reiter's syndrome***.
2. **Psoriatic arthropathy***.

AP

Claw Osteophytes
Arising from the vertebral margin with no gap and having an obvious claw appearance.

1. **Stress response** — but in the absence of disc space narrowing does not indicate disc degeneration.

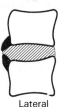

Lateral

Traction Spurs
Osteophytes with a gap between the end-plate and the base of the osteophyte and with the tip not protruding beyond the horizontal plane of the vertebral end-plate.

1. **Shear stresses across the disc** — more likely to be associated with a degenerative disc.

Lateral

Undulating Anterior Ossification
Undulating ossification of the anterior longitudinal ligament, intervertebral disc and paravertebral connective tissue.

1. **Diffuse idiopathic skeletal hyperostosis (DISH).**

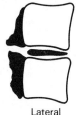

Lateral

Further Reading
Jones M.D., Pais M.J. & Omiya B. (1988) Bony overgrowths and abnormal calcifications about the spine. *Radiol. Clin. North Am.*, 26: 1213–34.

2.14 Coronal Cleft Vertebral Bodies

When occurring singly they may be seen in the normal spine.
When seen as part of a bone dysplasia they are usually
obliterated in the first few months of life.

1. **Chondrodysplasia punctata** — rhizomelic type.
2. **Kniest syndrome.**
3. **Metatropic dwarfism.**

2.15 Anterior Vertebral Body Beaks

Central   Lower third

Involves 1–3 vertebral bodies at the thoracolumbar junction
and usually associated with a kyphosis. Hypotonia is
probably the common denominator which leads to an
exaggerated thoraco-lumbar kyphosis, anterior herniation of
the nucleus pulposus and subsequently an anterior vertebral
body defect.

Central
1. Morquio's syndrome*.

Lower Third
1. Hurler's syndrome*.
2. Achondroplasia*.
3. Pseudoachondroplasia.
4. Cretinism*.
5. Down's syndrome*.
6. Neuromuscular diseases.

Further Reading
Swischuk L.E. (1970) The beaked, notched or hooked vertebra.
 Its significance in infants and young children. *Radiology*,
 95: 661–4.

2.16   Posterior Scalloping of Vertebral Bodies

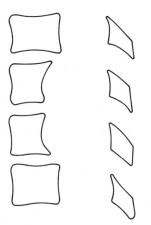

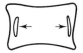

May be associated with
flattening of the pedicles
on the AP view

Scalloping is most prominent (a) at either end of the spinal
canal, (b) with large and slow growing lesions and (c) with
those lesions which originate during the period of active
growth and bone modelling.

1. **Tumours in the spinal canal** — ependymoma (especially
   of the filum terminale and conus), dermoid, lipoma,
   neurofibroma and less commonly meningioma.
2. **Neurofibromatosis*** — scalloping is due to a mesodermal
   dysplasia and is associated with dural ectasia. Localized
   scalloping can also result from pressure resorption by a
   neurofibroma, in which case there may also be enlargement
   of an intervertebral foramen and flattening of one pedicle
   ('dumb-bell tumour'). However, multiple wide thoracic
   intervertebral foramina are more likely due to lateral
   meningocoeles than to local tumours.
3. **Acromegaly*** — other spinal changes include increased AP
   and transverse diameters of the vertebral bodies giving
   a spurious impression of decreased vertebral height,
   osteoporosis, spur formation and calcified discs.
4. **Achondroplasia*** — with spinal stenosis and anterior
   vertebral body beaks.
5. **Communicating hydrocephalus** — if severe and untreated.
6. **Syringomyelia** — especially if the onset is before 30 years
   of age.

7. **Other congenital syndromes**
   (a) Ehlers-Danlos ⎫
   (b) Marfan's*.   ⎬ both associated with dural ectasia.
   (c) Hurler's*.
   (d) Morquio's*.
   (e) Osteogenesis imperfecta tarda*.

Further Reading
Mitchell G.E., Lourie H. & Berne A.S. (1967) The various causes of scalloped vertebrae and notes on their pathogenesis. *Radiology*, 89: 67–74.

2.17 Anterior Scalloping of Vertebral Bodies

1. **Aortic aneurysm** — intervertebral discs remain intact. Well-defined anterior vertebral margin. ± calcification in the wall of the aorta.
2. **Tuberculous spondylitis** — with marginal erosions of the affected vertebral bodies. Disc space destruction. Widening of the paraspinal soft tissues.
3. **Lymphadenopathy** — pressure resorption of bone results in a well-defined anterior vertebral body margin unless there is malignant infiltration of the bone.
4. **Delayed motor development** — e.g. Down's syndrome.

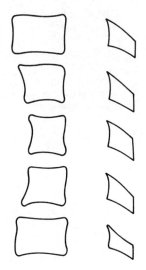

2.18   Anterior Scalloping of the Sacrum

1. **Metastases** (q.v.).
2. **Multiple myeloma***.
3. **Posterior soft tissue pelvic tumours** — invading bone or causing pressure resorption.
4. **Chordoma** — the majority of chordomas occur at this site. A bulky tumour. ± calcification.
5. **Anterior sacral meningocoele** — a round or oval defect in the anterior wall of the sacrum associated with a soft-tissue mass. The diagnosis is confirmed by myelography and/or C.T.

2.19   Syndromes with a Narrow Spinal Canal

1. **Achondroplasia***.
2. **Hypochondroplasia** — AD. Large calvarium, short stature and long fibula.
3. **Pseudohypoparathyroidism*** and **pseudopseudohypopara-thyroidism***.
4. **Diastrophic dwarfism.**
5. **Kniest syndrome.**
6. **Acrodysostosis.**

2.20 Widened Interpedicular Distance

Most easily appreciated by comparison with adjacent vertebrae. ± flattening of the inner side of the pedicles.

1. **Meningomyelocoele** — fusiform distribution of widened interpedicular distances with the greatest separation at the midpoint of the involved segment. Disc spaces are narrowed and bodies appear to be widened. Spinous processes and laminae are not identifiable. Facets may be fused into a continuous mass. Scoliosis (congenital or developmental) in 50–70% of cases ± kyphosis.
2. **Intraspinal mass** (q.v.) — especially ependymoma.
3. **Diastematomyelia** — 50% occur between L1 and L3; 25% between T7 and T12. Widened interpedicular distances are common but not necessarily at the same level as the spur. The spur is visible in 33% of cases and extends from the neural arch forward. Laminar fusion associated with a neural arch defect at the same or adjacent level are important signs in predicting the presence of diastemato-myelia. ± associated meningocoele, neurenteric cyst or dermoid.

2.21   Spinal Block

May be extradural, intradural or intramedullary.

1. Widespread malignancy — 42%.
2. Neural tumours — 20%.
3. Disorders of intervertebral joints — 15%.
4. Primary bone disorders — 13%.
5. Arachnoiditis — 6.5%.
6. Others — 4%.
    (a) Widespread infection.
    (b) Angioma.
    (c) Lipoma of cord.
    (d) Congenital cyst.
    (e) Spontaneous haemorrhage.

Further Reading
O'Carroll M.P. & Witcome J.B. (1979) Primary disorders of bone with spinal block. *Clin. Radiol.*, 30: 299–306.

2.22 Extradural Spinal Masses

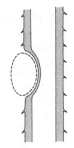

1. **Disc** — commonly lower cervical and lower lumbar. Rarely in thoracic region but even a small disc protrusion in this region may produce symptoms as the epidural space is smallest here. Congenital spinal stenosis may precipitate symptoms.

2. **Bone**
   (a) Osteophyte.
   (b) Metastases — breast and bronchus commonest. (NB disc destruction may occasionally occur in lymphoma and myeloma.)
   (c) Trauma — fracture or haematoma.
   (d) Paget's disease* — vertebral body enlarged with thickened cortex ('picture frame'). Neural arch may be involved. Paraspinal mass (osteoid tissue) may occur and may be calcified.
   (e) Osteomyelitis
       (i) TB (disc destruction and calcified paraspinal mass).
       (ii) Pyogenic.
       (iii) Hydatid — extradural extension of disease in 30% of those with spinal involvement. In the early stages there is a well defined lucency in the vertebral body often extending into the pedicle, lamina or transverse process. Later there is vertebral body collapse.
   (f) Primary bone tumours
       (i) Haemangioma* — due to compression fracture or chronic haemorrhage.
       (ii) Aneurysmal bone cyst*.
       (iii) Osteoblastoma*.
       (iv) Chordoma.
3. **Abscess** — commonly at the thoracolumbar junction. No bony abnormality if acute.
4. **Haematoma** — secondary to trauma or bleeding angioma.
5. **Arachnoid cyst** — commonly thoracic. Contains pulsatile CSF and scallops the posterior vertebra, flattens pedicles, and widens the interpedicular distance over several vertebral segments.

2.23 Intradural, Extramedullary Spinal Masses

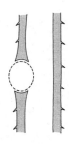

1. **Neurofibroma** — any level. Bony erosion, expansion of the intervertebral foramina, splaying of ribs, posterior scalloping of vertebral body. Scoliosis in 40%. Paraspinal mass. No calcification. Equal sex incidence.
2. **Meningioma** — commonly thoracic. Only 10% show bony erosion and this is usually minimal. 90% occur on the lateral aspect of the dura. Can calcify, but difficult to see on X-ray. May cause paraspinal mass. 80% occur in females over 40.
3. **Lipoma** — commonly lower cervical/upper thoracic. Slow growth causes bony erosion. May extend over several vertebral segments. Associated with spinal dysraphism. Occurs in early adulthood.
4. **Dermoid** — commonly conus/cauda equina. Associated with spinal dysraphism.
5. **Angioma** — no bony abnormality.
6. **Ependymoma** — commonly filum terminale and so appears as an intradural mass. Can be enormous and cause bone erosion and expansion.
7. **Metastases from CNS tumour** — particularly medulloblastoma, glioblastoma, pinealoma, ependymoma and primitive neuroectodermal tumours (PNET).

2.24 Intradural, Intramedullary Spinal Masses

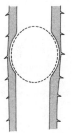

Most commonly due to (**1.**) tumour or (**2.**) syringomyelia. Helpful differentiating features are:

Syringomyelia	Tumour
Chiari malformation — this effectively establishes the diagnosis	—
Usually no bony abnormality	Bone erosion and expansion which is more marked with ependymomas than gliomas
Smooth outline of cord	Irregular outline
No dilated vessels on the surface of the cord	May have dilated vessels on the surface of the cord
—	Focal or asymmetrical expansion of the cord is more typical of tumours, especially when the cervical region is not involved

3. **Post-radiation myelopathy** — can cause symmetrical expansion of the cord which may extend beyond the irradiated segment, and may be indistinguishable from an intrinsic tumour.
4. **Haematoma** — due to contusion of the cord.

Further Reading

Moseley I.F. (1984) Myelography. In: du Boulay G.H. (ed.) *A Textbook of Radiological Diagnosis*, 5th edn, Vol. 1, Chapter 18, p. 530. London: H.K. Lewis.

Bibliography

Allen E.H., Cosgrove D. & Millard F.J.C. (1978) The radiological changes in infections of the spine and their diagnostic value. *Clin. Radiol.*, 29: 31–40.

Bradford D.S. & Hensinger R.M. (1985) *The Pediatric Spine*. New York: Thieme Inc.

Epstein B. (1976) *The Spine: A Radiological Text and Atlas*, 4th edn. Philadelphia: Lea & Febiger.

Felson B. (ed.) (1972) The spinal canal. *Semin. Roentgenol.*, 7(3).

Felson B. (ed.) (1979) Localised diseases of the spinal column. *Semin. Roentgenol.*, 14(1).

Lewtas N. (1980) The spine and myelography. In: Sutton D. (ed.) *Textbook of Radiology and Imaging*, 3rd edn. Edinburgh: Churchill Livingstone.

Reeder M. & Felson B. (1975) *Gamuts in Radiology*. Oxford: Pergamon Press.

Sandrock A.R. (ed.) (1977) The spine. *Radiol. Clin. North Am.*, 15(2).

Notes

Notes

Chapter 3
Joints

3.1 Monoarthritis

1. **Trauma** — pointers to the diagnosis are (a) the history, (b) the presence of a fracture and (c) a joint effusion, especially a lipohaemarthrosis.
2. **Osteoarthritis.**
3. **Crystal induced arthritis**
   (a) Gout*.
   (b) Calcium pyrophosphate dihydrate deposition disease*.
   (c) Calcium hydroxyapatite deposition disease.
4. **Rheumatoid arthritis*** — occasionally. Also juvenile chronic arthritis.
5. **Pyogenic arthritis** — commonest joints affected are the hip, knee and small joints of the hands and feet. 15% of those due to *Staphylococcus aureus* and 80% of those of gonococcal aetiology involve two or more joints. The joint may be radiologically normal at first clinical examination. Initially there is soft-tissue swelling due to effusion and synovial enlargement. Periarticular erosions progress to involve all of the articular cartilage and subchondral bone. Periosteal reaction. Osteoporosis follows the destructive changes.
6. **Tuberculous arthritis** — sometimes associated with pulmonary or renal tuberculosis. Similar sites of predilection to pyogenic arthritis. Insidious onset with radiological changes present at the time of first examination. Slowly developing osteoporosis precedes the destructive changes. Erosions first develop at peripheral non-contact points of the joint.
7. **Pigmented villonodular synovitis** — most commonly at the knee.
8. **Sympathetic** — a joint effusion can occur as a response to a tumour in the adjacent bone.

3.2 The Major Polyarthritides

Inflammatory		Chondropathic		Depositional
Periarticular (synovial) erosions **Osteoporosis** **Tendon-related erosions** **Periosteal reaction** **Syndesmophytes** **Malalignment**		**Subchondral erosions** **Subchondral sclerosis** **Osteophytes** **Chondrocalcinosis** **Normal bone density**		**Soft tissue masses** **Extra-articular erosions** — well defined — roofed — mass-related **Normal bone density**
Rheumatoid & its variants	*Seronegative*	*Degenerative*	*Metabolic*	
Symmetrical Small joints — esp. MCPJ & PIPJ Osteoporosis	Asymmetrical Large joints — SIJs, spine & DIPJs of hand Osteoporosis less marked Periosteal reaction Syndesmophytes	Weight bearing joints, DIPJs & first CMCJs Localized cartilage loss Marginal calcification	Atypical distribution Uniform cartilage loss Diffuse chondrocalcinosis Large subchondral cysts Greater destruction	
Rheumatoid arthritis Systemic lupus erythematosus Scleroderma Dermatomyositis	Ankylosing spondylitis Reiter's syndrome Psoriatic arthropathy Enteropathic arthritis Juvenile chronic arthritis	Osteoarthritis Neuropathic Haemophilic	Calcium pyrophosphate Haemochromatosis Alkaptonuria Hyperparathyroidism Wilson's disease	Gout Hypercholesterolaemia Reticulohistiocytosis Amyloidosis

3.3 Arthritis with Osteoporosis

1. **Rheumatoid arthritis***.
2. **Systemic lupus erythematosus***.
3. **Pyogenic arthritis.**
4. **Reiter's syndrome*** — in the acute phase.
5. **Scleroderma***.
6. **Haemophilia***.

3.4 Arthritis with Preservation of Bone Density

1. **Osteoarthritis.**
2. **Calcium pyrophosphate arthropathy** — see Calcium pyro-phosphate dihydrate deposition disease*.
3. **Gout***.
4. **Psoriatic arthropathy***.
5. **Ankylosing spondylitis.**
6. **Reiter's syndrome*** — in chronic or recurrent disease.
7. **Neuropathic arthropathy*** — especially in the spine and lower extremities.
8. **Pigmented villonodular synovitis.**

3.5 Arthritis with a Periosteal Reaction

1. **Juvenile chronic arthritis***.
2. **Reiter's syndrome***.
3. **Pyogenic arthritis.**
4. **Psoriatic arthropathy***.
5. **Rheumatoid arthritis*** — in less than 5% of patients.
6. **Haemophilia***.

3.6 Arthritis with Preserved or Widened Joint Space

1. **Early infective or inflammatory arthritis** — because of joint effusion.
2. **Psoriatic arthropathy*** — due to deposition of fibrous tissue.
3. **Acromegaly*** — due to cartilage overgrowth.
4. **Gout***.
5. **Pigmented villonodular synovitis.**

3.7   Arthritis Mutilans

A destructive arthritis of the hands and feet with resorption of bone ends and telescoping joints (main-en-lorgnette).

1. Rheumatoid arthritis*.
2. Juvenile chronic arthritis*.
3. Psoriatic arthropathy*.
4. Diabetes.
5. Leprosy.
6. Neuropathic arthropathy*.
7. Reiter's syndrome* — in the feet.

3.8   Diffuse Terminal Phalangeal Sclerosis

1. Normal variant — in 10% of normal individuals.
2. Rheumatoid arthritis* — most commonly in association with erosive arthropathy but may occur in its absence.
3. Scleroderma*.
4. Systemic lupus erythematosus*.
5. Sarcoidosis*.

Further Reading

Goodman N. (1967) The significance of terminal phalangeal osteosclerosis. *Radiology*, 89: 709–12.
Williams M. & Barton E. (1984) Terminal phalangeal sclerosis in rheumatoid arthritis. *Clin. Radiol.*, 35: 237–8.

3.9   Erosion (Enlargement) of the Intercondylar Notch of the Distal Femur

1. Juvenile chronic arthritis*.
2. Haemophilia*.
3. Psoriatic arthropathy*.
4. Tuberculous arthritis.
5. Rheumatoid arthritis*.

3.10 Calcified Loose Body (Single or Multiple) in a Joint

1. **Detached osteophyte** — larger and more variable in size than synovial osteochondromata. Other signs of degenerative arthritis.
2. **Osteochondral fracture.**
3. **Osteochondritis dissecans** — most commonly the knee, talus and elbow. A corresponding defect in the parent bone may be visible.
4. **Neuropathic arthropathy*** — joint disorganization.
5. **Synovial osteochondromatosis** — knee most commonly; hip, ankle, wrist and shoulder less commonly. Multiple small nodules of fairly uniform size. Faintly calcified initially; later ossified. Secondary erosion of intracapsular bone, joint space narrowing and osteophyte formation may occur later in the disease.

3.11 Calcification of Articular (Hyaline) Cartilage (Chondrocalcinosis)

1. **Calcium pyrophosphate dihydrate deposition disease*.**
2. **Hyperparathyroidism*.**
3. **Haemochromatosis*.**
4. **Acromegaly*.**
5. **Gout*.**
6. **Wilson's disease.**

Further Reading

Jensen P. (1988) Chondrocalcinosis and other calcifications. *Radiol. Clin. North Am.*, 26: 1315–25.

3.12 Sacroiliitis

1. Changes initially in the lower and middle thirds of the joint and the iliac side is more severely affected than the sacral side.
2. Periarticular osteoporosis, superficial erosions and sclerosis of subchondral bone.
3. Further erosion leads to widening of the joint space.
4. Subchondral sclerosis progresses to bony ankylosis.
5. Eventual return of the bones to normal density.

The most typical patterns of distribution are:

Bilateral Symmetrical
1. **Ankylosing spondylitis*** — may be asymmetrical early in the disease. Radiological signs as above.
2. **Inflammatory bowel disease** — ulcerative colitis, Crohn's disease and Whipple's disease. Identical appearances to ankylosing spondylitis.
3. **Psoriatic arthropathy*** — ankylosis is less frequent than in ankylosing spondylitis. Occurs in 30–50% of patients with arthropathy. Less commonly is asymmetrical or unilateral.
4. **Osteitis condensans ilii** — predominantly in young, multiparous women. A triangular segment of bone sclerosis on the inferior aspect of the iliac side of the joint is associated with a well-defined joint margin and a normal joint space.
5. **Hyperparathyroidism*** — subchondral bone resorption and joint-space widening only.
6. **Paraplegia** — joint-space narrowing and osteoporosis.

Bilateral Asymmetrical
1. **Reiter's syndrome***.
2. **Psoriatic arthropathy*** — this pattern in 40% of cases.
3. **Rheumatoid arthritis*** — rare. Minimal sclerosis and no significant bony ankylosis.
4. **Gouty arthritis** (see Gout*) — large well-defined erosions with surrounding sclerosis.
5. **Osteoarthritis** — the articular margins are smooth and well defined. Joint-space narrowing, subchondral sclerosis and anterior osteophytes are observed.

Unilateral
1. **Infection**.

3.13 Protrusio Acetabuli

1. **Rheumatoid arthritis*** — including juvenile chronic arthritis.
2. **Osteoporosis** (q.v.).
3. **Osteomalacia and rickets** (q.v.)*.
4. **Paget's disease***.
5. **Ankylosing spondylitis***.
6. **Osteoarthritis** — occasionally.
7. **Trauma** — acetabular fractures.
8. **Familial or idiopathic.**
9. **Marfan's syndrome*** — 45% show evidence of protrusio acetabulae. Of these, 50% are unilateral and 90% have an associated scoliosis.

Further Reading

Kuhlman J.E., Scott W.W., Fishman E.K., Pyeritz R.E. & Siegelman S.S. (1987) Acetabular protrusion in the Marfan Syndrome. *Radiology*, 164: 415–17.

3.14 Widening of the Symphysis Pubis (>7 mm)

Secondary

1. **Pregnancy** — resolves by the 3rd post partum month.
2. **Trauma.**
3. **Osteitis pubis** — one or more months following parturition or pelvic surgery, especially prostatic surgery. It may also be observed as a chronic stress reaction in athletes. Symmetrical bone resorption with subchondral bony irregularity and sclerosis. Ankylosis may be a late finding.
4. **Osteolytic metastases.**
5. **Infection** — low-grade osteomyelitis shows similar radiological features to osteitis pubis.
6. **Hyperparathyroidism*** — due to subperiosteal bone resorption.

Primary

1. **Bladder extrophy.**
2. **Epispadias** — the degree of widening correlates well with the severity of the epispadias.
3. **Other urogenital and anorectal anomalies** — have an increased incidence of this sign.
4. **Cleidocranial dysplasia*** — due to delayed or absent ossification.

Further Reading

Abramson D., Roberts S.M. & Wilson P.D. (1934) Relaxation of pelvic joints in pregnancy. *Surg. Gyneac & Obstet.*, 58: 595–613.

Muecke E.C. & Currarino G. (1968) Congenital widening of the pubic symphysis. *Am. J. Roentgenol.*, 103: 179–85.

3.15   Fusion or Bridging of the Symphysis Pubis

1. **Post-traumatic.**
2. **Post-infective.**
3. **Osteitis pubis** — see section 3.14.
4. **Osteoarthritis.**
5. **Ankylosing spondylitis***.
6. **Alkaptonuria***.
7. **Fluorosis.**

Bibliography

Forrester D.M., Brown J.C. & Nesson J.W. *The Radiology of Joint Disease*, 3rd edn, Philadelphia: Saunders.

Resnick D. & Niwayama G. (1988) *Diagnosis of Bone and Joint Disorders*, 2nd edn. Philadelphia: Saunders.

Notes

Chapter 4
Respiratory Tract

4.1 Acute Upper Airway Obstruction

Most commonly in infants, because of the small calibre of
the airways. Small or normal volume lungs with distension
of the upper airway proximal to the obstruction during
inspiration.

1. **Choanal atresia** — bilateral (33%) or unilateral, bony
   (90%) or membranous, complete or incomplete. When
   bilateral and complete presentation is with severe respiratory distress at birth. Incomplete obstruction is associated
   with respiratory difficulty during feeding. Diagnosis is
   by failure to pass a catheter through the nose and
   nasopharyngography or CT.
2. **Laryngo-tracheobronchitis** — narrowing of the glottic and
   subglottic regions. Indistinct tracheal margin because of
   oedema.
3. **Acute epiglottitis** — the epiglottis is swollen and may be
   shortened. Other components of the supraglottic region —
   aryepiglottic folds, arytenoids, uvula and prevertebral soft
   tissues — are also swollen. The hypopharynx and pyriform
   sinuses are distended with air.
4. **Retropharyngeal abscess** — enlargement of the prevertebral
   soft tissues which may contain gas or an air-fluid level.
5. **Oedema** — due to angio-oedema (allergic, anaphylactic
   or hereditary), inhalation of noxious gases or trauma.
   Predominantly laryngeal oedema.
6. **Foreign body** — more commonly produces a major
   bronchial occlusion rather than upper airway obstruction.
7. **Retropharyngeal haemorrhage** — due to trauma, neck
   surgery, direct carotid arteriography and bleeding disorders. Widening of the retropharyngeal soft-tissue space.

4.2   Chronic Upper Airway Obstruction in a Child

May be associated with overinflation of the lungs.

Nasal
1. **Choanal atresia** — bilateral (33%) or unilateral, bony (90%) or membranous, complete or incomplete. When bilateral and complete presentation is with severe respiratory distress at birth. Incomplete obstruction is associated with respiratory difficulty during feeding. Diagnosis is by failure to pass a catheter through the nose and nasopharyngography or CT.
2. **Nasal angiofibroma** — adolescent males. Symptoms of nasal obstruction and/or epistaxis. Plain films may show (1) anterior bowing of the posterior wall of the maxillary antrum, (2) deviation of the nasal septum and (3) a nasopharyngeal soft tissue mass with erosion of contiguous bony structures.
3. **Antrochoanal polyp.**

Supraglottic
1. **Grossly enlarged tonsils and adenoids.**
2. **Laryngomalacia** — presents at or shortly after birth, persists for several months and usually resolves by 2 years. Diagnosis is confirmed by direct laryngoscopy but fluoroscopy reveals anterior motion of the aryepiglottic folds and distension of the hypopharynx.
3. **Micrognathia** — in the Pierre Robin syndrome.
4. **Cysts** — of the epiglottis or aryepiglottic folds. The degree of obstruction depends on the size and location.

Glottic
1. **Laryngeal polyp, papilloma or cyst.**

Subglottic and Tracheal
1. **Tracheomalacia** — weakness of tracheal wall which may be primary or secondary:
   PRIMARY   Premature infants — probably related to intubation normal infants.

SECONDARY With innominate artery compression — persistent narrowing of the anterior tracheal wall at the level of the thoracic inlet.

With tracheo-oesophageal fistula/oesophageal atresia.

With vascular ring — most commonly a double aortic arch.

With external compression by tumour etc.

2. **Subglottic hemangioma** — the most common subglottic soft tissue mass in infancy. Occurs before 6 months. 50% have associated cutaneous hemangiomas. Characteristically it produces an asymmetrical narrowing of the subglottic airway.

3. **Following prolonged tracheal intubation** — see section 4.3.

4. **External compression from other mediastinal structures** — e.g. lymphadenopathy or thymic enlargement.

5. **Respiratory papillomatosis** — occurs anywhere from the nose to the lungs. Irregular soft-tissue masses around the glottis or in the trachea mostly. (Papillomata in adults are usually single).

Further Reading

Kushner, D.C. & Clifton Harris, G.B. (1978) Obstructing lesions of the larynx and trachea in infants and children. *Radiol. Clin. North Am.*, 16: 181–94.

Strife, J.L. (1988) Upper airway and tracheal obstruction in infants and children. *Radiol. Clin. North Am.*, 26: 309–22.

4.3 Chronic Upper Airway Obstruction in an Adult

May be associated with overinflation of the lungs.

Supraglottic
1. **Supraglottic carcinoma of the larynx** — involving the posterior surface of the epiglottis, the ventricle or the superolateral part of the vestibule. Dyspnoea is a late feature.

Glottic
1. **Vocal cord paralysis** — airway obstruction is most likely with bilateral recurrent nerve paresis and this most commonly occurs as a result of a thyroidectomy or malignant disease in the neck.
2. **Carcinoma of the glottis** — accounts for more than two-thirds of laryngeal carcinomas. Occurs mostly in the anterior two-thirds of the cords. Morphologically it can be proliferative or infiltrative.

Subglottic and Tracheal
1. **Extrinsic compression** — due to lymph nodes or local invasion from carcinomas of the bronchus, thyroid or oesophagus.
2. **Following prolonged tracheal intubation** — occurs in 5% of cases. The stenosis occurs most commonly at the level of the stoma. Less common sites are at the level of the inflatable cuff and where the tip impinged on the mucosa.
3. **Infraglottic carcinoma of the larynx** — either arising de novo at this site or as an extension from a glottic growth.
4. **Tracheal malignancy** — squamous cell carcinoma is the commonest tracheal primary.

Further Reading
Weber A.L. (ed.)(1978) The larynx and trachea. *Radio. Clin. North Am.*, **16**(2).

4.4 Unequal Lung Size, Lucency and Vascularity. Which is the Abnormal Side?

If Vascularity is Decreased, The Lung is Abnormal

If Vascularity is Normal or Increased, The Lung is Probably Normal

A Small Completely Opaque Hemithorax is Abnormal

When the small hemithorax is *completely* opaque the diagnosis is total collapse or agenesis. Furthermore the atelectasis can be presumed to be resorptive (i.e. secondary to obstruction) rather than compressive (i.e. from an overdistended contralateral lung) because *on the fully inspired film* an overexpanded lung will never compress the other lung to the extent of obliterating the costophrenic angle.

With Inspiration – Expiration, The Lung Changing Least or Not At All, is Abnormal

Further Reading
Swischuk L.E. (1984) *Differential Diagnosis in Paediatric Radiology*, pp. 7–12. Baltimore: Williams & Wilkins.

4.5   Unilateral Hypertransradiant Hemithorax

Exclude *contralateral* increased density, e.g. pleural effusion in a supine patient or pleural thickening.

Rotation
1. **Poor technique** } the hypertransradiant hemithorax is the
2. **Scoliosis** } side to which the patient is turned.

Chest Wall
1. **Mastectomy** — absent breast ± absent pectoral muscle shadows.
2. **Poliomyelitis** — atrophy of pectoral muscles ± atrophic changes in the shoulder girdle and humerus.
3. **Poland's syndrome** — unilateral congenital absence of pectoral muscles ± rib defects. Occurs in 10% of patients with syndactyly.

Pleura
1. **Pneumothorax** — note the lung edge and absent vessels peripherally.

Lung
1. **Compensatory emphysema** — following lobectomy (rib defects and opaque bronchial sutures indicate previous surgery) or lobar collapse.
2. **Obstructive emphysema** — due to bronchial stenosis or occlusion (q.v.). Air trapping on expiration results in increased lung volume and shift of the mediastinum to the contralateral side.
3. **Unilateral bullae** — vessels are absent rather than attenuated. May mimic pneumothorax.
4. **Macleod's syndrome** — the late sequela of childhood bronchiolitis. Small lung with small main and peripheral arteries. Air trapping occurs on expiration. Decreased number of bronchial divisions (5–10).
5. **Congenital lobar emphysema** — one-third present at birth. Marked overinflation of a lobe, most commonly the left upper lobe, right upper lobe or right middle lobe. The ipsilateral lobes are compressed and there is mediastinal displacement to the contralateral side.

Pulmonary Vessels

1. **Pulmonary embolus** (see Pulmonary embolic disease*) — to a major pulmonary artery (at least lobar in size). The pulmonary artery is dilated proximally and the affected lung shows moderate loss of volume.

4.6   Bilateral Hypertransradiant Hemithoraces

With Overexpansion of the Lungs

1. **Chronic obstructive emphysema** — with large central pulmonary arteries and peripheral arterial pruning. ± bullae.
2. **Asthma** — overinflation is secondary to bronchial constriction and mucus plugs.
3. **Acute bronchiolitis** — particularly affects children in the first year of life. Overexpansion is due to bronchial obstruction, secondary to mucosal swelling and this produces bronchial wall thickening on the radiograph. Collapse or consolidation are not a primary feature of the condition but are frequent complications of it.
4. **Tracheal, laryngeal or bilateral bronchial stenoses** (q.v.).

With Normal or Small Lungs

1. **Congenital heart disease producing oligaemia** — includes those conditions with right heart obstruction and right-to-left shunts. The hila are usually small except when there is post-stenotic dilatation of the pulmonary artery.
2. **Pulmonary artery stenosis** — if due to valvar stenosis there will be post-stenotic dilatation. 60% of congenital lesions have other associated cardiovascular abnormalities.
3. **Multiple pulmonary emboli**
4. **Primary pulmonary hypertension**
5. **Schistosomiasis**
6. **Metastatic trophoblastic tumour**

} identical radiological picture of big hilar vessels with peripheral pruning. History is most important. PPH occurs predominantly in young females and may be familial. Schistosomiasis more usually presents as a diffuse reticulonodular pattern.

Further Reading

Hodson M.E., Simon G. & Batten J.C. (1974) Radiology of uncomplicated asthma. *Thorax.*, 29: 296–303.
Thurlbeck W.M. & Simon G. (1978) Radiographic appearance of the chest in emphysema. *Am. J. Roentgenol.*, 130: 427–40.

4.7 Bronchial Stenosis or Occlusion

In the Lumen
1. **Foreign body** — air trapping is more common than atelectasis. The lower lobe is most frequently affected. The foreign body may be opaque.
2. **Mucus plug** — in asthma or cystic fibrosis.
3. **Misplaced endotracheal tube.**
4. **Aspergillosis** — with thickened bronchial walls.

In the Wall
1. **Carcinoma of the bronchus** — tapered narrowing ± irregularity.
2. **Bronchial adenoma** — usually a smooth, rounded filling defect, convex toward the hilum.
3. **Sarcoid granuloma.**
4. **Fibrosis** — e.g. tuberculosis and fungi. Can mimic carcinoma but usually produces a longer constriction.
5. **Bronchial atresia** — most commonly the apico-posterior segment of the left upper lobe.
6. **Fractured bronchus.**

Outside the Wall
1. **Lymph nodes**
2. **Mediastinal tumour**
3. **Enlarged left atrium** } smooth, eccentric narrowing.
4. **Aortic aneurysm**
5. **Anomalous origin of left pulmonary artery from right pulmonary artery** — producing compression of the right main bronchus as it passes over it, between the trachea and oesophagus to reach the left hilum. PA chest X-ray shows the right side of the trachea to be indented and the vessel is seen end-on between the trachea and oesophagus on the lateral view.

4.8   Increased Density of a Hemithorax

With Central Mediastinum

1. **Consolidation** — ± air bronchogram. Includes pneumonia, unilateral oedema (q.v.), aspiration pneumonia and radiation pneumonitis.
2. **Pleural effusion** — when the patient is supine a small or moderate effusion gravitates posteriorly producing a generalized increased density with an apical cap of fluid. Erect or decubitus films confirm the diagnosis.
3. **Mesothelioma** — often associated with a pleural effusion which obscures the tumour. Encasement of the lung limits mediastinal shift. ± pleural calcification.

With Mediastinal Displacement away from the Dense Hemithorax

1. **Pleural effusion** (q.v.) — N.B. a large effusion with no mediastinal shift implies underlying collapse which, in an older person, is often secondary to a bronchial carcinoma.
2. **Diaphragmatic hernia** — on the right side with herniated liver; on the left side the hemithorax is not usually opaque because of air within the herniated bowel. The left hemithorax may be opaque in the early neonatal period when air has not yet had time to reach the herniated bowel.

With Mediastinal Displacement towards the Dense Hemithorax

1. **Collapse.**
2. **Post-pneumonectomy** — rib resection ± opaque bronchial sutures.
3. **Lymphangitis carcinomatosa** — unilateral disease is uncommon. Linear and nodular opacities ± ipsilateral hilar and mediastinal lymphadenopathy. Septal lines.
4. **Pulmonary agenesis and hypoplasia** — usually asymptomatic. Absent or hypoplastic pulmonary artery.

N.B. 70% of unilateral diffuse *lung* opacities involve the right lung. Pneumonia, aspiration, pulmonary oedema, lymphangitis carcinomatosa and radiotherapy account for 90% (Youngberg 1977).

Further Reading

Youngberg A.S. (1977) Unilateral diffuse lung opacity. *Radiology.*, 123: 277–82.

4.9 Pneumatocoeles

One or more air-filled, thin-walled 'cysts'. They are usually
infective in origin and are thought to result from a check
valve obstruction of a communication between a cavity and
a bronchus. They appear during the first two weeks of the
pneumonia and resolve within several months. They may
contain fluid levels.

Infections
1. *Staphylococcus aureus* — a characteristic feature of
   childhood staphylococcal pneumonia, developing in
   40–60% of cases.
2. *Streptococcus pneumoniae.*
3. *Escherichia coli.*
4. *Klebsiella pneumoniae.*
5. *Haemophilus influenzae.*
6. *Legionella pneumophila* (Legionnaire's disease).

Traumatic
1. **Interstitial emphysema** — may be followed by thin-walled
   air-containing cysts.

4.10 Slowly Resolving or Recurrent Pneumonia

1. **Bronchial obstruction** (q.v.) — especially neoplasm or
   foreign body.
2. **Inappropriate chemotherapy** — especially for tuberculosis,
   Klebsiella and mycoses.
3. **Repeated aspiration**
   (a) Pharyngeal pouch.
   (b) Achalasia.
   (c) Scleroderma*.
   (d) Hiatus hernia.
   (e) 'H'-type tracheo-oesophageal fistula.
   (f) Paralytic or neuromuscular disorders.
   (g) Chronic sinusitis.
4. **Underlying lung pathology**
   (a) Abscess.
   (b) Bronchiectasis — see section 4.14.
   (c) Cystic fibrosis*.

5. **Immunological incompetence**
   (a) Cachexia.
   (b) Steroids and immunosuppressives.
   (c) Diabetes.
   (d) White-cell and immunoglobulin deficiency states.
6. **Pneumonias that resolve by fibrosis**
   (a) Tuberculosis.
   (b) Fungi.

4.11 Pneumonia with an Enlarged Hilum

Hilar lymph-node enlargement may be secondary to the pneumonia or pneumonia may be secondary to bronchial obstruction by a hilar mass. Signs suggestive of a secondary pneumonia are:
   (a) Segmental or lobar consolidation which is better defined than a primary pneumonia.
   (b) Slow resolution.
   (c) Recurrent consolidation in the same part of the lung.
   (d) Associated collapse.

Secondary Pneumonias
See section 4.7, but note particularly 'Carcinoma of the bronchus'.

Primary Pneumonias
1. **Primary tuberculosis** — lymph-node enlargement is unilateral in 80% and involves the hilar (60%), or combined hilar and paratracheal (40%) nodes.
2. **Viral pneumonias** — especially pertussis.
3. **Mycoplasma** — lymph-node enlargement is common in children but rare in adults. May be uni- or bilateral.
4. **Primary histoplasmosis** — in endemic areas. Hilar lymphadenopathy is common, particularly in children. During healing the lymph nodes calcify and may cause bronchial obstruction thereby initiating distal infection.
5. **Coccidioidomycosis** — in endemic areas. The pneumonic type consists of predominantly lower lobe consolidation which is frequently associated with hilar lymph-node enlargement.

See also section 4.30.

4.12 Lobar Pneumonia

Consolidation involving the air spaces of an anatomically recognizable lobe. The entire lobe may not be involved and there may be a degree of associated collapse.

1. *Streptococcus pneumoniae* — the commonest cause. Usually unilobar. Cavitation rare. Pleural effusion is uncommon. Little or no collapse.
2. *Klebsiella pneumoniae* — often multilobar involvement. Great propensity for cavitation and lobar enlargement.
3. *Staphylococcus aureus* — especially in children. 40–60% of children develop pneumatocoeles. Effusion (empyema) and pneumothorax are also common. Bronchopleural fistula may develop. No lobar predilection.
4. Tuberculosis — in primary or post-primary tuberculosis, but more common in the former. Associated collapse is common. The right lung is affected twice as often as the left and primary tuberculosis predilects the anterior segment of the upper lobe or the medial segment of the middle lobe.
5. *Streptococcus pyogenes* — affects the lower lobes predominantly. Often associated with pleural effusion.

4.13 Consolidation with Bulging of Fissures

Homogeneous or inhomogeneous air space opacification with bulging of the bounding fissures.

1. Infection with abundant exudates — *Klebsiella pneumoniae* (Friedländer's pneumonia), *Streptococcus pneumoniae*, *Mycobacterium tuberculosis* and *Yersinia pestis* (Plague pneumonia).
2. Abscess — when an area of consolidation breaks down. Organisms which commonly produce abscesses are *Staphylococcus aureus*, *Klebsiella* spp. and other Gram-negative organisms.
3. Carcinoma of the bronchus — this can fill and expand a lobe.

4.14 Bronchiectasis

1. Peribronchial thickening and retained secretions.
2. Crowded vessels, i.e. loss of volume.
3. Compensatory emphysema.
4. Cystic spaces ± air fluid levels.
5. Coarse honeycomb pattern in very severe disease.
6. Normal radiograph in 7%.

1. **Secondary to childhood infections** — especially measles and pertussis.
2. **Secondary to bronchial obstruction** — foreign body, neoplasm, mucus plugs (cystic fibrosis and asthma) and aspergillosis.
3. **Chronic aspiration.**
4. **Congenital structural defects**
   (a) Kartagener's syndrome — bronchiectasis with immobile cilia, dextro cardia and absent frontal sinuses. 5% of patients with dextrocardia will eventually develop bronchiectasis.
   (b) Williams–Campbell syndrome — bronchial cartilage deficiency.
5. **Immune deficiency states** — e.g. hypogammaglobulinaemia, chronic granulomatous disease and Chédiak–Higashi syndrome.

4.15 Widespread Air-space (Acinar) Disease

This is commonly referred to as alveolar shadowing but the term is incorrect because the lung densities are due to the anatomically larger acinus. The general term 'air space' shadow, nodule or disease is recommended. The signs of air space disease are:
1. Acinar nodules, 4–10 mm diameter.
2. Ill-defined margins.
3. Coalescence.
4. Mostly non-segmental.
5. Air bronchogram. N.B This sign may also be a feature of relaxation atelectasis (e.g. collapsed lung behind a large pneumothorax), cicatrisation atelectasis (e.g. bronchiectasis and radiation fibrosis) and adhesive atelectasis (e.g. acute radiation pneumonitis and hyaline membrane disease).
6. Air bronchiologram and alveologram — lucencies due to residual air in bronchioles and alveoli.

1. **Oedema** (q.v.).
2. **Pneumonia** — most often the unusual types
   (a) Tuberculosis.
   (b) Histoplasmosis.
   (c) Pneumocystis carinii.
   (d) Influenza — particularly in patients with mitral stenosis or who are pregnant.
   (e) Chicken pox — may be confluent in the central areas of the lungs. ± hilar lymph-node enlargement.
   (f) Other viral pneumonias.
3. **Haemorrhage**
   (a) Trauma (contusion).
   (b) Anticoagulants, haemophilia, leukaemia and disseminated intravascular coagulopathy.
   (c) Goodpasture's syndrome.
   (d) Idiopathic pulmonary haemosiderosis — in the acute stage.
4. **Fat emboli** — 1–2 days post-trauma. Predominantly peripheral. Resolves in 1–4 weeks.
5. **Alveolar cell carcinoma** — effusions are common. Mediastinal lymph nodes are uncommon. Diagnosis by sputum cytology or lung biopsy.
6. **Haematogenous metastases** — especially chorioncarcinoma. Others are rare.
7. **Lymphoma*** — usually with hilar or mediastinal lymphadenopathy.
8. **Sarcoidosis*** — often associated with a reticulonodular pattern elsewhere.
9. **Löffler's** — peripheral ('reversed bat's wing'), often in the upper zones.

Further Reading

Fraser R.G., Peter Paré J.A., Paré P.D., Fraser R.S. & Genereux G.P. (1988) *Diagnosis of Diseases of the Chest*. Philadelphia: Saunders. pp. 459–72.

4.16   Localized Air-space Disease

See 'Widespread airspace disease, section 4.15.

1. **Pneumonia.**
2. **Infarction** (see Pulmonary embolic disease*) — usually in the lower lobes. Often indistinguishable from pneumonia.
3. **Contusion** — ± rib fractures or other signs of trauma.
4. **Oedema** (q.v.)
5. **Radiation** — several weeks following radiotherapy. May have a straight margin, corresponding to the field of treatment.
6. **Alveolar cell carcinoma.**
7. **Lymphoma*.**

4.17 Pulmonary Oedema

1. Heart failure.
2. **Fluid overload** — excess i.v. fluids, renal failure and excess hypertonic fluids, e.g. contrast media.
3. **Cerebral disease** — cerebrovascular accident, head injury or raised intracranial pressure.
4. **Near drowning** — radiologically no significant differences between fresh-water and sea-water drowning.
5. **Aspiration (Mendelson's syndrome).**
6. **Radiotherapy** — several weeks following treatment. May have a characteristic straight edge.
7. **Rapid re-expansion of lung following thoracentesis.**
8. **Liver disease and other causes of hypoproteinaemia.**
9. **Transfusion reaction.**
10. **Drugs**
    (a) Those which induce cardiac arrhythmias or depress myocardial contractility.
    (b) Those which alter pulmonary capillary wall permeability, e.g. overdoses of heroin, morphine, methadone, dextropropoxyphene and aspirin. Hydrochlorothiazide, phenylbutazone, aspirin and nitrofurantoin can cause oedema as an idiosyncratic response.
    N.B. Contrast media can induce arrhythmias, alter capillary wall permeability and produce a hyperosmolar load.
11. **Poisons**
    (a) Inhaled — NO_2, SO_2, CO, Phosgene, hydrocarbons and smoke.
    (b) Circulating — Paraquat and snake venom.
12. **Mediastinal tumours** — producing venous or lymphatic obstruction.
13. **Shock lung (adult respiratory distress syndrome)** — 24–72 hours post insult.

Further Reading

Milne E.N.C., Pistolesi M., Miniati M. & Giuntini C. (1985) The radiological distinction of cardiogenic and noncardiogenic edema. *Am. J. Roentgenol.*, 144: 879–94.

4.18 Unilateral Pulmonary Oedema

Pulmonary *Oedema on the Same Side as a Pre-existing Abnormality*
1. Prolonged lateral decubitus position.
2. Unilateral aspiration.
3. Pulmonary contusion.
4. Rapid thoracentesis of air or fluid.
5. Bronchial obstruction.
6. Systemic artery to pulmonary artery shunts — e.g. Waterston (on the right side). Blalock–Taussig (left or right side) and Pott's procedure (on the left side).

Pulmonary *Oedema on the Opposite Side to a Pre-existing Abnormality*
i.e. oedema on the side opposite a lung with a perfusion defect.
1. Congenital absence or hypoplasia of a pulmonary artery.
2. Macleod's syndrome.
3. Thromboembolism.
4. Unilateral emphysema.
5. Lobectomy.
6. Pleural disease.

Further Reading
Calenoff L., Kruglik G.D. & Woodruff A. (1978) Unilateral pulmonary oedema. *Radiology.*, 126: 19–24.

4.19 Septal Lines (Kerley B Lines)

1. Due to visible interlobular lymphatics and their surrounding connective tissue.
2. 1–3 cm long, less than 1 mm thick, extending from and perpendicular to the pleural surface.
3. Best seen in the costophrenic angles.

Pulmonary Venous Hypertension
1. Left ventricular failure.
2. Mitral stenosis.

Lymphatic Obstruction
1. **Pneumoconioses** — surrounding tissues may contain a heavy metal, e.g. tin, which contributes to the density.
2. **Lymphangitis carcinomatosa.**
3. **Sarcoidosis*** — septal lines are uncommon.

4.20 'Honeycomb Lung'

1. A generalized reticular pattern or miliary mottling which when summated produces the appearance of air containing 'cysts' 0.5–2.0 cm in diameter.
2. Obscured pulmonary vasculature.
3. Late appearance of radiological signs after the onset of symptoms.
4. Complications
   (a) pneumothorax is frequent;
   (b) cor pulmonale later in the course of the disease.

1. **Collagen disorders**
   (a) Rheumatoid lung — most pronounced at the bases and may be preceded by basal infiltrates. ± small effusions.
   (b) Scleroderma* — predominantly basal. Less regular 'honeycomb' pattern, which is preceded by fine, linear, basal streaks. Cor pulmonale is unusual.
2. **Extrinsic allergic alveolitis*** — predominantly in the upper zones.
3. **Sarcoidosis*** — sparing of extreme apices. Hilar lymphadenopathy usually resolved by this stage but if present it is a useful sign.
4. **Pneumoconiosis** — particularly frequent in asbestosis*, but also in other reactive dusts.
5. **Cystic bronchiectasis** (q.v.) — in lower and middle lobes especially. Bronchial-wall thickening. ± localized areas of consolidation.
6. **Cystic fibrosis*.**
7. **Drugs** — nitrofurantoin, busulphan, cyclophosphamide, bleomycin and melphalan.
8. **Histiocytosis X*** — 'honeycomb' pattern probably always preceded by disseminated nodules. May be predominantly in the mid and upper zones. Cor pulmonale is uncommon.
9. **Tuberous sclerosis*** — lung involvement in 5% of patients. Symptoms first in adult life. Differentiated clinically.
10. **Idiopathic interstitial fibrosis (cryptogenic fibrosing alveolitis)** — no specific differentiating features. More marked in the lower half of the lungs initially and progresses to involve the whole of the lungs.
11. **Neurofibromatosis*** — ± rib notching, 'ribbon' ribs and/or scoliosis. In 10%, but not before adulthood.

4.21 Pneumoconioses

Inorganic Dusts

WITHOUT FIBROSIS
1. **Ferric oxide** — siderosis.
2. **Ferric oxide + silver** — argyrosiderosis.
3. **Tin oxide** — stannosis.
4. **Barium** — barytosis.
5. **Calcium.**

WITH FIBROSIS
1. **Free silica** — silicosis*.
2. **Coal dust** — coal miner's pneumoconiosis*.
3. **Silicates** — asbestosis*, china clay, talc and mica.

WITH CHEMICAL PNEUMONITIS
1. **Beryllium.**
2. **Manganese.**
3. **Vanadium.**
4. **Osmium.**
5. **Cadmium.**

CARCINOGENIC DUSTS
1. **Radioactive dusts** — e.g. uranium.
2. **Asbestos** — see Asbestos inhalation.
3. **Arsenic.**

Organic Dusts (Extrinsic Allergic Alveolitis*)
1. **Mouldy hay** — farmers' lung.
2. **Bagasse (sugar cane dust)** — bagassosis.
3. **Cotton or linen dust** — byssinosis.
4. **Mouldy vegetable compost** — mushroom workers' lung.
5. **Pigeon and budgerigar excreta** — pigeon breeder's and budgerigar fancier's lung.

Further Reading
Felson B (ed.) (1967) The pneumoconioses. *Semin. Roentgenol.*, 2 (3).
Fraser R.G. & Pare J.A.P. (1975) Extrinsic allergic alveolitis. *Semin. Roentgenol.*, 10: 31–42.

4.22   Multiple Pin-point Opacities

Must be of very high atomic number to be rendered visible.

1. **Post lymphogram** — iodized oil emboli. Contrast medium may be visible at the site of termination of the thoracic duct.
2. **Silicosis*** — usually larger than pin-point but can be very dense, especially in goldminers.
3. **Stannosis** — inhalation of tin oxide. Even distribution throughout the lungs. With Kerley A and B lines.
4. **Barytosis** — inhalation of barytes. Very dense, discrete opacities. Generalized distribution but bases and apices usually spared.
5. **Limestone and marble workers** — inhalation of calcium.
6. **Alveolar microlithiasis** — familial. Lung detail obscured by miliary calcifications. Few symptoms but may progress to cor pulmonale eventually. Pleura, heart and diaphragm may be seen as negative shadows.

4.23   Multiple Opacities (0.5–2 mm)

Soft-tissue Density

1. **Miliary tuberculosis** — widespread. Uniform size. Indistinct margins but discrete. No septal lines. Normal hila unless superimposed on primary tuberculosis.
2. **Fungal diseases** — miliary histoplasmosis, coccidioido-mycosis, blastomycosis and cryptococcosis (torulosis). Similar appearance to miliary tuberculosis.
3. **Coal miner's pneumoconiosis*** — predominantly mid zones with sparing of the extreme bases and apices. Ill defined and may be arranged in a circle or rosette. Septal lines.
4. **Sarcoidosis*** — predominantly mid zones. Ill defined. Often with enlarged hila.
5. **Acute extrinsic allergic alveolitis*** — micronodulation in all zones, but predominantly basal.
6. **Fibrosing alveolitis** — initially most prominent in the lower halves of the lungs and later spreads upwards. Poorly defined. Obliteration of vascular markings.

Greater than Soft-tissue Density

1. **Haemosiderosis** — secondary to chronic raised venous pressure (seen in 10–15% of patients with mitral stenosis), repeated pulmonary haemorrhage (e.g. Goodpasture's disease) or idiopathic. Septal lines. Smaller than miliary TB.
2. **Silicosis*** — relative sparing of bases and apices. Very well defined and dense when due to pure silica: ill defined and of lower density when due to mixed dusts. Septal lines.
3. **Siderosis** — lower density than silica. Widely disseminated. Asymptomatic.
4. **Stannosis** ⎫
5. **Barytosis** ⎭   see section 4.22.

4.24 Multiple Opacities (2–5 mm)

Remaining Discrete

1. **Carcinomatosis** — breast, thyroid, sarcoma, melanoma, prostate, pancreas or bronchus (eroding a pulmonary artery). Variable sizes and progressive increase in size. ± lymphatic obstruction.
2. **Lymphoma*** — nearly always with hilar or mediastinal lymphadenopathy.
3. **Sarcoidosis*** — predominantly mid zones. Often with enlarged hila.

Tending to Confluence and Varying Rapidly

1. **Multifocal pneumonia** — including aspiration pneumonia and tuberculosis.
2. **Pulmonary oedema** (q.v.).
3. **Extrinsic allergic alveolitis*** — predominantly basal.
4. **Fat emboli** — predominantly peripheral.

4.25   Solitary Pulmonary Nodule

Granulomas

1. **Tuberculoma** — more common in the upper lobes and on the right side. Well defined. 0.5–4 cm. 25% are lobulated. Calcification frequent. 80% have satellite lesions. Cavitation is uncommon and when present is small and eccentric. Usually persist unchanged for years.

2. **Histoplasmoma** — in endemic areas (Mississippi and the Atlantic coast of USA). More frequent in the lower lobes. Well defined. Seldom larger than 3 cm. Calcification is common and may be central producing a target appearance. Cavitation is rare. Satellite lesions are common.

Malignant Neoplasms

1. **Carcinoma of the bronchus** — usually greater than 2 cm. Accounts for less than 15% of all solitary nodules at 40 years: almost 100% at 80 years. Appearances suggesting malignancy are
   (a) Recent appearance or rapid growth (previous CXRs are very helpful here).
   (b) Size greater than 4 cm.
   (c) The lesion crosses a fissure (although some fungus diseases also do so).
   (d) Ill-defined margins.
   (e) Umbilicated or notched margin (if present it indicates malignancy in 80%).
   (f) Corona radiata (spiculation). (But also seen in PMF and granulomas.)
   (g) Peripheral line shadows.
   (h) Calcification is very rare, except in scar carcinomas.

2. **Metastasis** — accounts for 3–5% of asymptomatic nodules. 25% of pulmonary metastases are solitary. Most likely primaries are breast, sarcoma, seminoma and renal cell carcinoma. Predilection for the lung periphery. Calcification is rare but occurs with metastatic osteosarcoma, chondrosarcoma and some other rarer metastases.

3. **Alveolar cell carcinoma** — when localized, a mass is the most common presentation. More commonly ill defined. Air bronchogram is common. No calcification. Pleural effusion in 5%. Mediastinal lymphadenopathy is much less common than with carcinoma of the bronchus.

Benign Neoplasms
1. **Adenoma** — 90% occur around the hilum: 10% are peripheral. Round or oval and well defined. 25% present as a solitary nodule; 75% present with the effects of bronchial stenosis. Calcification and cavitation are rare. Histologically, 80–90% are carcinoids and 10–20% are cylindromas. The former may metastasize to bone (sclerotic secondaries) or to liver and may produce the carcinoid syndrome.
2. **Hamartoma** — 96% occur over 40 years. 90% are intrapulmonary and usually within 2 cm of the pleura. 10% produce bronchial stenosis. Usually less than 4 cm diameter. Well defined. Lobulated rather than smooth. Calcification in 30%, although the incidence increases with the size of the lesion (in 75% when greater than 5 cm). Calcification is 'popcorn', craggy or punctate.

Infections
1. **Pneumonia** — simple consolidation, especially pneumococcal. Air bronchogram.
2. **Hydatid** — in endemic areas. Most common in the lower lobes and more frequent on the right side. Well defined. 1–10 cm. Solitary in 70%. May have a bizarre shape. Rupture results in the 'water lily' sign.

Congenital
1. **Sequestration** — usually more than 6 cm. Two-thirds occur in the left lower lobe, one-third in the right lower lobe and contiguous to the diaphragm. Well defined, round or oval. Diagnosis confirmed by aortography and venous drainage is via the pulmonary veins (intralobar type) or bronchial veins (extralobar type).
2. **Bronchogenic cyst** — peak incidence in the 2nd and 3rd decades. Two-thirds are intrapulmonary and occur in the medial one-third of the lower lobes. Round or oval. Smooth walled and well defined.

Vascular

1. **Pulmonary infarction** (see Pulmonary embolic disease*) — most frequent in the lower lobes. With a pleural effusion and elevation of the hemidiaphragm.
2. **Haematoma** — peripheral, smooth and well defined. 2–6 cm. Slow resolution over several weeks.
3. **Arteriovenous malformation** — 66% are single. Well defined, lobulated ('bag of worms'). Tomography may show feeding or draining vessels. Calcification is rare.

4.26 Multiple Pulmonary Nodules (greater than 5 mm)

Neoplastic

1. **Metastases** — most commonly from breast, thyroid, kidney, gastrointestinal tract and testes. In children, Wilms' tumour, Ewing's tumour, neuroblastoma and osteosarcoma. Predilection for lower lobes and more common peripherally. Range of sizes. Well defined. Ill-definition suggests prostrate, breast or stomach. Hilar lymphadenopathy and effusions are uncommon.

Infections

1. **Abscesses** — widespread distribution but asymmetrical. Commonly *Staphylococcus aureus*. Cavitation common. No calcification.
2. **Coccidioidomycosis** — in endemic areas. Well defined with a predilection for the upper lobes. 0.5–3 cm. Calcification and cavitation may be present.
3. **Histoplasmosis** — in endemic areas. Round, well defined and few in number. Sometimes calcify. Usually unchanged for many years.
4. **Hydatid** — more common on the right side and in the lower zones. Well defined unless there is surrounding pneumonia. Often 10 cm or more. May rupture and show the 'water lily' sign.

Immunological

1. **Wegener's granulomatosis** — widespread distribution. 0.5–10 cm. Round and well defined. No calcification. Cavitation in 30–50% of cases. ± focal pneumonitis.

2. **Rheumatoid nodules** — peripheral and more common in the lower zones. Round and well defined. No calcification. Cavitation common.
3. **Caplan's syndrome** — well defined. Develop rapidly in crops. Calcification and cavitation occur. Background stippling of pneumoconiosis.

Inhalational
1. **Progressive massive fibrosis** — mid and upper zones. Begin peripherally and move centrally. Peripheral emphysema. Oval in shape. Calcification and cavitation occur. Background nodularity of pneumoconiosis.

Vascular
1. **Arteriovenous malformations** — 33% are multiple. Well defined. Lobulated. Tomography may show feeding or draining vessels. Calcification is rare.

4.27 Lung Cavities

Infective, i.e. Abscesses
1. *Staphylococcus aureus* — thick walled with a ragged inner lining. No lobar predilection. Associated with effusion and empyema ± pyopneumothorax — almost invariable in children, not so common in adults. Pneumatocoeles (q.v.). Multiple.
2. *Klebsiella pneumoniae* — thick walled with a ragged inner lining. More common in the upper lobes. Usually single but may be multilocular. ± effusion.
3. **Tuberculosis** — thick walled and smooth. Upper lobes and apical segment of lower lobes mainly. Usually surrounded by consolidation. ± fibrosis.
4. **Aspiration** — look for foreign body, e.g. tooth.
5. **Others** — Gram-negative organisms, actinomycosis, nocardiosis, histoplasmosis, coccidioidomycosis, aspergillosis, hydatid and amoebiasis.

Neoplastic

1. **Carcinoma of the bronchus** — thick walled with an eccentric cavity. Predilection for the upper lobes. Found in 2–10% of carcinomas and especially if peripheral. More common in squamous cell carcinomas and may then be thin walled.
2. **Metastases** — thin or thick walled. May only involve a few of the nodules. Seen especially in squamous cell, colon and sarcoma metastases.
3. **Hodgkin's disease** — thin or thick walled and typically in an area of infiltration. With hilar or mediastinal lymphadenopathy.

Vascular

1. **Infarction** — three situations may be encountered. *Primary* infection due to a septic embolus almost invariably results in cavitation. There may be *secondary* infection of an initially sterile infarct. An aseptic cavitating infarct may subsequently become infected — *tertiary infection*. Aseptic cavitation is usually solitary and arises in a large area of consolidation after about 2 weeks. If localized to a segment the commonest sites are apical or posterior segment of an upper lobe or apical segment of lower lobe (*cf.* lower lobe predominance with noncavitating infarction). Majority have scalloped inner margins and cross cavity band shadows. ± effusion.

Abnormal Lung

1. **Cystic bronchiectasis** (q.v.) — thin walled. More common in the lower lobes.
2. **Infected emphysematous bulla** — thin walled. ± air fluid level.
3. **Sequestrated lung** — thick or thin walled. 66% in the right lower lobe, 33% in the left lower lobe. ± air fluid level. ± surrounding pneumonia.
4. **Bronchogenic cyst** — in medial third of lower lobes. Thin walled. ± air fluid level. ± surrounding pneumonia.

Granulomas

1. **Wegener's granulomatosis** — widespread. Cavitation in some of the nodules. Thick walled, becoming thinner with time. Can be transient.
2. **Rheumatoid nodules** — thick walled with a smooth inner lining. Especially in the lower lobes and peripherally. Well defined. Become thin walled with time.
3. **Progressive massive fibrosis** — predominantly in the mid and upper zones. Thick walled and irregular. Background nodularity.
4. **Sarcoidosis*** — thin walled. In early disease due to a combination of central necrosis of areas of coalescent granulomas and a check-valve mechanism beyond partial obstruction of airways by endobronchial sarcoidosis.

Traumatic

1. **Haematoma** — peripheral. Air fluid level if it communicates with a bronchus.
2. **Traumatic lung cyst** — thin walled and peripheral. Single or mutiple. Uni- or multilocular. Distinguished from cavitating haematomas as they present early, within hours of the injury.

Further Reading

Jones D.K., Dent R.G., Rimmer M.J. & Flower C.D.R. (1984) Thin-walled ring shadows in early pulmonary sarcoidosis. *Clin. Radiol.*, 35: 307–10.

Wilson, A.G., Joseph A.E.A. & Butland R.J.A. (1986) The radiology of aseptic cavitation in pulmonary infarction. *Clin. Radiol.*, 37: 327–33.

4.28   Opacity with an Air Bronchogram

Infective
1. Pneumonia.

Inflammatory
1. Radiation pneumonitis.
2. Progressive massive fibrosis.

Neoplastic
1. Alveolar cell carcinoma.
2. Lymphoma*.
3. Lymphosarcoma.

4.29   Pulmonary Calcification or Ossification

Localized Calcification
1. **Tuberculosis** — demonstrable in 10% of those with a positive tuberculin test. Small central nidus of calcification. Calcification ≠ healed.
2. **Histoplasmosis** — in endemic areas, calcification due to histoplasmosis is demonstrable in 30% of those with a positive histoplasmin test. Calcification may be laminated producing a target lesion. ± multiple punctate calcifications in the spleen.
3. **Coccidioidomycosis.**
4. **Blastomycosis** — rare.

Calcification Within a Solitary Nodule
Calcification within a nodule equates with a benign lesion. The exceptions are:
   (a) Carcinoma engulfing a pre-existing calcified granuloma (eccentric calcification).
   (b) Solitary calcifying/ossifying metastasis — osteosarcoma, chondrosarcoma, mucinous adenocarcinoma of the colon or breast, papillary carcinoma of the thyroid, cystadenocarcinoma of the ovary and carcinoid.
   (c) $1°$ peripheral squamous cell or papillary adenocarcinoma.

Diffuse or Multiple Calcifications
1. Infections.
   (a) Tuberculosis — healed miliary.
   (b) Histoplasmosis.
   (c) Varicella — following chicken pox pneumonia in adulthood. 1–3 mm. Numbered in 10s.
2. **Chronic pulmonary venous hypertension** — especially mitral stenosis. Up to 8 mm. Most prominent in mid and lower zones. ± ossification.
3. **Silicosis** — in up to 20% of those showing nodular opacities.
4. **Metastases** — as above.
5. **Alveolar microlithiasis** — often familial. Myriad minute calcifications in alveoli which obscure all lung detail. Because of the lung's increased density, the heart, pleura and diaphragm may be evident as negative shadows.
6. **Metastatic due to hypercalcaemia** — chronic renal failure, 2° hyperparathyroidism and multiple myeloma*. Predominantly in the upper zones.
7. **Lymphoma following radiotherapy.**

Interstitial Ossification
Branching calcific densities extending along the bronchovascular distribution of the interstitial space.
1. **Fibrosing alveolitis.**
2. **Long-term busulphan therapy.**
3. **Chronic pulmonary venous hypertension.**
4. **Idiopathic.**

Further Reading
Jacobs A.N., Neitzschman H.R. & Nice C.M. Jr. (1973) Metaplastic bone formation in the lung. *Am. J. Roentgenol.*, 118: 344–6.
Kuplic J.B., Higley C.S., Niewoehner D.E. (1972) Pulmonary ossification associated with long-term busulfan therapy in chronic myeloid leukaemia. Case report. *Am. Rev. Resp. Dis.*, 106: 759.
Maile C.W., Rodan B.A., Godwin J.D., Chen J.T.T. & Ravin C.E. (1982) Calcification in pulmonary metastases. *Br. J. Radiol.*, 55: 108–13.
Mendeloff J. (1971) Disseminated nodular pulmonary ossification in the Hamman–Rich lung. *Am. Rev. Resp. Dis.*, 103: 269.

4.30   Unilateral Hilar Enlargement

Lymph Nodes
1. **Carcinoma of the bronchus** — the hilar enlargement may be due to the tumour itself or involved lymph nodes.
2. **Lymphoma*** — unilateral is very unusual; involvement is usually bilateral and asymmetrical.
3. **Infective**
   (a) Primary tuberculosis.
   (b) Histoplasmosis.
   (c) Coccidioidomycosis.
   (d) Mycoplasma.
   (e) Pertussis.
4. **Sarcoidosis*** — unilateral disease in only 1–5%.

Pulmonary Artery
1. **Post-stenotic dilatation** — on the left side.
2. **Pulmonary embolus** (see Pulmonary embolic disease*) — massive to one lung. Peripheral oligaemia.
3. **Aneurysm** — in chronic pulmonary arterial hypertension. ± egg-shell calcification.

Others
1. **Mediastinal mass** (q.v.) — superimposed on a hilum.
2. **Perihilar pneumonia** — ill defined, ± air bronchogram.

See also section 4.11.

4.31 Bilateral Hilar Enlargement

Due to lymph node enlargement or pulmonary artery enlargement.

Idiopathic
1. Sarcoidosis* — symmetrical and lobulated. Bronchopulmonary ± unilateral or bilateral paratracheal lymphadenopathy.

Neoplastic
1. Lymphoma* — asymmetrical.
2. Lymphangitis carcinomatosa.

Infective
1. Viruses — most common in children.
2. Primary tuberculosis — rarely bilateral and symmetrical.
3. Histoplasmosis.
4. Coccidioidomycosis.

Vascular
1. Pulmonary arterial hypertension — see section 5.15.

Immunological
1. Extrinsic allergic alveolitis* — in mushroom workers.

Inhalational
1. Silicosis* — symmetrical.
2. Chronic berylliosis — only in a minority of cases. Symmetrical.

4.32 'Eggshell' Calcification of Lymph Nodes

The criteria for diagnosis were listed by Gross *et al.* and Jacobsen *et al.* as:

1. Shell-like calcifications up to 2 mm thick in the periphery of at least two lymph nodes.
2. Calcifications may be solid or broken.
3. In at least one of the lymph nodes the ring of calcification must be complete.
4. The central part of the lymph node may show additional calcifications.
5. One of the affected lymph nodes must be at least 1 cm in its greatest diameter.

1. **Silicosis*** — seen in approximately 5% of silicotics. Predominantly hilar lymph nodes but may also be observed in the anterior and posterior mediastinal lymph nodes, cervical lymph nodes and intraperitoneal lymph nodes. More frequently seen in complicated pneumoconiosis. Lungs show multiple small nodular shadows or areas of massive fibrosis.
2. **Coal miner's pneumoconiosis*** — occurs in only 1% of cases. Associated pulmonary changes include miliary shadowing or massive shadows.
3. **Sarcoidosis*** — calcification of lymph nodes occurs in approximately 5% of patients and is occasionally 'eggshell' in appearance. There may be extensive lymph-node involvement throughout the mediastinum. Calcification appears about 6 years after the onset of the disease and is almost invariably associated with advanced pulmonary disease and in some cases with steroid therapy. The pulmonary manifestations include reticulonodular, acinar or fibrotic changes in the mid to upper zones.
4. **Lymphoma following radiotherapy** — appears 1–9 years post radiotherapy.

Differential Diagnosis
1. **Pulmonary artery calcification** — a rare feature of pulmonary arterial hypertension.
2. **Aortic calcification** — especially in the wall of a saccular aneurysm.
3. **Anterior mediastinal tumours** — teratodermoids and thymomas may occasionally exhibit rim calcification.

Further Reading
Gross B.H., Schneider H.J. & Proto A.V. (1980) Eggshell calcification of lymph nodes: an update. *Am. J. Roentgenol.*, 135: 1265.
Jacobsen G., Felson B., Pendergrass E.P., Flinn R.H. & Lainhart W.S. (1967) Eggshell calcification in coal and metal miners. *Semin. Roentgenol.*, 2: 276–82.

4.33 Upper Zone Fibrosis

1. **Tuberculosis** — calcification frequent.
2. **Radiotherapy** — no calcification. ± evidence of the cause, e.g. mastectomy for carcinoma, or radiation osteonecrosis of ribs or clavicle.
3. **Sarcoidosis*** — no calcification. ± 'eggshell' calcification of lymph nodes.
4. **Chronic extrinsic allergic alveolitis***.
5. **Histoplasmosis** — similar to tuberculosis.
6. **Progressive massive fibrosis** — conglomerate infiltrates with peripheral emphysema. Background nodularity. ± 'eggshell' calcification of lymph nodes.
7. **Ankylosing spondylitis*** — resembles tuberculosis. Cavitation frequent with mycetoma. Disease is almost invariably bilateral and associated with severe spondylitis.

Further Reading
Howarth F.H., Kendall M.J., Lawrence D.S & Whitfield A.G.W. (1975) Chest radiograph in ankylosing spondylitis. *Clin. Radiol.* 26:455–60.

4.34   Pleural Effusion

Transudate (protein <30 gl^{-1})
1. Cardiac failure.
2. Hepatic failure.
3. Nephrotic syndrome.
4. Meigs' syndrome.

Exudate (protein >30 gl^{-1})
1. Infection.
2. Malignancy.
3. Pulmonary infarction — see Pulmonary embolic disease*.
4. Collagen vascular diseases.
5. Subphrenic abscess.
6. Pancreatitis.

Haemorrhagic
1. Carcinoma of the bronchus.
2. Trauma.
3. Pulmonary infarction — see Pulmonary embolic disease*.
4. Bleeding disorders.

Chylous
1. Obstructed thoracic duct — due to trauma, malignant invasion or filariasis.

4.35 Pleural Effusion due to Extrathoracic Disease

1. **Pancreatitis** — acute, chronic or relapsing. Effusions are predominantly left-sided. Elevated amylase content.
2. **Subphrenic abscess** — with elevation and restriction of movement of the ipsilateral diaphragm and basal atelectasis or consolidation.
3. **Following abdominal surgery** — most often seen on the side of the surgery and larger after upper abdominal surgery. Disappears after 2 weeks.
4. **Meigs syndrome** — pleural effusion + ascites + benign pelvic tumour (most commonly an ovarian fibroma, thecoma, granulosa cell tumour or cystadenoma).
5. **Nephrotic syndrome.**
6. **Fluid overload** — e.g. due to renal disease.
7. **Cirrhosis.**

4.36 Pleural Effusion with an Otherwise Normal Chest X-ray

Effusion may be the only abnormality or other signs may be obscured by the effusion.

Infective
1. **Primary tuberculosis** — more common in adults (40%) than children (10%). Rarely bilateral.
2. **Viruses and mycoplasma** — effusions occur in 10–20% of cases but are usually small.

Neoplastic
1. **Carcinoma of the bronchus** — effusion occurs in 10% of patients and a peripheral carcinoma may be hidden by the effusion.
2. **Metastases** — most commonly from breast; less commonly pancreas, stomach, ovary and kidney.
3. **Mesothelioma** — effusion in 90%; often massive and obscures the underlying pleural disease.
4. **Lymphoma*** — effusion occurs in 30% but is usually associated with lymphadenopathy or pulmonary infiltrates.

Immunological
1. **Systemic lupus erythematosus*** — effusion is the sole manifestation in 10% of cases. Usually small but may be massive. Bilateral in 50%. 35–50% of those with an effusion have associated cardiomegaly.
2. **Rheumatoid disease** (see Rheumatoid arthritis*) — observed in 3% of patients. Almost exclusively males. Usually unilateral and may antedate joint disease. Tendency to remain unchanged for a long time.

Extrathoracic Diseases
See section 4.35.

Others
1. **Pulmonary embolus** (see Pulmonary embolic disease*) — effusion is a common sign and it may obscure an underlying area of infarction.
2. **Closed chest trauma** — effusion may contain blood, chyle or food (due to oesophageal rupture). The latter is almost always left-sided.
3. **Asbestosis*** — mesothelioma and carcinoma of the bronchus should be excluded but an effusion may be present without these complications. Effusion is frequently recurrent and usually bilateral. Usually associated with pulmonary disease.

4.37 Pneumothorax

1. **Spontaneous** — M:F, 8:1. Especially those of tall thin stature. ? due to ruptured blebs or bullae. 20% are associated with a small pleural effusion.
2. **Iatrogenic** — e.g. postoperative, after chest aspiration, during artificial ventilation, after lung biopsy or following attempted insertion of a subclavian venous line.
3. **Traumatic** — ± rib fractures, haemothorax, surgical emphysema or mediastinal emphysema.
4. **Secondary to mediastinal emphysema** (q.v.).
5. **Secondary to lung disease**
   (a) Emphysema.
   (b) 'Honeycomb lung' (q.v.).
   (c) Cystic fibrosis*.
   (d) Pneumonia.
   (e) Broncho-pleural fistula, e.g. due to lung abscess or carcinoma.
   (f) Lung neoplasms — especially metastases from osteogenic sarcomas and other sarcomas.
6. **Pneumoperitoneum** — air passes through a pleuroperitoneal foramen.

4.38 Pneumomediastinum

May be associated with pneumothorax and subcutaneous emphysema.

1. **Lung tear** — a sudden rise in intra-alveolar pressure, often with airway narrowing, causes air to dissect through the interstitium to the hilum and then to the mediastinum.
   (a) Spontaneous — the most common cause and may follow coughing or strenuous exercise.
   (b) Asthma.
   (c) Diabetic ketoacidosis related to severe and protracted vomiting.
   (d) Childbirth — because of repeated Valsalva manoeuvres.
   (e) Artificial ventilation.
   (f) Chest trauma.
2. **Perforation of oesophagus, trachea or bronchus** — ruptured oesophagus is often associated with a hydrothorax or hydropneumothorax, usually on the left side.
3. **Perforation of a hollow abdominal viscus** — with extension of gas via the retroperitoneal space.

Further Reading

Fraser R.G. & Paré J.A.P. (1979) Pneumomediastinum. In: Fraser R.G. & Paré J.A.P. (Eds) *Diagnosis of Diseases of the Chest*, 2nd edn pp. 1810–17. Philadelphia: Saunders.

4.39 Right Sided Diaphragmatic Humps

At Any Site
1. Collapse/consolidation of adjacent lung.
2. Localized eventration.
3. Loculated effusion.
4. Subphrenic abscess.
5. Hepatic abscess.
6. Hydatid cyst.
7. Hepatic metastasis.

Medially
1. Pericardial fat pad.
2. Aortic aneurysm.
3. Pleuro-pericardial (spring water cyst).
4. Sequestrated segment.

Anteriorly
1. Morgagni hernia.

Posteriorly
1. Bochdalek hernia.

Further Reading
Baron R.L., Lee J.K.T. & Melson G.L. (1980) Sonographic evaluation of right juxtadiaphragmatic masses in children using transhepatic approach. *J. Clin. Ultrasound*, 8: 156–8.

Kangerloo H., Sukov R., Sample F., Lipson M. & Smith L. (1977) Ultrasonic evaluation of juxtadiaphragmatic masses in children. *Radiology*, 125: 785–7.

Khan A.N. & Gould D.A. (1984) The primary role of ultrasound in evaluating right sided diaphragmatic humps and juxtadiaphragmatic masses: a review of 22 cases. *Clin. Radiol.*, 35: 413–18.

4.40 Unilateral Elevated Hemidiaphragm

Causes Above the Diaphragm

1. **Phrenic nerve palsy** — smooth hemidiaphragm. No movement on respiration. Paradoxical movement on sniffing. The mediastinum is usually central. The cause, e.g. bronchial carcinoma or mediastinal nodes, may be evident on the X-ray.
2. **Pulmonary collapse.**
3. **Pulmonary infarction** — see Pulmonary embolic disease*.
4. **Pleural disease** — especially old pleural disease, e.g. haemothorax, empyema or thoracotomy.
5. **Splinting of the diaphragm** — associated with rib fractures or pleurisy.
6. **Hemiplegia** — an upper motor neurone lesion.

Diaphragmatic Causes

1. **Eventration** — more common on the left side. The heart is frequently displaced to the contralateral side. Limited movement on normal respiration and paradoxical movement on sniffing. Stomach may show a partial volvulus.

Causes Below the Diaphragm

1. **Gaseous distension of the stomach or splenic flexure** — left hemidiaphragm only.
2. **Subphrenic inflammatory disease** — subphrenic abscess, hepatic or splenic abscess and pancreatitis.

Scoliosis

The raised hemidiaphragm is on the side of the concavity.

Decubitus Film

The raised hemidiaphragm is on the dependent side.

Differential Diagnosis

1. **Subpulmonary effusion** — movement of fluid is demonstrable on a decubitus film. On the left side there is increased distance between lung and stomach fundal gas.
2. **Ruptured diaphragm** — more common on the left. Barium meal confirms the diagnosis.

4.41   Bilateral Elevated Hemidiaphragms

Poor Inspiratory Effort

Obesity

Causes Above the Diaphragms
1. Bilateral basal pulmonary collapse — which may be secondary to infarction or subphrenic abscesses.
2. Small lungs — fibrotic lung disease, e.g. fibrosing alveolitis.

Causes Below the Diaphragms
1. Ascites.
2. Pregnancy.
3. Pneumoperitoneum.
4. Hepatosplenomegaly.
5. Large intra-abdominal tumour.
6. Bilateral subphrenic abscesses.

Differential Diagnosis
1. Bilateral subpulmonary effusions.

4.42   Pleural Calcification

1. Old empyema
2. Old haemothorax
} Amorphous bizarre, plaques, often with a vacuolated appearance near the inner surface of greatly thickened pleura. Usually unilateral.

3. Asbestos inhalation — small curvilinear plaques in the parietal pleura. More delicate than (1) and (2). Often multiple and bilateral and found over the domes of the diaphragms and immediately deep to the ribs. Observed in 50% of people exposed to asbestos but not before 20 years have elapsed. Not necessarily associated with asbestosis, i.e. pulmonary disease.
4. Silicosis*
5. Talc exposure
} similar appearances to asbestos exposure.

4.43   Local Pleural Masses

1. **Loculated pleural effusion.**
2. **Metastases** — from bronchus or breast. Often multiple.
3. **Malignant mesothelioma** — nearly always due to asbestos exposure. Extensive thickening of the pleura which may be partly obscured by an effusion. Little mediastinal shift. Adjacent bone destruction in 12%.
4. **Pleural fibroma (local benign mesothelioma)** — a smooth lobular mass, 2–15 cm diameter, arising more frequently from the visceral pleura than the parietal pleura. Tendency to change position with respiration as 30–50% are pedunculated. They form an obtuse angle with the chest wall which indicates their extrapulmonary location. Usually found in patients over 40 years of age and usually asymptomatic. However it causes hypertrophic osteo-arthropathy in a greater proportion of cases than any other disease.
5. **Fibrin balls** — develop in a serofibrinous pleural effusion and become visible following absorption of the fluid. They are small and tend to be situated near the lung base. They may disappear spontaneously or remain unchanged for many years.

Differential Diagnosis

1. **Extrapleural masses** — see section 4.44.
2. **Plombage** — the insertion of foreign material into the extrapleural space as a treatment for tuberculosis. The commonest materials used were solid Lucite spheres, hollow 'ping-pong' balls (which may have fluid levels in them) or crumpled cellophane. They produce a well-defined, smooth pleural surface, convex inferiorly and medially and displacing the lung apex. The pleura makes an acute angle with the chest wall.

4.44 Rib Lesion with an Adjacent Soft-tissue Mass

Neoplastic

1. **Bronchogenic carcinoma** — solitary site unless metastatic.
2. **Metastases** — solitary or multiple.
3. **Multiple myeloma*** — classically multiple sites and bilateral.
4. **Mesothelioma** — rib destruction occurs in 12%.
5. **Lymphoma*.**
6. **Fibrosarcoma** — similar appearances to mesothelioma.
7. **Neurofibroma** — rib notching.

Infective

1. **Tuberculous osteitis** — commonest inflammatory lesion of a rib. Second only to malignancy as a cause of rib destruction. Clearly defined margins ± abscess.
2. **Actinomycosis** ⎫ usually a single rib. Adjacent consoli-
3. **Nocardiosis** ⎭ dation.
4. **Blastomycosis** — adjacent patchy or massive consolidation ± hilar lymphadenopathy.

Inflammatory

1. **Radiation osteitis.**

Metabolic

1. **Renal osteodystrophy** ⎫ rib fractures and osteopenia
2. **Cushing's syndrome** ⎬ associated with a subpleural hae-
⎭ matoma.

Further Reading

Steiner R.M., Cooper M.W. & Brodovsky H. (1982) Rib destruction: a neglected finding in malignant mesothelioma. *Clin. Radiol.* 33: 61–5.

4.45 The Chest Radiograph Following Chest Trauma

Soft Tissues
1. Foreign bodies.
2. Surgical emphysema.

Ribs
1. Simple fracture
2. Flail chest

may be associated with surgical emphysema, pneumothorax, extrapleural haematoma or haemothorax. First-rib fractures have a high incidence of other associated injuries.

Sternum
1. Fracture — may be associated with an unsuspected dorsal spine fracture.

Clavicles
1. Fracture.

Spine
1. Fracture.
2. Cord trauma.
3. Nerve root trauma — especially to the brachial plexus.

Pleura
1. Pneumothorax — simple or tension.
2. Haemothorax.

Lung
1. Contusion — non-segmental alveolar opacities. Resolve in a few days.
2. Haematoma — usually appears following resolution of contusion. Round, well-defined nodule. Resolution in several weeks.
3. Aspiration pneumonitis.
4. Foreign bodies.
5. Pulmonary oedema — following blast injuries.

6. **Adult respiratory distress syndrome** — widespread alveolar shadowing appearing 24–72 hours after injury.
7. **Fat embolism.**

Trachea and Bronchi

1. **Laceration or fracture** — initially surgical emphysema and pneumomediastinum followed by collapse of the affected lung or lobe.

Diaphragm

1. **Rupture** — 90% occur on the left side. ± herniation of stomach or colon.

Mediastinum

1. **Aortic dissection** — widening of the mediastinum, blurring of the aortic shadow, apical effusion, tracheal shift and depression of the left main bronchus.
2. **Traumatic aortic aneurysm** — usually saccular.
3. **Mediastinal haematoma** — blurring of the mediastinal outline.
4. **Mediastinal emphysema** (q.v.).
5. **Haemopericardium.**
6. **Oesophageal rupture.**

Further Reading

Dow J., Roebuck E.J. & Cole F. (1970) Dissecting aneurysms of the aorta. *Br. J. Radiol.*, 39: 915–27.
Joffe N. (1974) The adult respiratory distress syndrome. *Am. J. Roentgenol.*, 122: 719–32.
Reynolds J. & Davis J.T. (1966) Thoracic injuries. The radiology of trauma. *Radiol. Clin. North Am.*, 4: 383–402.

4.46　Neonatal Respiratory Distress

Pulmonary Causes

A.　WITH NO MEDIASTINAL SHIFT

1. **Hyaline membrane disease** — in premature infants. Fine granular pattern throughout both lungs, air bronchograms and, later, obscured heart and diaphragmatic outlines. Often cardiomegaly. May progress to a complete 'white-out'. Interstitial emphysema, pneumomediastinum and pneumothorax are frequent complications of ventilator therapy.
2. **Transient tachypnoea of the newborn** — prominent interstitial markings and vessels, thickened septa, small effusions and mild cardiomegaly. Resolves within 24 hours.
3. **Meconium aspiration syndrome** — predominantly post-mature infants. Coarse linear and irregular opacities of uneven size, generalized hyperinflation and focal areas of collapse and emphysema. Spontaneous pneumothorax and effusions in 20%. No air bronchograms.
4. **Pneumonia** — segmental or lobar consolidation. May resemble hyaline membrane disease or meconium aspiration syndrome, but should be suspected if unevenly distributed.
5. **Pulmonary haemorrhage** — 75% are less than 2.5 kg. Onset at birth or delayed several days. Resembles meconium aspiration syndrome or hyaline membrane disease.
6. **Upper airway obstruction** — e.g. choanal atresia and micrognathia.
7. **Mikity–Wilson syndrome (pulmonary dysmaturity)** — always premature infants and usually less than 1.5 kg. Initially well but there is an insidious onset of respiratory distress between 1 and 6 weeks. Streaky opacities radiating from both hila with small bubbly areas of focal hyperaeration throughout both lungs. Moderate hyperinflation. Severe disease leads to death but infants may recover fully. Resolution over a period of 12 months. Bases clear before apices and hyperinflation is the last feature to disappear.
8. **Abnormal thoracic cage** — e.g. osteogenesis imperfecta and Jeune's thoracic dysplasia.

B. WITH MEDIASTINAL SHIFT AWAY FROM THE
ABNORMAL SIDE

1. **Diaphragmatic hernia** — 6 × more common on the left
   side. Multiple lucencies due to gas containing bowel in
   the chest. Herniated bowel may appear solid if X-rayed
   too early but there will still be a paucity of gas in the
   abdomen.
2. **Congenital lobar emphysema** — involves the left upper,
   right upper and right middle lobes (in decreasing order
   of frequency) with compression of the lung base (cf.
   pneumothorax which produces symmetrical lung compression).
3. **Cystic adenomatoid malformation** — translucencies of
   various shapes and sizes scattered throughout an area of
   opaque lung with well-defined margins.
4. **Pleural effusion (empyema, chylothorax)** — rare.

C. WITH MEDIASTINAL SHIFT TOWARDS THE
ABNORMAL SIDE

1. **Atelectasis** — most commonly due to incorrect placement
   of an endotracheal tube down a major bronchus. Much
   less commonly primary atelectasis may occur without any
   other abnormality.
2. **Agenesis** — rare. May be difficult to differentiate from
   collapse but other congenital defects especially hemivertebrae are commonly associated.

Cardiac Causes (q.v.)

Cerebral Causes
Haemorrhage, oedema and drugs. After cardiopulmonary
causes these account for 50% of the remainder.

Metabolic Causes
Metabolis acidosis, hypoglycaemia and hypothermia.

Abdominal Causes
Massive organomegaly, e.g. polycystic kidneys, elevating the
diaphragms.

4.47   Ring Shadows in a Child

Neonate
1. **Diaphragmatic hernia** — unilateral.
2. **Interstitial emphysema** — secondary to ventilator therapy. Bilateral.
3. **Cystic adenomatoid malformation** — unilateral.
4. **Mikity–Wilson syndrome** — bilateral.

Older Child.
1. **Cystic bronchiectasis** (q.v.).
2. **Cystic fibrosis***.
3. **Pneumatocoeles** (q.v.).
4. **Histiocytosis X*** ⎱ see 'Honeycomb lung', section 4.20.
5. **Neurofibromatosis*** ⎰

See also section 4.46.

4.48   Drug-induced Lung Disease

Lung Parenchyma
1. **Diffuse pneumonitis** — methotrexate, procarbazine, azathioprine, amiodarone.
2. **Diffuse pneumonitis progressing to fibrosis** — nitrofurantoin, melphalan, busulphan, cyclophosphamide and bleomycin.
3. **Pneumonitis associated with drug-induced systemic lupus erythematosus** — procainamide, hydralazine and isoniazid.
4. **Pulmonary haemorrhage** — anticoagulants and those drugs which produce an idiosyncratic thrombocytopenia.
5. **Pulmonary eosinophilia** — sulphonamides, chlorpropamide, sulphasalazine and imipramine.
6. **Allergic alveolitis** — pituitary snuff.

Pulmonary Vasculature
1. **Pulmonary oedema**
   (a) Excess intravenous fluids.
   (b) Altered capillary wall permeability — heroin, dextro-propoxyphene, methyldopa, hydrochlorothiazide, aspirin, nitrofurantoin and contrast media.
   (c) Drug-induced cardiac arrhythmias or impaired myo-cardial contractility.
2. **Pulmonary emboli** — high oestrogen oral contraceptives causing thromboemboli and oily emboli following lymphangiography.

Bronchospasm
1. β-blockers.
2. **Histamine liberators** — iodine containing contrast media and morphine.
3. **Drugs as antigens** — antisera, penicillins and cephalosporins.
4. **Others** — aspirin, anti-inflammatory agents, paracetamol.

Hilar Enlargement or Mediastinal Widening
Phenytoin and steroids.

Increased Opportunistic Infections
1. **Antimitotics.**
2. **Steroids.**
3. **Actinomycin C.**
4. **Drug-induced neutropenia or aplastic anaemia** — idiosyncratic or dose-related.

Further Reading
Millar J.W. (1982) Drugs and the lungs. *Medicine International*, **1**(20):944–7.
Morrison D.A. & Goldman A.L. (1979) Radiographic patterns of drugs induced lung disease. *Radiology*, **131**:299–304.

4.49 Anterior Mediastinal Masses

Anterior to the pericardium and trachea. Superiorly the retrosternal air space is obliterated. For ease of discussion it can be divided into three regions:

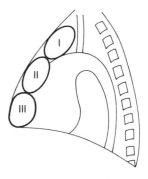

Region I

1. **Retrosternal goitre** — goitre extends into the mediastinum in 1–3% of cases. On a PA chest X-ray it appears as an inverted truncated cone with its base uppermost. It is well defined, smooth or lobulated. The trachea may be displaced posteriorly and laterally and may be narrowed. Calcification is common. Uptake by ^{131}I is diagnostic when positive but they are seldom functioning.

2. **Tortuous innominate artery** — a common finding in the elderly.

3. **Lymph nodes** — due to reticuloses, metastases or granulomas.

4. **Thymus** — at birth, the thymus is largest in proportion to overall body size than at any other time of life although it reaches its largest absolute size at puberty. The normal thymus is visible up to 2–3 years and may be seen in older chidren. CT may demonstrate a normal thymus in adulthood. The frontal X-ray may reveal a 'sail' sign or 'wave' sign and the thymus may be more prominent on one side of the mediastinum. A large normal thymus may be seen in:
   (a) Well-nourished children.
   (b) Following recovery from illness (rebound overgrowth following previous involution).
   (c) Hyperthyroidism and euthyroid children following treatment for hypothyroidism.

Pathological thymic enlargement may occur in lymphoma and leukaemia. Intrathymic haemorrhage is suggested by a rapidly enlarging mediastinal mass. In neonates it may accompany birth trauma whilst in older children haemorrhage occurs into normal glands, thymic cysts, cystic thymomas and cystic teratomas.

Thymic tumours are uncommon but occur in 15% of adult patients with myasthenia gravis. They are round or oval and smooth or lobulated. They may contain nodular or rim calcification. If it contains a large amount of fat (thymolipoma) then it may be very large and soft and reach the diaphragm, leaving the superior mediastinum clear.

5. **Aneurysm of the ascending aorta.**

Region II

1. **Germinal cell neoplasms** — including dermoids, teratomas, seminomas, choriocarcinomas, embryonal carcinomas and endodermal sinus tumours. More than 80% are benign and they occur with equal incidence to thymic tumours. Usually larger than thymomas (but not thymolipomas). Round or oval and smooth. They usually project to one or other side of the mediastinum on the PA view. Calcification, especially rim calcification, and fragments of bone or teeth may be demonstrable, the latter being diagnostic.
2. **Thymic tumours** — see Thymic masses (above).
3. **Sternal tumours** — metastases (breast, bronchus, kidney and thyroid) are the most common. Of the primary tumours, malignant (chondrosarcoma, myeloma, reticulum cell sarcoma and lymphoma) are more common than benign (chondroma, aneurysmal bone cyst and giant cell tumour).

Region III (Anterior Cardiophrenic Angle Masses)

1. **Pericardiac fat pad** — especially in obese people. A triangular opacity in the cardiophrenic angle on the PA view. It appears less dense than expected because of the fat content. CT is diagnostic. Excessive mediastinal fat can be due to steroid therapy.

2. **Diaphragmatic hump** — or localized eventration. Commonest on the anteromedial portion of the right hemidiaphragm. A portion of liver extends into it and this can be confirmed by ultrasound or isotope examination of the liver.

3. **Morgagni hernia** — through the defect between the septum transversum and the costal portion of the diaphragm. It is almost invariably on the right side but is occasionally bilateral. It usually contains a knuckle of colon or, less commonly, colon and stomach. Appears solid if it contains omentum and/or liver. US and/or barium studies will confirm the diagnosis.

4. **Pericardial cysts** — either a true pericardial cyst ('spring water' cyst) or a pericardial diverticulum. The cyst is usually situated in the right cardiophrenic angle and is oval or spherical. CT confirms the liquid nature of the mass.

4.50 Middle Mediastinal Masses

Between the anterior and posterior mediastinum and containing the heart, great vessels and pulmonary roots. Causes of cardiac enlargement are excluded.

1. **Lymph nodes** — the paratracheal, tracheobronchial, bronchopulmonary and/or subcarinal nodes may be enlarged. This may be due to neoplasm (most frequently metastatic bronchial carcinoma), reticuloses (most frequently Hodgkin's disease), infection (most commonly tuberculosis, histoplasmosis or coccidioidomycosis) or sarcoidosis.
2. **Carcinoma of the bronchus** — arising from a major bronchus.
3. **Aneurysm of the aorta** — CT scanning after i.v. contrast medium or, if this is not available, aortography is diagnostic. Peripheral rim calcification is a useful sign if present.
4. **Bronchogenic cyst** — round or oval, homogeneous, water-density mass with well-defined borders. There may be airway obstruction and secondary infection, both within the cyst and in the surrounding lung. Communication with the tracheo-bronchial tree, resulting in a cavity, is not common. Four groups may be defined according to location.
   (a) *Paratracheal* cysts are attached to the tracheal wall above the carina.
   (b) *Carinal* cysts are the most common and are attached to the carina ± anterior oesophageal wall.
   (c) *Hilar* cysts are attached to a lobar bronchus and appear to be intrapulmonary.
   (d) *Paraoesophageal* cysts may be attached or communicate with the oesophagus but have no connection with the bronchial tree.

Further Reading

DuMontier C., Graviss E.R., Silberstein M.J. & McAlister W.H. (1985) Bronchogenic cysts in children. *Clin. Radiol.*, 36: 431–6.

4.51   Posterior Mediastinal Masses

Posterior to the posterior pericardial surface. For ease of
discussion it can be divided
into three regions:

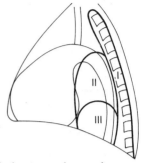

Region I (Paravertebral)

1. **Neurogenic tumours** — usually benign and more frequent
   in children and young adults. All the different tumour
   types look very similar: well defined, round or oval and
   smooth, lying in the paravertebral region. Ganglioneur-
   omas are said to have a broader base towards the
   mediastinum. Calcification is rare but more common in
   malignant tumours. Benign tumours may cause pressure
   erosion of adjacent vertebral bodies, transverse processes
   or ribs; malignant tumours produce irregular bone destruction.
2. **Other paravertebral masses** (q.v.) — usually elongated and
   bilateral.
   (a) Abscess — with disc space and vertebral body
       destruction.
   (b) Extramedullary haemopoiesis — with splenomegaly
       ± bone changes of specific disease entities, e.g.
       haemolytic anaemias.
   (c) Reticuloses, myeloma and metastases — bone destruc-
       tion with preserved discs.
3. **Anterior thoracic meningocoele** — mainly in patients with
   neurofibromatosis. A well-defined mass anterior to the
   spine which projects laterally into the lung fields. The
   spine shows hemivertebra, 'butterfly' vertebra or other
   congenital abnormalities. The diagnosis is confirmed by
   myelography in the prone position.

Region II

1. **Dilated oesophagus** — especially achalasia. Contains
   mottled gas shadows ± an air fluid level. Diagnosis is
   confirmed by barium swallow.

2. **Aorta** — unfolded, dilated or ruptured.
3. **Enteric cyst** — an intestinal duplication cyst related to the oesophagus. Usually to the right of the midline. May be an incidental finding or produce symptoms, usually during infancy, related to tracheal or oesophageal compression. US and CT show a cystic structure but some cysts have a higher mucus content resulting in increased echogenicity or attenuation. There are no vertebral anomalies and there is no splaying of the posterior ribs. The cyst may contain acid-secreting mucosa and erosion into the tracheo-bronchial tree or oesophagus may produce life-threatening haemmorrhage. Imaging with 99m-Tc Pertechnetate may be useful.
4. **Neurenteric cyst** — a special type of duplication cyst associated with vertebral anomalies. It is most frequently dorsal and prevertebral but may be partly or completely intraspinal. The vertebral anomaly is usually higher than the cyst.

Region III

1. **Hiatus hernia** — often contains an air fluid level which is projected through the cardiac shadow on a penetrated PA view.
2. **Bochdalek hernia** — most present shortly after birth but 5% present after the neonatal period, previous radiographs having been normal. Rarely, it may complicate Group B streptococcal infection. Bochdalek hernias include:
   (a) Persistence of the pleuroperitoneal canal with a posterior lip of diaphragm.
   (b) Larger defects with no diaphragm.
   (c) Herniation through the costo-lumbar triangles.
   The appearance of herniated liver may provoke thoracentesis and herniated bowel may mimic a pneumothorax or pneumatocoeles.

Further Reading

Berman L., Stringer D.A., Ein S. & Shandling B. (1988) Childhood diaphragmatic hernias presenting after the neonatal period *Clin. Radiol.*, 39: 237–44.
Lien H.H., Kolbenstvedt A. & Lund G. (1984) The thoracic paraspinal shadow: a review of the appearances in pathological conditions. *Clin. Radiol.*, 35: 215–21.

4.52   CT Mediastinal Mass containing Fat

1. **Teratodermoid** — well defined soft tissue mass containing fat and calcification.
2. **Diaphragmatic hernia** — bowel, liver, kidney or stomach may also be present. Anterior (Morgagni) hernias are usually on the right, and posterior (Bochdalek) hernias usually on the left. Linear soft tissue densities representing omental vessels help to distinguish hernias which only contain omental fat from pericardial fat pads.
3. **Lipoma** — relatively rare. Can occur anywhere in mediastinum.
4. **Liposarcoma** — can contain calcification, and may also appear as a soft tissue mass with no visible fat, due to excess soft tissue component of the sarcoma.
5. **Thymolipoma** — occurs in children and young adults. Accounts for 2–9% of thymic tumours. Usually asymptomatic.
6. **Mediastinal lipomatosis** — associated with Cushing's, steroid treatment and obesity.
7. **Hamartoma.**
8. **Chylolymphatic cyst** — fat/fluid level in cyst.
9. **Neurofibroma** — can have a negative CT attentuation due to myelin content.

Further Reading

Phillips G.W.L., Serapati A. & Young A.E. (1988) Chylolymphatic mesenteric cyst: a diagnostic appearance on computed tomography. *Br. J. Radiol.*, 61: 413–14.

Reed D.H. (1988) The changing mediastinum. *Br. J. Radiol.*, 61: 695–6.

Shirkhoda A., Chasen M.H., Eftekhari F., Goldman A.M. & Decaro L.F. (1987) M.R. imaging of mediastinal thymolipoma. *J. Comput. Assist. Tomogr.*, 11: 364–5.

4.53 CT Mediastinal Cysts

1. Congenital
   (a) Bronchogenic cyst — usually subcarinal or right paratracheal site. 50% homogenous water density, 50% soft tissue density due to mucous or milk of calcium content. Occasional calcification in cyst wall, and air in cyst if communicates with airway.
   (b) Enteric cyst — paraoesophageal site.
   (c) Neuroenteric cyst — associated anomaly of spine.
2. **Pericardial cyst** — usually cardiophrenic angle.
3. **Thymic cyst** — can develop following radiotherapy for Hodgkin's.
4. **Cystic tumours**
   (a) Lymphangioma.
   (b) Teratoma.
   (c) Teratodermoid.
5. **Pancreatic pseudocyst** — can track up into mediastinum.
6. **Meningocoele** — 75% association with neurofibromatosis.
7. **Chronic abscess.**
8. **Old haematoma.**

Further Reading

DuMontier C., Graviss E.R., Silberstein M.J. & McAlister W.H. (1985) Bronchogenic cysts in children. *Clin. Radiol.*, 36: 431–6.

Nakata H, Sato Y., Nakayama T., Yoshimatsu H. & Kobayashi T. (1986) Bronchogenic cyst with high C.T. numbers: analysis of contents. *J. Comput. Assist. Tomogr.*, 10 (2): 360–2.

4.54 CT Thymic Mass

Normal shape of thymus is an arrowhead with maximum length less than 2 cm and maximum width less than 1.8 cm if age less than 20 years, and 1.3 cm if age greater than 20 years. However measurements are misleading, and a multilobular appearance or focal alteration in shape is abnormal at any age. Fatty involution occurs after the age of 30.

1. **Thymoma** — occurs in 15% of myasthenia gravis (usually occurring in the 4th decade) and 40% of these will be malignant. If malignant it is usually locally invasive and can extend along pleura to involve diaphragm and even spread into abdomen. Can contain calcification.
2. **Thymic hyperplasia**
   (a) Lymphoid — occurs in 65% of myasthenia gravis. Only medulla enlarges and this is not sufficient to be visible on CT.
   (b) True hyperplasia — occurs in myasthenia gravis, post chemotherapy rebound, Graves thyrotoxicosis, Addison's and acromegaly. Thymus increases in size but is normal in shape.
3. **Germ cell tumour** — teratodermoid, benign and malignant teratomas.
4. **Lymphoma** — thymus is infiltrated in 35% Hodgkin's, but there is always associated lymphadenopathy.
5. **Thymolipoma** — usually children or young adults. Asymptomatic.

Further Reading

Heron C.W., Husband J.E. & Williams M.P. (1988) Hodgkin's disease: C.T. of the thymus. *Radiology*, 167: 647–51;.
Moore N.R. (1989) Imaging in myasthenia gravis. *Clin. Radiol.*, 40: 115–16.
Williams M.P. (1989) Problems in Radiology: C.T. assessment of the thymus. *Clin. Radiol.*, 40: 113–14.

Bibliography

General

Felson B. (1973) *Chest Roentgenology*. Philadelphia: Saunders.

Fraser R.G., Paré J.A.P., Paré P.D., Fraser R.S. & Genereux G.P. (1988) *Diagnosis of Diseases of the Chest,* 3rd edn. Philadelphia: Saunders.

Reeder M. & Felson B. (1975) *Gamuts in Radiology.* Oxford: Pergamon Press.

Simon G. (1978) *Principles of Chest X-Ray Diagnosis,* 4th edn. London: Butterworths.

Sutton D. (ed.)(1980) *Textbook of Radiology and Imaging,* 3rd edn, chaps 11–21. Edinburgh: Churchill Livingstone.

Diffuse Pulmonary Disease, Emphysema and Pneumoconiosis

Crofton J. (1978) Diffuse pulmonary abnormalities: clinical correlations. *Clin. Radiol.,* 29: 353–62.

Cunningham C.D.B. & Hugh A.E. (1973) Pneumoconiosis in women. *Clin. Radiol.,* 24: 491–3.

Felson B. (ed.)(1967) The pneumoconioses. *Semin. Roentgenol.,* 2 (3).

Felson B. (1979) A new look at pattern recognition of diffuse pulmonary disease. *Am. J. Roentgenol.,* 133: 183–9.

Fraser R.G. (1974) The radiologist and obstructive airway disease. *Am. J. Roentgenol.,* 120: 737–75.

Thurlbeck W.M. & Simon G. (1978) Radiographic appearance of the chest in emphysema. *Am. J. Roentgenol.,* 130: 427–40.

Infections

Balikian J.P. & Mudarris F.F. (1974) Hydatid disease of the lungs. A roentgenological study of 50 cases. *Am. J. Roentgenol.,* 122: 692–707.

Connell J.V. & Muhim J.R. (1976) Radiographic manifestations of pulmonary histoplasmosis. *Radiology,* 121: 281–5.

Felson B. (ed.)(1970) Fungus diseases of the lungs. *Semin. Roentgenol.,* 5 (1).

Felson B. (ed.)(1979) Thoracic tuberculosis. *Semin. Roentgenol.,* 16 (3).

Felson B. (ed.)(1980) The acute pneumonias. *Semin. Roentgenol.,* 15 (1).

Felson B. (ed.)(1980) Lobar collapse. *Semin. Roentgenol.,* 15 (2).

Forrest J.V. & Potchen E.J. (eds)(1973) Radiology of the chest. *Radiol. Clin. North Am.,* 11 (1).

Freundlich I.M. & Israel H.L. (1973) Pulmonary aspergillosis. *Clin. Radiol.,* 24: 246–53.

Gordonson J., Birnbaum W., Jacobson G. & Sargent E.N. (1974) Pulmonary cryptococcosis. *Radiology*, 112: 557–61.
Klein, D.L. & Gamsu G. (1980) Thoracic manifestations of aspergillosis. *Am. J. Roentgenol.*, 134: 543–52.
Vaněk J. & Schwarz J. (1971) The gamut of histoplasmosis. *Am J. Med.*, 50: 89–104.

Neoplasms

Bateson E.M. (1964) The solitary bronchogenic carcinoma, 100 cases. *Br. J. Radiol.*, 37: 598–607.
Felson B. (ed.)(1977) Pulmonary neoplasms. *Semin. Roentgenol.*, 12 (3).
Grainger R.G. (1975) Benign tumours of the respiratory tract. Clinical presentation and radiological features. In: Lant A.F (ed.) Eleventh Symposium of Advanced Medicine, pp. 353–63. London: Royal College of Physicians.
Higgins G.A., Shields T.W. & Keehn R.J. (1975) The solitary pulmonary nodule. Ten year follow-up V.A.S.A.G. study. *Arch. Surg.*, 110: 570–5.
Libschitz H.I. & North L.B. (1982) Pulmonary metastases. *Radiol. Clin. North Am.*, 20 (3), 437–51.
Rigler, L.G. (1955) The roentgen signs of carcinoma of the lung. *Am. J. Roentgenol.*, 74: 415–28.

Miscellaneous

Fataar S. & Schulman A. (1979) Diagnosis of diaphragmatic tears. *Br. J. Radiol.*, 52: 375–81.
Felson B. (ed.)(1975) Immunology and the lung. *Semin. Roentgenol.*, 10 (1).
Goodman L.R. (1980) Post-operative chest radiograph: I. Alterations after abdominal surgery. *Am. J. Roentgenol.*, 134: 533–41.
Goodman L.R. (1980) Post-operative chest radiograph: II. Alterations after major intrathoracic surgery. *Am. J. Roentgenol.*, 134: 803–13.
Joffe N. (1974) The adult respiratory distress syndrome. *Am. J. Roentgenol.*, 122: 719–32.
McGregor M.B.B. & Sandler G. (1964) Wegener's granulomatosis. *Br. J. Radiol.*, 37: 430–9.

Notes

Notes

Chapter 5
Cardiovascular System

5.1 Gross Cardiac Enlargement

1. **Multiple valvular disease** — aortic and mitral valve disease, particularly with regurgitation.
2. **Pericardial effusion** — no recognizable chamber enlargement. Flask-shaped heart on the erect film which becomes globular on the supine film. Acute angle between right heart border and right hemidiaphragm. The effusion masks ventricular wall movement; therefore, unusually sharp cardiac outline on the chest radiograph and poor pulsation on the fluoroscopy. Rapid change in size on serial films. Diagnosis best made by echocardiography.
3. **ASD** — with pulmonary pleonaemia or an Eisenmenger situation.
4. **Cardiomyopathy** — including ischaemia.
5. **Ebstein's anomaly** — the posterior or septal cusp of the tricuspid valve arises distally from the wall of the right ventricle. Marked tricuspid incompetence. Marked right atrioventricular enlargement. Small aorta. Oligaemic lungs. Sharp cardiac outline.

5.2 Small Heart

1. **Normal variant.**
2. **Emphysema.**
3. **Addison's disease.**
4. **Dehydration/malnutrition.**
5. **Constrictive pericarditis.**

5.3   Enlarged Right Atrium

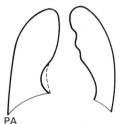

PA
Prominent right heart
border

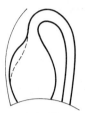

Lateral
Prominent anterosuperior
part of cardiac shadow

Volume Overload
1. **ASD.**
2. **AV canal.**
3. **Tricuspid incompetence** — including Ebstein's anomaly, endocardial fibroelastosis and endomyocardial fibrosis. In 9% of patients following mitral valve replacement. In Uhl's disease there is a thin walled, dilated right ventricle due to focal or complete absence of right ventricular myocardium.
4. **Anomalous pulmonary venous drainage.**

Pressure Overload
1. **Tricuspid stenosis** — N.B. in tricuspid atresia a shunt must exist to preserve life. This decompresses the right atrium, so that it is not large (typically a straight right heart border).
2. **Myxoma of the right atrium** — may cause tricuspid obstruction.

Secondary to Right Ventricular Failure
See section 5.4.

Further Reading
Rubin S.A., Hightower C.W. & Flicker S. (1987) Giant right atrium after mitral valve replacement: plain film findings in 15 patients. *Am. J. Roentgenol.*, 149: 257–60.

5.4 Enlarged Right Ventricle

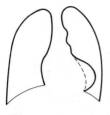

PA
Prominent left heart
border
Elevated apex

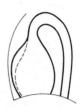

Lateral
Prominent anterior part
of cardiac shadow

Secondary to Left Heart Failure/Mitral Valve Disease
See section 5.6.

Pulmonary Arterial Hypertension
1. **Diffuse lung disease** — e.g. chronic obstructive airways disease, interstitial fibrosis, cystic fibrosis etc.
2. **Pulmonary emboli** — see Pulmonary embolic disease*.
3. **Chronic left to right shunt** — with pulmonary hypertension and right ventricular failure.
4. **Vasculitis** — e.g. polyarteritis nodosa.
5. **Idiopathic** — mostly young females.

Pressure Overload
1. Pulmonary stenosis.

Volume Overload
1. ASD.
2. VSD.

5.5   Enlarged Left Atrium

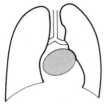

PA
1 Prominent left atrial appendage
2 'Double' right heart border
3 Increased density due to left atrium
4 Splaying of carina and elevated
   left main bronchus

Lateral
1 Prominent
   posterosuperior
   part of cardiac
   shadow
2 Prominent left
   atrial impression
   on oesophagus
   during barium
   swallow

Volume Overload
1. Mitral incompetence.
2. VSD.
3. PDA.
4. ASD with shunt reversal — Eisenmenger's complex or tricuspid atresia.

Pressure Overload
1. Mitral stenosis.
2. Myxoma of the left atrium.

Secondary to Left Ventricular Failure

5.6   Enlarged Left Ventricle

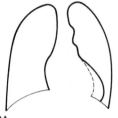

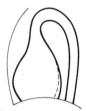

PA
1   Prominent left heart border
2   Rounding of left heart border
3   Apex displaced inferiorly

Lateral
Prominent posteroinferior
part of cardiac shadow

Myocardial
1. Ischaemia.
2. Cardiomyopathy/myocarditis.

Volume Overload
1. Aortic incompetence.
2. Mitral incompetence.
3. VSD.
4. PDA.

High Output States
1. Anaemia.
2. Hyperthyroidism.
3. Paget's disease*.
4. AV fistula.

Pressure Overload (dilatation is end stage)
1. Aortic stenosis.
2. Hypertension.
3. Coarctation of the aorta.

5.7 Bulge on the Left Heart Border

1. Enlarged left atrial appendage.
2. Ventricular aneurysm.
3. Pericardial cyst.
4. Pericardial sac defect.
5. Myocardial mass — e.g. neoplasm, hydatid.
6. Coronary artery aneurysm.

5.8 Cardiac Calcification

Pericardial
Primarily located over the right sided chambers and in the atrio-ventricular grooves; less frequently over the base of the left ventricle and rarely over the apex of the left ventricle. When the left ventricle is involved there is always more extensive calcification elsewhere in the pericardium.
1. **Post-pericarditis** — TB, rheumatic fever, pyogenic, viral.
2. **Post-traumatic/postoperative.**
3. **Uraemia.**
4. **Asbestosis***   } may appear to be 'pericardial'.
5. **Coronary artery**

Myocardial
Predominantly in the apex of the left ventricle or, uncommonly, in the posterior wall of the left ventricle.
1. **Calcified infarct.**
2. **Aneurysm.**
3. **Post-myocarditis** — especially rheumatic fever.
4. **Hydatid.**

Intracardiac
1. **Calcified valve** — see section 5.9.
2. **Calcified thrombus** — overlying an infarct or in an aneurysm.
3. **Atrial myxoma** — larger, more mobile and lobulated than a calcified thrombus.

Further Reading

MacGregor J.H., Chen J.T.T., Chiles C., Kier R., Godwin J.D. & Ravi C.E. (1987) The radiographic distinction between pericardial and myocardial calcifications. *Am. J. Roentgenol.*, 148: 675–7.

Shawdon H.H. & Dinsmore R.E. (1967) Pericardial calcification: radiological features and clinical significance in twenty-six patients. *Clin. Radiol.*, 18: 205–14.

5.9   Valve Calcification

Aortic Valve

1. Bicuspid aortic valve.
2. Rheumatic heart disease.
3. Ageing.
4. Syphilis.
5. Ankylosing spondylitis*.

Mitral Valve

1. Rheumatic heart disease.

Pulmonary Valve

1. Pulmonary valve stenosis
2. Fallot's tetralogy   } in middle age
3. Pulmonary hypertension.
4. Homograft — for severe Fallot's tetralogy or pulmonary atresia.

Tricuspid Valve

1. Pulmonary valve stenosis (with high systolic pressures).
2. ASD.
3. Isolated tricuspid regurgitation.

5.10 Large Aortic Arch

1. **Unfolded** (atherosclerotic) **aorta** — parallel walls ± calcification.
2. **Hypertension** — on its own only leads to slight unfolding with left ventricular enlargement.
3. **Aortic incompetence** — prominent ascending aorta.
4. **Aortic stenosis** — post-stenotic dilation. ± aortic valve calcification.
5. **Aneurysm** — loss of parallelism of walls. Aetiologies include
   (a) Atherosclerosis — calcification prominent.
   (b) Trauma.
   (c) Infection — e.g. syphilis, subacute bacterial endocarditis.
   (d) Intrinsic abnormality — e.g. Marfan's syndrome.
   Macroscopically the aneurysm may be
   (a) Fusiform.
   (b) Saccular.
   (c) Dissecting — signs on the plain chest X-ray include
       (i) Ill-defined aortic outline (because of mediastinal haematoma).
       (ii) Tracheal shift.
       (iii) Left pleural effusion (haemothorax).
       (iv) Left apical cap (also due to effusion).
       (v) Sudden increase in size of the aorta when compared with a previous film.
6. **PDA.**

Further Reading
Dow J., Roebuck E.J. & Cole F. (1970) Dissecting aneurysms of the aorta. *Br. J. Radiol.*, 39: 915–27.

5.11 Small Aortic Arch

1. **Decreased cardiac output** — e.g. mitral stenosis, HOCM.
2. **Intracardiac left to right shunt.**
3. **Coarctation** — long segment 'infantile' type.
4. (**Transposition of great arteries** — rotated but not small.)

5.12 Right-sided Aortic Arch

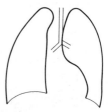

1. Aortic knuckle on right side.
2. Absent left sided aortic knuckle.
3. Trachea central or slightly to left side.

1. Fallot's tetralogy — a feature in 25% of cases.
2. Pulmonary atresia with a VSD — 25% .
3. Transposition of the great vessels — 20%.
4. Uncomplicated VSD — 3%.
5. Tricuspid atresia — 5%.
6. Truncus arteriosus — 50%.

5.13 Enlarged Superior Vena Cava

Volume Overload
1. Tricuspid incompetence.
2. TAPVD — if supracardiac. 'Cottage loaf' cardiac configuration, with pulmonary pleonaemia.

Obstruction
1. Carcinoma of the bronchus.
2. Mediastinal mass.
3. Mediastinal fibrosis — radiotherapy, idiopathic.
4. Constrictive pericarditis.

5.14 Enlarged Azygos Vein

If greater than 1 cm. in diameter. (A normal or abnormal azygos vein will decrease in size in the erect position, on deep inspiration, and during a Valsalva manoeuvre.)

1. Heart failure.
2. Portal hypertension.
3. Superior or inferior vena cava obstruction.
4. Pregnancy.
5. Constrictive pericarditis/pericardial effusion.

Differential Diagnosis
1. Sinus venosus defect — Right upper and middle lobe pulmonary veins drain into the superior vena cava (+ASD).

5.15 Enlarged Pulmonary Arteries

Volume Overload (enlarged central and peripheral vessels)
1. Left-to-right shunt — the sign is apparent when the shunt reaches 3:1.
2. Hyperdynamic circulation — e.g. thyrotoxicosis, severe anaemia, beri-beri and Paget's disease.

Peripheral Arterial Vasoconstriction (enlarged central vessels only)
1. Hypoxia — e.g. due to chronic obstructive airways disease or cystic fibrosis.
2. Secondary to pulmonary venous hypertension — e.g. mitral stenosis or left ventricular failure.
3. Secondary to left-to-right shunts.

Peripheral Arterial Obliteration (enlarged central vessels only)
1. Secondary to left-to-right shunts.
2. Thromboembolic disease (see Pulmonary embolic disease*).
3. Tumour emboli.
4. Schistosomiasis.
5. Vasculitides — e.g. polyarteritis nodosa.
6. Idiopathic pulmonary arterial hypertension — typically in young females.

5.16   Enlarged Pulmonary Veins

Left Ventricular Failure

Obstruction at Mitral or Atrial Level
1. Mitral stenosis.
2. Left atrial myxoma.
3. Ball-valve thrombus.
4. Cor triatriatum.

Obstruction Proximal to the Atrium
1. TAPVD.
2. Constrictive pericarditis — rarely.
3. Mediastinal fibrosis.

5.17   Neonatal Pulmonary Venous Congestion

1. Prominent interstitial markings.
2. Indistinct vessels.
3. Perihilar haze.
4. Pleural effusions.
5. Cardiomegaly — in all except the infradiaphragmatic type of TAPVD.

1st Week
1. Overhydration — delayed clamping of the cord and twin-twin transfusion.
2. Asphyxia — the most common cause of cardiomegaly on the first day.
3. Hypoplastic left heart.
4. Critical aortic stenosis.
5. TAPVD (obstructed).

2nd–3rd Weeks
1. Coarctation of the aorta.
2. Interrupted aortic arch.
3. Critical aortic stenosis.

4th–6th Weeks
1. Coarctation.
2. Critical aortic stenosis.
3. Endocardial fibroelastosis.
4. Anomalous left coronary artery.

N.B. Left-to-right shunts are usually asymptomatic during the neonatal period because of the high pulmonary vascular resistance. However, pulmonary vascular resistance in premature infants is lower, so shunts may present earlier in this particular group. Patent ductus arteriosus is the commonest shunt to cause heart failure in premature infants.

5.18 Neonatal Cyanosis

With Pleonaemia
Cyanosis and congestive cardiac failure — either may predominate.

1. Transposition.
2. Truncus arteriosus.
3. TAPVD.
4. Single ventricle.
5. Hypoplastic left ventricle } predominantly congestive cardiac failure, but may be cyanosed.
6. Interrupted aortic arch

With Oligaemia and Cardiomegaly
All have an ASD.

1. Pulmonary stenosis.
2. Ebstein's anomaly.
3. Pulmonary atresia with an intact ventricular septum.
4. Tricuspid atresia.

With Oligaemia but no Cardiomegaly
Signs appear towards the end of the first week due to closure of the ductus arteriosus.

1. Fallot's tetralogy.
2. Pulmonary atresia with a VSD.
3. Tricuspid atresia.

See also 'Neonatal respiratory distress', section 4.46.

5.19 Cardiovascular Involvement in Syndromes

Cri-du-chat	Variable.
Down's*	AV canal, VSD, PDA, ASD, and aberrant right subclavian artery.
Ehlers-Danlos	Mitral valve prolapse, aortic root dilatation, dissecting aortic aneurysm and intracranial aneurysm.
Ellis-Van Creveld	ASD and common atrium.
Friedreich's ataxia	Hypertrophic cardio-myopathy.
Holt-Oram	ASD and VSD.
Homocystinuria*	Medial degeneration of the aorta and pulmonary artery causing dilatation. Arterial and venous thromboses.
Hurler's/Hunter's*	Intimal thickening of coronary arteries and valves.
Kartagener's	Situs inversus ± septal defects.
Marfan's*	Cystic medial necrosis of the wall of the aorta, and less commonly the pulmonary artery, leading to dilatation and predisposing to dissection. Aortic and mitral regurgitation.
Morquio's*	Late onset of aortic regurgitation.
Noonan's	Pulmonary valve stenosis, and branch stenosis of pulmonary arteries septal defects.
Osteogenesis imperfecta*	Aortic and mitral regurgitation. Ruptured chordae.
Rubella	Septal defects, PDA, pulmonary artery branch stenoses and myocardial disease.
Trisomy 13	VSD, ASD, PDA and dextroposition.
Trisomy 18	VSD, ASD and PDA.
Tuberous sclerosis*	Cardiomyopathy and rhabdomyoma of the heart.
Turner's	Coarctation, aortic and bicuspid aortic valve stenosis.

5.20   Complications of Subclavian Vein Catheterization (after Gibson *et al.*)

Major
1. **Pneumothorax** — in up to 6% of cases and 30% of all major complications.
2. **Vascular injury** — haemomediastinum, haemothorax, arteriovenous fistula.
3. **Extravascular infusion** — intrapleural, mediastinal.
4. **Thrombosis.**
5. **Air embolism.**
6. **Catheter embolism.**
7. **Nerve injury** — e.g. brachial plexus.
8. **Cardiac** — arrhythmias, myocardial perforation, tamponade.

Minor
1. **Failed catheterization.**
2. **Catheter malposition.** ⎫
3. **Subclavian artery puncture.** ⎬ potentially major complications.
4. **Local haematoma.** ⎭
5. **Subcutaneous infusion.**
6. **Occluded catheter.**
7. **Dislodged catheter.**

Further Reading
Gibson R.N., Hennessy O.F., Collier N. & Hemingway A.P. (1985) Major complications of central venous catheterization: a report of five cases and a brief review of the literature. *Clin. Radiol.* 36: 205–8.

Mitchell S.E. & Clark R.A. (1979) Complications of central venous catheterization. *Am. J. Roentgenol.*, 138: 467–76.

Bibliography

Felson B. (ed.)(1969) The myocardium. *Semin. Roentgenol.*, 4 (4).
Felson B. (ed.)(1979) Acquired valvular disease of the heart. *Semin. Roentgenol.*, 14 (2).
Hipona F.A. (ed.)(1971) Cardiac radiology, medical aspects. *Radiol. Clin. North Am.*, 9 (3).
Hipona F.A. (ed.)(1971) Cardiac radiology, surgical aspects. *Radiol. Clin. North Am.*, 9 (2).
Jefferson, K. (1970) The plain chest radiograph in congenital heart disease. *Br. J. Radiol.*, 43: 753–70.
Jefferson K. & Rees S. (1980) *Clinical Cardiac Radiology*, 2nd edn. London: Butterworths.
Möes, C.A.F. (1975) Analysis of the chest in the neonate with congenital heart disease. *Radiol. Clin. North Am.*, 13: 251–76.
Sutton D. (ed.)(1980) *Textbook of Radiology and Imaging*, 3rd edn, chaps 22–28. Edinburgh: Churchill Livingstone.

Notes

Notes

Chapter 6

Abdomen and Gastrointestinal Tract

6.1 Extraluminal Intra-abdominal Gas

1. **Pneumoperitoneum** (q.v.) — see section 6.2.
2. **Gas in bowel wall**
   (a) Pneumatosis coli.
   (b) Linear pneumatosis intestinalis — infarction (e.g. due to vascular disease, volvulus, necrotizing enterocolitis).
3. **Bilary tree gas** (q.v.) — see section 7.3.
4. **Portal vein gas** (q.v.) — see section 7.4.
5. **Urinary tract gas** (q.v.) — see section 8.4.
6. **Abscess** — mottled gas which may mimic gas within colonic faeces. A homogeneous gas distribution (less common) may mimic gas in normal bowel. Lack of mucosal pattern helps to differentiate it.
7. **Necrotic tumour** — especially following chemotherapy, radiotherapy and therapeutic embolization.
8. **Retroperitoneal gas** — small 'bubbles' or linear translucencies. Secondary to perforation or post-nephrectomy.

Further Reading
Rice R.P., Thompson W.M. & Gedgandas R.K. (1982) The diagnosis and significance of extraluminal gas in the abdomen. *Radiol. Clin. North Am.*, 20: 819–37.

6.2 Pneumoperitoneum

1. Erect — free gas under diaphragm or liver. Can detect 10 ml of air. Can take 10 min for all gas to rise.
2. Supine — Gas outlines both sides of bowel wall, which then appears as a white line. In infants a large volume of gas will collect centrally producing a rounded, relative translucency over the central abdomen. The falciform ligament may also be outlined by free gas. This is seen as a characteristic curvilinear white line in the right upper abdomen.

1. **Perforation**
   (a) Peptic ulcer — 30% do not have free air visible.
   (b) Inflammation — diverticulitis, appendicitis, toxic megacolon, necrotizing enterocolitis.
   (c) Infarction.
   (d) Malignant neoplasms.
   (e) Obstruction.
   (f) Pneumatosis coli — the cysts may rupture.
2. **Iatrogenic (surgery; peritoneal dialysis)** — may take 3 weeks to reabsorb (faster in obese and children), but serial views will show progressive diminution in volume of free air.
3. **Pneumomediastinum** (q.v.) — see section 4.38.
4. **Introduction per vaginam** — e.g. douching.
5. **Pneumothorax** — due to a congenital pleuroperitoneal fistula.
6. **Idiopathic.**

6.3   Gasless Abdomen

Adult
1. **High obstruction.**
2. **Ascites** (q.v.) — see section 6.4.
3. **Pancreatitis** (Acute) — due to excess vomiting.
4. **Fluid-filled bowel** — closed-loop obstruction, total active colitis, mesenteric infarction (early), bowel wash-out.
5. **Large abdominal mass** — pushes bowel laterally.
6. **Normal.**

Child
1. **High obstruction**
   (a) Oesophageal atresia, without a fistula distally
   (b) Duodenal atresia.
   (c) Annular pancreas.
   (d) Volvulus (secondary to malrotation).
   (e) Hypertrophic pyloric stenosis.
   (f) Choledochal cyst.
2. **Vomiting** — including excess naso-gastric aspiration.
3. **Fluid filled bowel** — see above.
4. **Congenital diaphragmatic hernia** — bowel in the chest.

6.4   Ascites

1. Hazy appearance of entire abdomen.
2. Bowel gas 'floats' centrally on supine film.
3. Bulging flank lines.

1. **Cirrhosis.**
2. **Tumours.**
   (a) Malignant — peritoneal metastases, primary carcinoma (particularly ovary and gastrointestinal tract).
   (b) Benign — fibroma of ovary (Meig's syndrome).
3. **Hypoalbuminaemia** — e.g. nephrotic syndrome.
4. **Peritonitis** — particularly TB.
5. **Increased pressure in vascular system distal to liver** — congestive cardiac failure, constrictive pericarditis, thrombosis of inferior vena cava.
6. **Lymphatic obstruction** — chylous ascites, lymphoma, radiation, trauma or filariasis.

6.5 Abdominal Mass in a Neonate

(After Kirks et al., 1981).

Renal (55%)(q.v.)
1. **Hydronephrosis** (25%) — e.g. pelviureteric junction obstruction, posterior urethral valves, ectopic ureteroele, prune-belly and ureterovesical junction obstruction.
2. **Multicystic kidney** (15%).
3. **Infantile polycystic kidneys** (see Polycystic disease*) — ± hepatic fibrosis.
4. **Mesoblastic nephroma** — benign hamartoma.
5. **Renal vein thrombosis** (q.v.) — complication of dehydration/sepsis.
6. **Renal ectopia.**
7. **Wilms' tumour.**

Genital (15%)
1. **Hydrometrocolpos** — dilated fluid-filled vagina and/or uterus, due to vaginal stenosis. ± Associated with imperforate anus or gastrointestinal fistula.
2. **Ovarian cyst.**

Gastrointestinal (15%) — commonly associated with obstruction.
1. **Duplication** — commonest bowel mass in neonate. Commonly in right lower quadrant.
2. **Mesenteric cyst.**

Non-renal Retroperitoneal (10%)
1. **Adrenal haemorrhage** — relatively common. Due to neonatal stress. ± asymptomatic.
2. **Neuroblastoma.**
3. **Teratoma.**

Hepato/spleno/biliary (5%)
1. **Hepatoblastoma.**
2. **Hepatic cyst.**
3. **Splenic haematoma.**
4. **Choledochal cyst.**

Further Reading

Kirks D.R., Merten D.F., Grossman H. & Bowie J.D. (1981) Diagnostic imaging of paediatric abdominal masses: an overview. *Radiol. Clin. North Am.*, 19: 527–45.

See also 'Renal mass in the newborn and young infant', section 8.14.

6.6   Abdominal Mass in a child

(After Kirks et al., 1981).

Renal (55%)

1. **Wilms' tumour** — second commonest primary abdominal neoplasm in childhood (just behind neuroblastoma).
   Age: peak incidence at 3 years.
   Site: bilateral in 5%.
   Clinical: usually asymptomatic; pain in 37%, fever in 23%, haematuria in 20%.
   Signs on IVU: 5% calcify; mass causes pelvicalyceal distortion; 10% non-functioning.
   Spread: lung commonest (10–15% at presentation); liver less common and bone is rare; 5% extend into renal vein and inferior vena cava.
   Associations: genitourinary anomalies (5%), hemihypertrophy (2%), aniridia (1%) and Beckwith-Wiedemann syndrome.
2. **Hydronephrosis** (20%) (q.v.).
3. **Cysts** (q.v.).

Non-renal Retroperitoneal (23%)

1. **Neuroblastoma** (21%) —
   Age: usually less than 3 years.
   Site: can occur anywhere in sympathetic chain; 65% in adrenal gland; 5% in pelvis; remainder in thoracic or cervical sympathetic chain.
   Clinical: often present with metastases; symptoms due to local invasion, metastases or catecholamine production.
   Signs on IVU: 50% calcify; mass causes pelvicalyceal displacement; commonly crosses the mid-line.
   Spread: bone, liver, skin, orbit, skull, sutures, nodes.
   Prognosis: poor; in 5% of patients aged less than 1 year, spontaneous cure may occur. A fully differentiated form (ganglioneuroma) may behave as a benign tumour.

2. **Teratoma** (1%) — presacral, 60% calcify. Benign, but malignant change can occur.

Gastrointestinal (18%)

1. **Appendix abscess** (10%) — particularly spreads to pouch anterior to rectum.

2. **Hepatoblastoma** — more commonly in right lobe, but 40% in both lobes. 40% calcify. Arteriography important to define lobar extent.

3. **Haemangioma** — commonly multiple, involving entire liver. Rarely calcify. ± associated with congestive heart failure, and cutaneous haemangiomas.

4. **Choledochal cyst** — the classical triad of mass, pain and jaundice is only present in 10%. Usually affects the supraduodenal portion of common duct. A radioisotope HIDA (hydroxyiminodiacetic acid) scan is diagnostic.

Genital (4%)

1. **Ovarian cysts or teratoma**

Further Reading

Kirks D.R., Merten D.F., Grossman H. & Bowie J.D. (1981) Diagnostic imaging of paediatric abdominal masses: an overview. *Radiol. Clin. North Am.*, 19: 527–45.

6.7   Intestinal Obstruction in a Neonate

Duodenal — most common
1. **Stenosis/atresia** — 'double bubble' sign, which may also be seen by ultrasound of fetus (+ hydramnios). Associated with annular pancreas (20%), mongolism (30%) and other abnormalities of gastrointestinal tract (60%).
2. **Annular pancreas** — if not associated with duodenal atresia it may not present until adulthood.
3. **Congenital fibrous band (of Ladd)** — connects caecum to posterolateral abdominal wall and commonly crosses the duodenum. May be complicated by malrotation and mid-gut volvulus.
4. **Congenital web.**
5. **Choledochal cyst.**
6. **Preduodenal portal vein.**

Jejunal
1. **Malrotation and volvulus.**
2. **Atresia** — 50% associated with atretic sites distally (ileum > colon).

Ileal
1. **Meconium ileus** — mottled lucencies due to gas trapped in meconium but only few fluid levels (since it is very viscous). Bowel loops of variable calibre. Rapid appearance of fluid levels suggests volvulus. Peritoneal calcification due to perforation occurring in-utero is seen in 30%. Secondary microcolon.
2. **Atresia.**
3. **Inguinal hernia.**
4. **Inspissated milk** — presents 3 days–6 weeks of age. Dense, amorphous intraluminal masses frequently surrounded by a rim of air, ± mottled lucencies within them. Usually resolves spontaneously.
5. **Paralytic ileus** — e.g. due to drugs administered during labour.

Colonic
1. **Hirschsprung's disease.**
2. **Functional immaturity** — including meconium plug syndrome and small left colon syndrome.
3. **Imperforate anus**
   (a) High — ± sacral agenesis and gas in the bladder (due to a recto-vesical fistula).
   (b) Low — ± perineal or urethral fistula.
4. **Atresia.**

Further Reading
Carty H. & Brereton R.J. (1983) The distended neonate. *Clin. Radiol.*, 34: 367–80.
LeQuesne G.W. & Reilly B.J. (1975) Functional immaturity of the large bowel. *Radiol. Clin. North Am.*, 13: 331–42.
Martin D.J. (1975) Experiences with acute surgical conditions. *Radiol. Clin. North Am.*, 13: 297–329.

6.8 Abnormalities of Bowel Rotation

1. **Exompholos** — total failure of the bowel to return to the abdomen from the umbilical cord. Bowel is contained within a sac. To be differentiated from gastroschisis in which bowel protrudes through a defect in the abdominal wall.
2. **Non-rotation** — usually an asymptomatic condition with the small bowel on the right side of the abdomen and the colon on the left side. Small and large bowel lie on either side of the superior mesenteric artery (SMA) with a common mesentery. CT or transverse US scans show the superior mesenteric vein (SMV) lying to the left of the SMA cf the normal arrangement in which the SMV lies to the right of the SMA.
3. **Malrotation** — the duodeno-jejunal flexure lies to the right and caudad to its usual position which is to the left of the midline and approximately in the same axial plane as the 1st part of the duodenum. The caecum is usually more cephalad than normal but is normally sited in 5%. Malrotation nearly always complicates left sided diaphragmatic hernia. US or CT show the SMV immediately anterior to the SMA. *This sign is not reliable when*

SMA lies to the left of the aorta e.g. in association with hepatomegaly, aortic aneurysm or scoliosis and a normal US does not exclude malrotation.

4. **Reverse rotation** — rare. Colon lies dorsal to the SMA with jejunum and duodenum anterior to it.
5. **Paraduodenal hernia** — rare.
6. **Extroversion of the cloaca** — rare. No rotation of the bowel and the ileum and colon open separately onto the extroverted area in the midline below the umbilical cord.

Further Reading

Gaines P.A., Saunders A.J.S. & Drake D. (1987) Midgut malrotation diagnosed by ultrasound. *Clin. Radiol.*, 38: 51–3.

Houston C.S. & Wittenborg M.H. (1965) Roentgen evaluation of anomalies of rotation and fixation of the bowel in children. *Radiology*, 84: 1–17.

Nichols D.M. & Li D.K. (1983) Superior mesenteric vein rotation: a CT sign of midgut malrotation. *Am. J. Roentgenol.*, 141: 707–8.

6.9   Haematemesis

Oesophagus
1. Hiatus hernia.
2. Varices — 20% of cases are bleeding from a coexisting peptic ulcer.
3. Neoplasms.
4. Mallory-Weiss tears.

Stomach
1. Ulcer.
2. Erosions — may be associated with steroids, analgesics or alcohol.
3. Carcinoma.

Duodenum
1. Ulcer.

Others
1. Blood dyscrasias.
2. Osler-Weber-Rendu (hereditary telangiectasia) — autosomal dominant. Telangiectasis not prominent until age 20. Epistaxis is often the first symptom.
3 Connective tissue disorders — Ehlers-Danlos syndrome, pseudoxanthoma elasticum.

6.10 Dysphagia — Adult

Intrinsic

1. **Reflux stricture.**
2. **Tumours** — carcinoma, lymphoma, leiomyoma.
3. **Ingestion** — corrosive, lye, foreign body.
4. **Iatrogenic** — radiotherapy, prolonged nasogastric intubation.
5. **Plummer-Vinson web** — narrow anterior indentation. Can occur from C4 to T1. Females with iron deficiency anaemia; males post-gastrectomy. Premalignant, but tumour can occur at different site.
6. **Schatzki ring** — marks the squamo-columnar junction lying above the diaphragm. Acute obstruction may occur if internal diameter is less than 6 mm.
7. **Monilia** — painful dysphagia. Can involve entire oesophagus — 'shaggy', ulcerated. Immunosuppression, long-term antibiotics, hypoparathyroidism and debilitation all predispose. Herpes simplex and CMV may cause identical changes.
8. **Skin disorders** — epidermolysis bullosa and pemphigus can produce strictures.

Extrinsic

1. **Tumours** — lymph nodes, mediastinal tumours.
2. **Vascular** — aortic aneurysm; aberrant right subclavian artery (posterior indentation); aberrant left pulmonary artery (anterior indentation); right-sided aortic arch (right lateral and posterior indentation).
3. **Pharyngeal pouch** — ± air/fluid level in neck. Can cause superior mediastinal mass. Signs of aspiration on chest X-ray.
4. **Goitre.**
5. **Enterogenous cyst** — adjacent to, but rarely communicates with, the oesophagus. Hemivertebra and anterior meningocoele may be associated (neuro-enteric cyst).
6. **Prevertebral abscess/haematoma.**

Neuromuscular
1. Achalasia.
2. Scleroderma*.
3. Chagas' disease.
4. Myasthenia gravis.
5. Bulbar/pseudobulbar palsy.

Psychiatric
1. Globus hystericus.

6.11 Dysphagia — Neonate

1. **Cleft palate.**
2. **Macroglossia/glossoptosis** — e.g. Beckwith-Wiedemann syndrome and Pierre Robin syndrome.
3. **Oesophageal atresia.**
4. **Vascular rings.**

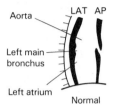

Normal

Aberrant right
subclavian artery

Right-sided
aortic arch

Aberrant left
pulmonary artery

5. **Choanal atresia.**
6. **Neuromuscular defects** — e.g. delayed maturation, prematurity and mental subnormality.

Further Reading

Illingworth R.S. (1969) Sucking and swallowing difficulties in infancy. Diagnostic problems of dysphagia. *Arch. Dis. Child.*, 44: 655–65.

6.12 Pharyngeal/Oesophageal 'Diverticula'

Upper Third

1. **Pouch (Zenker's)** — posteriorly, usually on left side, between the fibres of the inferior constrictor and cricopharyngeus. Can cause dysphagia, regurgitation, aspiration and hoarseness ± an air/fluid level. If large, can appear as a superior mediastinal mass. Food residue with it seen as 'mobile' filling defects.
2. **Lateral pharyngocoele**
   (a) Congenital — remnant of the second branchial arch. Wide mouth (may not retain barium and so may only be seen in recumbent position).
   (b) Acquired — glassblower, trumpeter, etc.

Middle Third

1. **Traction** — at level of carina. May be related to fibrosis after treatment for TB. Asymptomatic.
2. **Developmental** — failure to complete closure of tracheo-oesophageal communication.
3. **Intramural** — very rare. Mutiple, tiny flask-shaped outpouchings. 90% have associated strictures, mainly in the upper third of the oesophagus.

Lower Third

1. **Epiphrenic.**
2. **Ulcer** — peptic or related to steroids, immunosuppression and radiotherapy.
3. **Mucosal tears** — Mallory-Weiss syndrome, post-oesophagoscopy.
4. **Post-Heller's operation.**

Further Reading

Levine M.S., Moolten D.N., Herlinger H. & Laufer I. (1986) Esophageal intramural pseudodiverticulosis: a reevaluation. *Am. J. Roentgenol.*, 147: 1165–70.

Schwartz E.E., Tucker J. and Holt G.P. (1981) Cervical dysphagia: pharyngeal protrusions and achalasia. *Clin. Radiol.*, 32: 643–50.

6.13 Oesophageal Ulceration

In addition to ulceration there may be non-specific signs of oesophagitis viz.
1. Thickening of longitudinal folds, (> 2 mm), which may be slightly scalloped.
2. Thickening of transverse folds resembling small bowel mucosal folds.
3. Reduced or absent peristalsis.

Inflammatory

1. **Reflux oesophagitis** — ± hiatus hernia. Signs characteristic of reflux oesophagitis are
   (a) a gastric fundal fold crossing the gastro-oesophageal junction and ending as a polypoid protruberance in the distal oesophagus,
   (b) erosions — dots or linear streaks of barium in the distal oesophagus,
   (c) ulcers which may be round or, more commonly, linear or serpiginous.
2. **Barrett's oesophagus** — to be considered in any patient with oesophageal ulceration or stricture but especially if the abnormality is in the body of the oesophagus.
3. **Moniliasis** — predominantly in immunosuppressed patients. Sudden onset of pain and dysphagia, not relieved by antacids. Early — small, plaque-like filling defects, often orientated in the long axis of the oesophagus. Advanced — cobblestone mucosal surface ± luminal narrowing. Ulceration is uncommon.
   Patients with mucocutaneous candidiasis or oesophageal stasis due to achalasia, scleroderma etc. may develop chronic infection which is characterized by a lacy or reticular appearance of the mucosa ± nodular filling defects.
4. **Viral** — herpes and CMV occurring mostly in immunocompromised patients. May manifest as discrete ulcers, ulcerated plaques or mimic monilial oesophagitis. Discrete ulcers on an otherwise normal background mucosa are strongly suggestive of a viral aetiology.
5. **Caustic ingestion** — ulceration is most marked at the sites of anatomical hold-up and progress to a long, smooth stricture.

6. **Radiotherapy** — ulceration is rare. Altered oesophageal motility is frequently the only abnormality.
7. **Crohn's disease*** — aphthous ulcers and, in advanced cases, undermining ulcers, intramural tracking and fistulae.
8. **Drug induced** — due to prolonged contact with tetracycline, quinidine and potassium supplements.
9. **Behçet's disease.**
10. **Intramural diverticulosis.**

Neoplastic
1. **Carcinoma.**
2. **Leiomyosarcoma and leiomyoma.**
3. **Lymphoma*.**
4. **Melanoma.**

Further Reading

Cynn W.S., Chon H.K., Gureghian P.A. & Levin B.L. (1975) Crohn's disease of the esophagus. *Am. J. Roentgenol.*, 125: 359–64.

Goldstein H.M., Rogers L.F. & Fletcher G.H. (1975) Radiological manifestations of radiation induced injury to the normal upper gastrointestinal tract. *Radiology*, 117: 145–40.

Heading R.C. (1987) Barrett's oesophagus. *Br. Med. J.* 294: 461–2.

Laufer I. (1982) Radiology of esophagitis. *Radiol. Clin. North Am.*, 20 (4): 687–99.

Levine M.S., Laufer I., Kressel H.Y. & Friedman H.M. (1981) Herpes esophagitis. *Am. J. Roentgenol.*, 136: 863–6.

Lewicki A.M. & Moore J.P. (1975) Eosophageal moniliasis. A review of common and less frequent characteristics. *Am. J. Roentgenol.*, 125: 218–25.

Shortsleeve M.J. Gauvin G.P. & Gardner R.C. (1981) Herpetic esophagitis. *Radiology*, 141: 611–17.

6.14   Oesophageal Strictures — Smooth

Inflammatory

1. **Peptic** — the stricture develops relatively late. Most frequently at the oesophagogastric junction and associated with reflux and a hiatus hernia. Less commonly, more proximal in the oesophagus and associated with heterotopic gastric mucosa (Barrett's oesophagus). ± ulceration.
2. **Scleroderma*** — reflux through a wide open cardia may produce stricture. Oesophagus is the commonest internal organ to be affected. Peristalsis is poor, cardia wide open and the oesophagus dilated (contains air in the resting state).
3. **Corrosives** — acute — oedema, spasm, ulceration and loss of mucosal pattern at 'hold-up' points (aortic arch and oesophago-gastric junction). Strictures are typically long and symmetrical, may take several years to develop and are more likely to be produced by alkalis than acid.
4. **Iatrogenic** — prolonged use of a naso-gastric tube. Stricture in distal oesophagus probably secondary to reflux.

Neoplastic

1. **Carcinoma** — squamous carcinoma may infiltrate submucosally. The absence of a hiatus hernia and the presence of an extrinsic soft-tissue mass should differentiate it from a peptic stricture but a carcinoma arising around the cardia may predispose to reflux.
2. **Mediastinal tumours** — carcinoma of the bronchus and lymph nodes. Localized obstruction ± ulceration and an extrinsic soft-tissue mass.
3. **Leiomyoma** — narrowing due to a smooth, eccentric, polypoid mass. ± central ulceration.

Others

1. **Achalasia** — 'rat-tail' tapering may mimic a stricture; this occurs below the diaphragm. Considerable oesophageal dilatation with food in the lumen.
2. **Skin disorders** — epidermolysis bullosa, pemphigus.

6.15 Oesophageal Strictures — Irregular

Neoplastic
1. **Carcinoma** — increased incidence in achalasia, Plummer-Vinson syndrome, Barrett's oesophagus, coeliac disease, asbestosis, lye ingestion and tylosis. Mostly squamous carcinomas; adenocarcinoma is rare. Appearances include
   (a) Irregular filling defect — annular or eccentric.
   (b) Extraluminal soft tissue mass.
   (c) Re-entrant angles at its margins (shouldering).
   (d) Ulceration.
   (e) Proximal dilatation.
2. **Leiomyosarcoma.**
3. **Carcinosarcoma** — big polypoid tumour ± pedunculated. Better prognosis than squamous carcinoma.
4. **Lymphoma*** — usually extension from gastric involvement.

Inflammatory
1. **Reflux** — rarely irregular.
2. **Crohn's disease*** — rare.

Iatrogenic
1. **Radiotherapy** — rare, unless treating an oesophageal carcinoma. Dysphagia post radiotherapy is usually due to a motility disorder. Acute oesophagitis may occur with a dose of 50–60 Gy (5000–6000 rad).
2. **Fundoplication.**

Further Reading
Levine M.S., Dillon E.C, Saul S.H. & Laufer I. (1986) Early esophageal cancer. *Am. J. Roentgenol.*, 146: 507–12.

6.16 Tertiary Contractions in the Oesophagus

Unco-ordinated, non-propulsive contractions.

1. **Reflux oesophagitis.**
2. **Presbyoesophagus** — impaired motor function due to muscle atrophy in the elderly. Occurs in 25% of people over 60 years.
3. **Obstruction at the cardia** — from any cause.
4. **Neuropathy**
   (a) Early achalasia — before dilatation occurs.
   (b) Diabetes.
   (c) Alcoholism.
   (d) Malignant infiltration.
   (e) Chagas' disease.

6.17 Stomach Masses and Filling Defects

Primary Malignant Neoplasms

1. **Carcinoma** — most polypoidal carcinomas are 1–4 cm in diameter. (Any polyp greater than 2 cm in diameter must be considered to be malignant.) Granular/lobulated surface pattern is suggestive of carcinoma. Asbestosis, adenomatous polyps and Peutz-Jeghers' syndrome predispose. Metastases may calcify and sclerotic or lytic bone metastases may occur.
2. **Lymphoma*** — primary gastric lymphoma is usually non-Hodgkin's. It can be ulcerative and infiltrative as well as polypoid. Often cannot distinguish it from carcinoma, but extension across the pylorus is suggestive of a lymphoma.

Polyps

1. **Hyperplastic** — accounts for most polyps. Usually multiple, small (less than 1 cm in diameter) and occur randomly throughout stomach but predominantly affect body and fundus. Associated with chronic gastritis.
2. **Adenomatous** — usually solitary, 1–4 cm in diameter, sessile and occur in antrum. High incidence of malignant transformation (particularly if greater than 2 cm in size) and carcinomas elsewhere in stomach (because of dysplastic epithelium). Associated with pernicious anaemia.

3. **Hamartomatous** — characteristically multiple, small and relatively spare the antrum. Occur in 30% of Peutz-Jeghers' syndrome, 40% of familiar polyposis coli and Gardner's syndrome.

Submucosal Neoplasms

Smooth, well-defined filling defect, with a re-entry angle.
1. **Leiomyoma** — commonest by far. Can be very large with a substantial exogastric component. Central ulceration and massive haematemesis may occur.
2. **Lipoma** — can change shape with position of patient and may be relatively mobile on palpation.
3. **Neurofibroma** — N.B. Leiomyomas and lipomas are more common, even in patients with generalized neurofibromatosis.
4. **Metastases** — Frequently ulcerate — 'bulls eye' lesion (q.v.). Usually melanoma, but bronchus, breast, lymphoma, Kaposi's sarcoma and any adenocarcinoma may metastasize to stomach. Breast primary often produces a scirrhous reaction in the distal part of the stomach which is indistinguishable from linitis plastica (q.v.).

Extrinsic Indentation

1. **Pancreatic tumour/pseudocyst.**
2. **Splenomegaly/hepatomegaly.**
3. **Retroperitoneal tumours.**

Others

1. **Nissen fundoplication** — may mimic a distorted mass in the fundus.
2. **Bezoar** — 'mass' is mobile. Tricho- (hair) or phyto (vegetable matter).
3. **Pancreatic rest** — ectopic pancreatic tissue causes a small filling defect, usually on the inferior wall of the antrum, and resembles a submucosal tumour. Central 'blob' of barium ('bull's eye' or target lesion) in 50%.

6.18   Thick Stomach Folds

Thickness greater than 1 cm.

Inflammatory
1. **Gastritis** — associated with peptic ulceration.
2. **Zollinger-Ellison syndrome** — suspect if post-bulbar ulcers. Ulceration in both 1st and 2nd parts of duodenum is suggestive, but ulceration distal to this is virtually diagnostic. Thick folds and small bowel dilatation may occur in response to excess acidity.

    Due to gastrinoma of non-beta cells of pancreas (no calcification, moderately vascular). 50% malignant — metastases to liver. (10% of gastrinomas may be ectopic — usually in medial wall of the duodenum.)
3. **Pancreatitis (acute).**
4. **Crohn's disease*** — mild thickening of folds with aphthous ulceration may occur in up to 40% of Crohn's. However, these signs are subtle, and more obvious disease (i.e deformity and narrowing of the antrum) only occurs in 2% of these.

Infiltrative/Neoplastic
1. **Lymphoma*** — usually non-Hodgkin's lymphoma and may be primary or secondary. Accounts for half of all gastro-intestinal lymphomas. The predominant features of early disease are shallow ulceration or uneven mucosa with enlarged, radiating folds. Features which may suggest the diagnosis of advanced disease are: multiple masses or ulcerations, diffuse thickening of folds, extensive submucosal infiltration, extension across the pylorus or the gastrooesophageal junction, large tumours over 10 cm in diameter and preservation of wall pliability.
2. **Carcinoma** — irregular folds with rigid wall.
3. **Pseudolymphoma** — benign reactive lymphoid hyperplasia. 70% have an ulcer near the centre of the area affected.
4. **Eosinophilic gastroenteritis.**

Others

1. **Ménétrier's disease** — smooth folds predominantly on greater curve. Rarely extend into antrum. No rigidity or ulcers. 'Weep' protein sufficient to cause hypoproteinaemia (effusion, oedema, thick folds in small bowel). Commonly achlorhydric — c.f. Zollinger-Ellison syndrome. In adults it pursues a chronic and unremitting course but in children resolution should be expected after weeks or months. In children the aetiology is likely to be cytomegalovirus infection.

2. **Varices** — occur in fundus and usually associated with oesophageal varices.

Further Reading

Coad N.A.G. & Shah K.J. (1986) Ménétrier's disease in childhood associated with cytomegalovirus infection: a case report and review of the literature. *Br. J. Radiol.*, 59: 615–20.

Hricak H., Thoeni R.F., Margulis A.R., Eyler W.R. & Francis I.R. (1980) Extension of gastric lymphoma into the esophagus and duodenum. *Radiology*, 135: 309–12.

Sato T., Sakai Y., Ishiguro S. & Furukawa H. (1986) Radiologic manifestations of early gastric lymphoma. *Am. J. Roentgenol.*, 146: 513–17.

6.19 Linitis Plastica

Neoplastic
1. **Gastric carcinoma.**
2. **Lymphoma*.**
3. **Metastases** — particularly breast.
4. **Local invasion** — pancreatic carcinoma.

Inflammatory
1. **Corrosives** — can cause rigid stricture of antrum extending up to the pylorus.
2. **Radiotherapy** — can cause rigid stricture of antrum with some deformity. Mucosal folds may be thickened or effaced. Large antral ulcers can also occur.
3. **Granulomata** — Crohn's disease, TB.
4. **Eosinophilic enteritis** — commonly involves gastric antrum (causing narrowing and nodules) in addition to small bowel. Blood eosinophilia. Occasionally spares the mucosa, so needs full thickness biopsy for confirmation.

6.20 Gastrocolic Fistula

Inflammatory
1. **Peptic ulcer.**
2. **Crohn's disease*.**
3. **Pancreatitis (chronic).**
4. **Infections** — tuberculosis, actinomycosis.

Neoplastic
1. **Carcinoma** — of stomach, colon or pancreas.
2. **Metastases.**

6.21 Gastric Dilatation

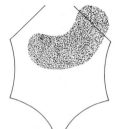

Gas- or food-filled stomach. Mottled translucencies (due to gas trapped in food residue) may be seen in gastric dilatation secondary to chronic obstruction. Resembles heavy faecal loading of the colon.

Mechanical Obstruction

1. **Fibrosis secondary to ulceration** — long history of dyspepsia.
2. **Malignancy** — shorter history, therefore dilatation is usually less marked. Often no abdominal pain.
3. **Volvulus** — 'organo-axial', associated with hiatus hernia. 'Vertical axis', not associated with hiatus hernia.
4. **Infantile hypertrophic pyloric stenosis** — the radiological signs on a barium meal are

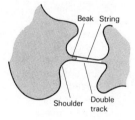

   (a) 'String sign' — barium in the narrowed pyloric canal.
   (b) 'Shoulder sign', the pyloric 'tumour' indenting the barium-filled antrum.
   (c) 'Beak sign' — incomplete extension of the barium into the narrowed pyloric channel.
   (d) 'Double track sign' — parallel mucosal folds in the pyloric channel.

   U.S. now replacing barium meal for diagnosis.
5. **Proximal small bowel obstruction** — gastric and small bowel dilatation.
6. **Bezoar**

Paralytic Ileus

1. **Postoperative.**
2. **Post-vagotomy.**
3. **Drugs** — e.g. anticholinergics.
4. **Metabolic** — uraemia, hypokalaemia, etc.
5. **Acute gastric dilatation** — see section 7.4.

6.22 'Bull's Eye' (Target) Lesion in the Stomach

Ulcer on apex of a nodule.

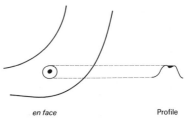

en face   Profile

1. **Submucosal metastases** — may be multiple
   (a) Melanoma — commonest.
   (b) Lymphoma*.
   (c) Carcinoma — breast, bronchus, pancreas.
   (d) Carcinoid.
2. **Leiomyoma.**
3. **Pancreatic 'rest'** — ectopic pancreatic tissue. Usually on inferior wall of antrum. A central 'blob' of barium is seen in 50% — collects in primitive duct remnant. Can also occur in duodenum, jejunum, Meckel's diverticulum, liver, gallbladder and spleen.
4. **Neurofibroma** — may be multiple. Other stigmata of neurofibromatosis.

6.23   Gas in the Stomach Wall

Interstitial Gastric Emphysema

Linear or curvilinear gas shadows in the wall of the stomach ± extension into the duodenum.

1. **Raised intragastric pressure** — obstruction and gastric distension.
2. **Post-gastroscopy.**
3. **Peptic ulceration** — with submucosal gas.
4. **Necrotizing enterocolitis.**

Emphysematous Gastritis

Due to gas-forming organisms in the stomach wall. Severe epigastric pain, haematemesis, prostration and toxaemic shock. Contracted stomach with mottled lucencies resembling interstitial emphysema.

1. **Diabetes.**
2. **Alcohol abuse.**
3. **Corrosive ingestion.**

Cystic Pneumatosis

Mild symptoms; usually in elderly patients and often associated with chronic obstructive airways disease.

Further Reading

Colquhoun J. (1965) Intramural gas in hollow viscera. *Clin. Radiol.*, 16: 71–86.

Tuck J.S. & Boobis L.H. (1987) Case report: interstitial emphysema of the stomach due to perforated appendicitis. *Clin Radiol.*, 38: 315–17.

6.24   Cobblestone Duodenal Cap

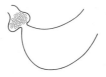

Big 'Polypoid'

1. **Oedema** — associated with an ulcer.
2. **Hypertrophied Brunner's glands** — can extend from pylorus to ampulla of Vater. Uniform in size.
3. **Crohn's disease*** — involved in 2% and may rarely present here. Usually signs present in gastric antrum also.
4. **Varices** — base of cap. Decrease in size in erect position. Invariably associated with oesophageal varices.
5. **Lymphoma*.**
6. **Carcinoma.**

Small

1. **Duodenitis** — ± central flecks of barium.
2. **Nodular lymphoid hyperplasia** — pinpoint (1–3 mm) nodules involving the entire duodenal loop. (Duodenum > jejunum.)
3. **Food residue/effervescent granules** — move around.
4. **Heterotopic gastric mucosa** — base of cap adjacent to pylorus.

Further Reading

Schulman A. (1970) The cobblestone appearance of the duodenal cap, duodenitis and hyperplasia of Brunner's glands. *Br. J. Radiol.*, 43: 787–95.

6.25   Decreased/absent Duodenal Folds

1. **Scleroderma*.**
2. **Crohn's disease*.**
3. **Strongyloides.**
4. **Cystic fibrosis*.**
5. **Amyloidosis.**

6.26 Thickened Duodenal Folds

Inflammatory
1. Duodenitis
2. Pancreatitis
3. **Crohn's disease*** — occurs before aphthous ulcers. Mild signs occur in duodenum in up to 40%, but severe involvement only occurs in 2%. Cap and proximal half of second part of duodenum predominantly affected.
4. **Zollinger-Ellison syndrome** — response to excess acidity.

Neoplastic
1. Lymphoma*.
2. Metastases — particularly melanoma, breast, ovary, gastro-intestinal tract (lung, kidney are rare).

Infiltrative
1. **Amyloidosis** — bowel commonly involved (primary gener-alized thickening; secondary — segmental thickening).
2. **Eosinophilic enteritis** — gastric antrum commonly involved. Blood eosinophilia.
3. **Mastocytosis** — dense bones. ± gastric polyps.
4. **Whipple's disease.**

Vascular
1. **Intramural haematoma** — due to trauma. Common in the duodenum because it is fixed to the posterior abdominal wall. 'Stacked coins' appearance. An extensive haematoma may occur in bleeding diatheses.
2. **Ischaemia** — widespread changes can occur in vasculitis secondary to radiotherapy, collagen diseases and Henoch-Schönlein purpura.

Oedema
1. **Hypoproteinaemia** — nephrotic syndrome, cirrhosis or protein-losing enteropathy.
2. **Venous obstruction** — cirrhosis, Budd-Chiari syndrome or constrictive pericarditis.
3. **Lymphatic obstruction.**
4. **Angioneurotic oedema.**

Infestations
1. **Worms**
   (a) Hookworm (*Ankylostoma duodenale*) — the head of the worm produces an inflammatory reaction.
   (b) Tapeworm (*Taenia saginata* or *T. solium*) — has a similar effect on the duodenum. The worm may be visible as a filling defect during a barium study.
   (c) Strongyloides — similar appearance to giardiasis (see below). Strictures in chronic cases.
2. **Giardiasis** — predominantly affects the duodenum and proximal jejunum. Thickened, blunted and distorted mucosal folds. Hypermotility leads to rapid transit. Spasm produces narrowing. May be associated with nodular lymphoid hyperplasia or hypogammaglobulinaemia.
See also sections 6.30 and 6.31.

6.27   Dilated Duodenum

Mechanical Obstruction
1. **Bands** — most frequent cause of neonatal duodenal obstruction. Associated with malrotation and midgut volvulus.
2. **Atresia, webs, stenosis** — often associated with Down's syndrome. 'Double bubble' sign in neonate due to dilated stomach and duodenum. Webs have a high incidence of incomplete rotation.
3. **Annular pancreas.**
4. **Superior mesenteric artery syndrome** — hold up of barium in third part of duodenum with some proximal dilatation and vigorous peristalsis (prior to muscle relaxant). Postprandial pain relieved by lying on left side. Associated with a plaster of Paris body cast. 20% have associated duodenal ulcer. Never occurs in obese people.

Paralytic Ileus
— particularly due to pancreatitis.

Scleroderma*

Further Reading
Anderson J.R., Earnshaw P.M. & Fraser G.M. (1982) Extrinsic compression of the third part of the duodenum. *Clin. Radiol.*, 33: 75–81.

6.28   Dilated Small Bowel

Calibre: proximal jejunum > 3.5 cm (4.5 cm if small
bowel enema)
mid-small bowel > 3.0 cm (4.0 cm if small
bowel enema)
ileum > 2.5 cm (3.0 cm if small bowel enema).

Normal Folds

1. **Mechanical obstruction** — ± dilated large bowel, depending on level of obstruction.
2. **Paralytic ileus** — dilated small and large bowel.
3. **Coeliac disease, tropical sprue, dermatitis herpetiformis** — can produce identical signs. Dilatation is the hallmark, and correlates well with severity, but it is relatively uncommon. ± dilution and flocculation of barium. See section 6.33.
4. **Scleroderma*.**
5. **Iatrogenic** — post-vagotomy and gastrectomy may produce dilatation due to rapid emptying of stomach contents. Dilatation may also occur proximal to a small bowel loop.

Thick Folds

1. **Ischaemia.**
2. **Crohn's disease*** — combination of obstructive and inflammatory changes.
3. **Radiotherapy.**
4. **Lymphoma*.**
5. **Zollinger-Ellison syndrome** — ileus due to excess acidity.
6. **Extensive small bowel resection** — compensatory dilatation and thickening of folds.
7. **Amyloidosis.**

6.29 Strictures in the Small Bowel

1. **Adhesions** — angulation of bowel which is constant in site. Normal mucosal folds.
2. **Crohn's disease*** — ± ulcers and altered mucosal pattern.
3. **Ischaemia** — ulcers are rare. Evolution is more rapid than Crohn's ± long strictures.
4. **Radiation enteritis** — see section 6.30.
5. **Tumours**
   (a) Lymphoma — usually secondary to contiguous spread from lymph nodes. Primary disease may occur and is nearly always due to non-Hodgkin's lymphoma.
   (b) Carcinoid — although the appendix is the commonest site, these never metastasize. Of those occurring in small bowel, 90% are in ileum (mostly distal 2 feet), and 30% are multifocal. A fibroblastic response to infiltration produces a stricture, ± mass. It is the commonest primary malignancy of small bowel, but only 30% metastasize (more likely if > 2 cm diam.) or invade. Carcinoid syndrome only develops with liver metastases — see section 6.35.
   (c) Carcinoma — if duodenal lesions are included this is the most common primary malignancy of the small bowel and the duodenum is the most frequent site. Ileal lesions are rare (unless associated with Crohn's disease). Short segment stricture with mucosal destruction, ulcerating or polypoidal lesion. High incidence of second primary tumours.
   (d) Sarcoma — lymphoma- or leiomyo-. Tick folds with an eccentric lumen. Leiomyosarcomas may present as a large mass displacing bowel loops with a large barium-filled cavity.
   (e) Metastases — usual sites of origin are malignant melanoma, ovary, pancreas, stomach, colon, breast, lung and uterus. Rounded deformities of the bowel wall with flattened mucosal folds. In patients with gynaecological malignancies duodenal or jejunal obstruction are most likely due to metastases; most radiation induced strictures are in the ileum.
6. **Enteric coated potassium tablets.**

Further Reading
Papadopoulos V.D. & Nolan D.J. (1985) Carcinoma of the small intestine. *Clin. Radiol.*, 36: 409–13.
Yuhasz M., Laufer I., Sutton G., Herlinger H. & Caroline D.F. (1985) Radiography of the small bowel in patients with gynaecological malignancies. *Am. J. Roentgenol.*, 144: 303–7.

6.30 Thickened Folds in Non-dilated Small Bowel — Smooth and Regular

Fold thickness: jejunum   > 2.5 mm
                 ileum   > 2.0 mm

Vascular
1. **Intramural haematoma**
   (a) Trauma — commonest in duodenum, since fixed to posterior abdominal wall ('stacked coin' appearance).
   (b) Bleeding diathesis — commonly localized to a few loops.
2. **Ischaemia**
   (a) Acute — embolus, Henoch-Schönlein purpura. Can produce ileus. May perforate. Ulcers rare.
   (b) Chronic — vasculitis (collagen, radiotherapy), atheroma, fibromuscular dysplasia. Present with post-prandial pain, and malabsorption.

Radiotherapy
Infrequently seen with tumour doses <45 Gy. Underlying pathological process is endarteritis obliterans and concomitant arterial disease will exacerbate the damage. Majority of cases are secondary to treatment of female genital tract malignancy. Acute symptoms during radiotherapy do not correlate with the development of chronic radiation enteritis which may have a latent period of up to 25 years. Distal jejunum and ileum are the commonest sites.
1. **Acute** — thickening of valvulae conniventes and poor peristalsis. Ulceration is rare.
2. **Chronic** — most common signs are submucosal thickening of valvulae conniventes and/or mural thickening. Stenoses, adhesions, sinuses and fistulae may also occur. (The absence of ulceration, cobblestoning and asymmetry differentiate it from Crohn's disease).

Oedema
1. **Adjacent inflammation** — focal.
2. **Hypoproteinaemia** — e.g. nephrotic, cirrhosis, protein losing enteropathy. Generalized.
3. **Venous obstruction** — e.g. cirrhosis, Budd-Chiari syndrome, constrictive pericarditis.
4. **Lymphatic obstruction** — e.g. lymphoma, retroperitoneal fibrosis, primary lymphangiectasia (child with leg oedema).
5. **Angioneurotic.**

Early Infiltration
1. **Amyloidosis** — gastrointestinal tract commonly involved. Primary amyloid tends to produce generalized thickening, whereas secondary amyloid produces focal lesions. Malabsorption is unusual.
2. **Eosinophilic enteritis** — focal or generalized. Gastric antrum frequently involved. No ulcers. Blood eosinophilia. Occasionally spare mucosa — therefore need full thickness biopsy for diagnosis.

Coeliac Disease
Thickening of folds is not common, and is probably a functional abnormality rather than true fold thickening. ± jeunal dilatation.

Abetalipoproteinaemia
Rare, inherited. Malabsorption, acanthocytosis, and CNS abnormality. ± dilated bowel.

Further Reading
Mendelson R.M. & Nolan D.J. (1985) The radiological features of chronic radiation enteritis. *Clin. Radiol.*, 36: 141–8.

6.31 Thickened Folds in Non-dilated Small Bowel — Irregular and Distorted

Fold   jejunum   < 2.5 mm
thickness: ileum   < 2.0 mm

Localized

Inflammatory
1. **Crohn's disease*** — occurs before aphthous ulcers.
2. **Zollinger-Ellison syndrome** — predominantly proximal small bowel. Dilatation may occur.

Neoplastic
1. **Lymphoma***.
2. **Metastases** — particularly melanoma, breast, ovary and gastrointestinal tract.
3. **Carcinoid** — commonest primary malignant small bowel tumour. 90% in the ileum and mostly in the distal 60 cm. It is more common in the appendix, where it is a benign tumour.

Infective
1. **Tuberculosis** — can look identical to Crohn's disease, but predominant caecal involvement may help to distinguish it. Less than 50% have pulmonary tuberculosis.

Widespread

Infiltrative
1. **Amyloidosis.**
2. **Eosinophilic enteritis.**
3. **Mastocytosis** — may have superimposed small nodules, uticaria pigmentosa and sclerotic bone lesions.
4. **Whipple's disease** — flitting arthralgia, lymphadenopathy and sacro-iliitis.

Inflammatory
1. **Crohn's disease***.

Infestations

1. **Giardiasis** — associates with hypogammaglobulinaemia and nodular lymphoid hyperplasia.
2. **Strongyloides** — ± absent folds in chronic cases.

Stomach Abnormality with Thickened Small Bowel Mucosal Folds

1. Lymphoma/metastases.
2. Zollinger-Ellison syndrome.
3. Ménétrier's disease.
4. Amyloidosis.
5. Eosinophilic enteritis.

Further Reading

Goldberg H.I. & Sheft D.J. (1976) Abnormalities in small intestine contour and calibre. *Radiol. Clin. North Am.*, 14: 461–75.

6.32 Multiple Nodules in the Small Bowel

Inflammatory

1. **Nodular lymphoid hyperplasia** — nodules 2–4 mm with normal fold thickness. Associated with hypogammaglobulinaemia (IgA and IgM). Produces malabsorption, and there is a high incidence of intestinal infections (particularly giardiasis, but strongyloides and monilia may also occur). Can also affect the colon, where in children it may be a normal variant, but in adults it may be an early sign of Crohn's disease.
2. **Crohn's disease*** — 'cobblestone' mucosa but other characteristic signs present.

Infiltrative

1. **Whipple's disease** — ± myriad of tiny (< 1 mm) nodules superimposed on thick folds.
2. **Waldenström's macroglobulinaemia** — ± myriad of tiny (< 1 mm) nodules. Folds usually normal, but may occasionally be thick.
3. **Mastocytosis** — nodules a little larger and folds usually thick.

Neoplastic
1. **Lymphoma*** — can produce diffuse nodules (2–4 mm) of varying sizes. Ulceration in the nodules is not uncommon.
2. **Polyposis**
   (a) Peutz-Jeghers' syndrome — autosomal dominant. Buccal pigmentation. Multiple hamartomas (± intussuscept) 'carpeting' the small bowel. Can also involve the colon (30%) and stomach (25%). Not in themselves premalignant, but associated with carcinoma of stomach, duodenum and ovary.
   (b) Gardner's syndrome — predominantly in the colon. Occasionally has adenomas in small bowel.
   (c) Canada-Cronkhite syndrome — predominantly stomach and colon, but may affect the small bowel.
3. **Metastases** — on antimesenteric border. Particularly melanoma, breast, gastrointestinal tract and ovary. (Rarely bronchus and kidney.) ± ascites.

Infective
1. **Typhoid** — hypertrophy of 'Peyer's patches'.
2. **Yersinia** — ± nodules in terminal ileum.

Further Reading
Marshak R.H., Lindner A.E. & Maklansky D. (1976) Immunoglobulin disorders of the small bowel. *Radiol. Clin. North Am.*, 14: 477–91.

6.33   Malabsorption

Mucosal

1. **Coeliac disease** — commonest cause of malabsorption. Not all have steatorrhea — can present with iron of folate deficiency. Jejunal biopsy shows subtotal villous atrophy (this can also occur in Whipple's disease, primary lymphoma and chronic ulcerative enteritis). Jejunal dilatation is the hallmark, but is relatively uncommon. It correlates well with severity. Fold thickness is normal in uncomplicated coeliac disease. An increase in ileal fold pattern ± a decrease of jejunal folds, i.e. a reversal of the normal fold pattern indicates long standing disease and should heighten awareness to potential malignant complications. Other signs, which are occasionally demonstrable on a barium follow through examination are

   (a) Dilution of barium, because of hypersecretion of fluid by the bowel.

   (b) Segmentation of the column of barium. This is most marked in the ileum.

   (c) Moulage sign. The appearance of barium in a featureless tube due to the complete effacement of mucosal folds.

   If bowel calibre increases while on a gluten free diet suspect a complication, i.e. lymphoma, carcinoma or intussusception (rare and non-obstructive). Tropical sprue and dermatitis herpetiformis can present with identical appearances.

2. **Inflammation**

   (a) Crohn's disease*.

   (b) Radiotherapy — if there is widespread involvement.

   (c) Scleroderma* — due to hypomotility.

3. **Ischaemia** — can cause mild malabsorption if chronic and widespread.

4. **Infiltration**

   (a) Whipple's disease.

   (b) Mastocytosis.

   (c) Amyloidosis — particularly in primary amyloidosis, since generalized bowel involvement is more common.

   (d) Eosinophilic enteritis — blood eosinophilia is common.

5. **Lymphangiectasia** — child. Blocked lymphatics interfere with the transport of fat. Hypoproteinaemia due to protein loss into the gut is common.
6. **Parasites** — particularly *Giardia* and *Strongyloides* spp.

Digestive
1. **Gastrectomy.**
2. **Biliary obstruction.**
3. **Pancreatic dysfunction** — pancreatitis, cystic fibrosis, carcinoma and pancreatectomy.
4. **Disaccharidase deficiency** — lactase deficiency is the commonest.

Anatomical
1. **Fistula** — even a small one to the colon allows bacterial colonization.
2. **Resection.**
3. **Stagnant loop/stricture.**
4. **Jejunal diverticulosis** — in the erect view may resemble obstruction with multiple fluid levels. However, the diverticula have smooth walls, i.e. no mucosal folds. Produces folate deficiency.

Further Reading
Bova J.G., Friedman A.C., Weser E., Hopens T.A. & Wytock D.H. (1985) Adaptation of the ileum in nontropical sprue: reversal of the jejunoileal fold pattern. *Am. J. Roentgenol.*, 144: 299–302.
Laws J.W. & Pitman R.G. (1960) The radiological investigation of the malabsorption syndromes. *Br. J. Radiol.*, 33: 211–22.

6.34   Protein-losing Enteropathy

Oedema in small bowel will occur if plasma albumin <20 gl^{-1}.

'Mucosal'
1. Coeliac disease.
2. Ménétrier's disease.
3. Sprue.

Inflammatory
1. Crohn's disease*.
2. Ulcerative colitis*.
3. Radiotherapy.

Ulceration
1. Carcinoma stomach/colon.
2. Villous adenoma.

Venous Obstruction
1. Cirrhosis.
2. Inferior vena cava thrombosis.
3. Constrictive pericarditis.

Chronic Arterial Obstruction

Lymphatic Obstruction
1. Lymphangiectasia.
2. Lymphoma*.
3. Retroperitoneal fibrosis (q.v.).

Infiltrative
1. Whipple's disease.
2. Eosinophilic enteritis.

Further Reading
Marshak R.H., Wolf B.S., Cohen N. & Janowitz H.D. (1961)
    Protein-losing disorders of the gastrointestinal tract: Roentgen
    features. *Radiology*, 77: 893–905.

6.35 Lesions in the Terminal Ileum

Inflammatory
1. **Crohn's disease***.
2. **Ulcerative colitis*** — 10% of those with total colitis have 'backwash' ileitis for up to 25 cm causing granular mucosa, ± dilatation. No ulcers.
3. **Radiation enteritis** — submucosal thickening of mucosal folds, mural thickening, symmetrical stenoses, adhesions, sinuses and fistulae. Ulceration and cobblestoning are not seen.

Infective
1. **Tuberculosis** — can look identical to Crohn's disease. Continuity of involvement with caecum and ascending colon can occur. Longitudinal ulcers are uncommon. Less than 50% have pulmonary TB. Caecum is predominantly involved — progressive contraction of caecal wall opposite the ileocaecal valve, and cephalad retraction of the caecum with straightening of the ileocaecal angle.
2. **Yersinia** — 'cobblestone' appearance and aphthous ulcers. No deep ulcers and spontaneous resolution, usually within 10 weeks, distinguishes it from Crohn's disease.
3. **Actinomycosis** — very rare. Predominantly caecum. ± associated bone destruction with periosteal reaction.
4. **Histoplasmosis** — very rare.

Neoplastic
1. **Lymphoma*** — may look like Crohn's disease.
2. **Carcinoid** — appendiceal carcinoid tumours are the most common and usually benign. Most ileal carinoids originate in the distal ileum and are invariably malignant if >2 cm. Radiological signs reflect the primary lesion (annular fibrotic stricture (± obstruction); intraluminal filling defect(s)), the mesenteric secondary mass (stretching of loops; rigidity and fixation), interference with the blood supply to the ileum by the secondary mass (thickening of mucosal folds) or the effects of fibrosis (sharp angulation of a loop; stellate arrangement of loops). The caecum may be involved and strictures may be multifocal.
3. **Metastases** — no ulcers.

Ischaemia

Rare site. Thickened folds, 'cobblestone' appearance and 'thumb printing', but rapid progression of changes helps to discriminate it from Crohn's disease.

Further Reading

Calenoff, L. (1970) Rare ileocaecal lesions. *Am. J. Roentgenol.*, 110: 343–51.

Jeffree M.A., Barter S.J., Hemingway A.P. & Nolan D.J. (1984) Primary carcinoid tumours of the ileum: the radiological appearances. *Clin. Radiol.*, 35: 451–5.

Mendelson R.M. & Nolan D.J. (1985) The radiological features of chronic radiation enteritis. *Clin. Radiol.*, 36: 141–8.

6.36 Colonic Polyps

Adenomatous

1. **Simple tubular adenoma — tubulovillous adenoma — villous adenoma** — these three form a spectrum both in size and degree of dysplasia. Villous adenoma is the largest, shows the most severe dysplasia and has the highest incidence of malignancy. Signs suggestive of malignancy are

   (a) Size —　　< 5 mm　　　　— 0% malignant
   　　　　　　　5 mm – 1 cm —　1% malignant
   　　　　　　　1–2 cm　　　— 10% malignant
   　　　　　　　> 2 cm　　　— 50% malignant.

   (b) Sessile — base greater than height.

   (c) 'Puckering' of colonic wall at base of polyp.

   (d) Irregular surface.

   Villous adenomas are typically fronded, sessile and are poorly coated by barium because of their mucous secretion. May cause a protein-losing enteropathy or hypokalaemia.

2. **Familial polyposis coli** — autosomal dominant. Starts in adolescence. Carpets the entire colon with adenomas. Always affects rectum and polyps are more numerous in distal colon. Carcinoma of colon develops in early adulthood. (Has occurred in 30% by 10 years after diagnosis made, and in 100% by 20 years.) 60% of those who present with colonic symptoms already have a carcinoma. The carcinoma is multifocal in 50%. Extra-colonic abnormalities may occur — hamartomas of stomach (40%) and adenomas of duodenum (25%).

3. **Gardner's syndrome** — autosomal dominant. Adenomas of colon (and occasionally small bowel), osteomas of skull and mandible, multiple skin tumours and epidermoid cysts. Same risk of colonic carcinoma as familial polyposis coli. Also, 12% develop carcinoma of duodenum (periampullary). Other tumours associated are carcinomas of thyroid and adrenal, carinoid, and hamartomas of the stomach. About 5% may develop desmoid tumours of the mesentery or anterior abdominal wall.

Hyperplastic
1. **Solitary/multiple** — most frequently found in rectum.
2. **Nodular lymphoid hyperplasia** — usually children. Filling defects are smaller than familial polyposis coli.

Hamartomatous
1. **Juvenile polyposis** — ± familial. Children under 10. Commonly solitary in rectum.
2. **Peutz-Jeghers' syndrome** — autosomal dominant. 'Carpets' small bowel, but also affects colon and stomach in 30%. Increased incidence of carcinoma of stomach, duodenum and ovary.

Inflammatory
1. **Ulcerative colitis** * — polyps can be seen at all stages of activity of the colitis (no malignant potential): acute — pseudo-polyps (i.e. mucosal hyperplasia); chronic — sessile polyp (resembles villous adenoma); quiescent — tubular/filiform ('wormlike') and can show a branching pattern.

   Dysplasia in colitic colons is usually not radiologically visible. When visible it appears as a solitary nodule, several separate nodules (both non-specific) or as a close grouping of multiple adjacent nodules with apposed, flattened edges (the latter appearance being associated with dysplasia in 50% of cases).
2. **Crohn's disease** * — polyps less common than in ulcerative colitis.

Infective
1. **Schistosomiasis** — predominantly involves rectum. ± strictures.
2 **Amoebiasis.**

Others
1. **Canada-Cronkhite syndrome** — not hereditary. Predominantly affects stomach and colon, but can occur anywhere in bowel. Increased incidence of carcinoma of colon. Other features are alopecia, nail atrophy and skin pigmentation.
2. **Turcot's syndrome** — autosomal recessive. Increased incidence of CNS malignancy.

Further Reading

Bresnihan E.R. & Simpkins K.C. (1975) Villous adenoma of the large bowel: Benign and malignant. *Br. J. Radiol.*, 48: 801–6.

Dodds W.J. (1976) Clinical and roentgen features of the intestinal polyposis syndromes. *Gastrointest. Radiol.*, 1: 127–42.

Dolan K.D., Seibert J. & Siebart R.W. (1973) Gardner's syndrome. *Am. J. Roentgenol.*, 119: 359–64.

Hooyman J.R., MacCarty R.L., Carpenter H.A., Schroeder K.W. & Carlison H.C. (1987) Radiographic appearance of mucosal dysplasia associated with ulcerative colitis. *Am. J. Roentgenol.*, 149: 47–51.

Morson, B.C. (1974) The polyp cancer sequence in the large bowel. *Proc. Roy. Soc. Med.*, 67: 451–7.

Morson, B.C. (1984) The evolution of colorectal carcinoma. *Clin. Radiol.*, 35: 425–31.

6.37 Colonic Strictures

Neoplastic
1. **Carcinoma** — mucosal destruction and 'shouldering'. Often shorter than 6 cm.
2. **Lymphoma***.

Inflammatory
Tend to be symmetrical, smooth and tapered.
1. **Ulcerative colitis*** — usually requires extensive involvement for longer than 5 years. Commonest in sigmoid colon. May be multiple. Beware malignant complications — these are commonly irregular, annular strictures (30% are multiple). Risk factors are: total colitis, length of history (risk starts at 10 years and increases by 10% per decade), epithelial dysplasia on biopsy.
2. **Crohn's disease*** — strictures occur in 25% of colonic Crohn's disease, and 50% of these are multiple.
3. **Pericolic abscess** — can look malignant, but relative lack of mucosal destruction.
4. **Radiotherapy** — occurs several years after treatment. Commonest site is rectosigmoid colon, which appears smooth and narrow and rises vertically out of pelvis due to thickening of surrounding tissue.

Ischaemia
Infarction heals by stricture formation relatively rapidly. Commonest site is splenic flexure, but 20% occur in other sites. It can be extensive and has tapering ends.

Infective
1. **Tuberculosis** — commonest in ileocaecal region. Short, 'hourglass' stricture.
2. **Amoeboma** — more common in descending colon. Occurs in 2–8% of amoebiasis and is multiple in 50%. Rapid improvement after treatment with metronidazole.
3. **Schistosomiasis** — commonly rectosigmoid region. Granulation tissue forming after the acute stage (oedema, fold-thickening and polyps) may cause a stricture.

4. **Lymphogranuloma venereum** — sexually transmitted chlamydia. Late complications are strictures which are characteristically long and tubular and affect the rectosigmoid region. Fistulate may occur.

Extrinsic masses — inflammatory, tumours (primary and secondary), and endometriosis.

Cathartic colon — pseudostrictures which alter their configuration during the barium enema. The colon may be atonic and dilated. Changes are initially in the ascending colon, but can progress to involve all of the colon.

Further Reading
Simpkins K.C. and Young A.C. (1971). The differential diagnoses of large bowel strictures. *Clin. Radiol.*, 22: 449–57.

6.38   Gas in the Wall of the Colon

1. **Toxic megacolon** (q.v.).
2. **Pneumatosis coli** — can produce 'polypoid' filling defects in barium enema which may be large enough to cause obstruction. Some are associated with chronic obstructive airways disease.
3. **Infarction.**
4. **Necrotizing enterocolitis** (neonate).
5. **Collagen disorders** — mainly scleroderma but also dermatomyositis and juvenile rheumatoid arthritis.
6. **Steroid and other immunosuppressive therapy.**
7. **Leukaemia.**

Further Reading
Bornes P.F. & Johnston T.A. (1973) Indulent pneumatosis of the bowel wall associated with suppressive therapy. *Ann Radiol.*, 16: 163–6.

Keats T.E. & Smith T. H. (1974) Benign pneumatosis intestinalis in childhood leukaemia. *Am. J. Roentgenol.*, 122: 150–2.

Mueller C.F., Morehead R., Alter A.J. & Michener W. (1972) Pneumatosis intestinalis in collagen disorders. *Am. J. Roentgenol.*, 115: 300–5.

6.39 Megacolon in an Adult

Colonic calibre greater than 5.5 cm.

Non-toxic (without mucosal abnormalities)
1. **Distal obstruction** — e.g. carcinoma.
2. **Ileus** — paralytic or secondary to electrolyte imbalance.
3. **Pseudo-obstruction** — symptoms and signs of large bowel obstruction but with no organic lesion identifiable by barium enema. A continuous, gas-filled colon with sharp, thin bowel wall, few fluid levels and gas or faeces in the rectum may differentiate from organic obstruction. Mortality is 25–30% and the risk of caecal necrosis and perforation is up to 15%.
4. **Purgative abuse.**

Toxic (with severe mucosal abnormalities)
Deep ulceration and inflammation produce a neuromuscular degeneration. Thick oedematous folds and extensive sloughing of the mucosa leaves mucosal islands. The underlying causes produce similar plain film changes. The presence of intramural gas indicates that perforation is imminent.
1. **Inflammatory**
   (a) Ulcerative colitis*.
   (b) Crohn's disease*.
   (c) Pseudomembranous colitis.
2. **Ischaemic colitis.**
3. **Dysentery**
   (a) Amoebiasis.
   (b) Salmonella.

Further Reading
Gilchrist A.M., Mills J.O.M. & Russell C.F.J. (1985) Acute large-bowel pseudo-obstruction *Clin. Radiol.*, 36: 401–4.

6.40 Megacolon in a Child

1. Hirschsprung's disease.
2. Functional/psychogenic — the rectum is distended with faeces.
3. Cretinism*.
4. Mechanical obstruction
   (a) Stricture — e.g. post necrotizing enterocolitis (25%).
   (b) Tumour — e.g. sacrococcygeal teratoma.
   (c) Imperforate anus — in a neonate.
5. Paralytic ileus — generalized large and small bowel distension.
6. Neurogenic — e.g. spina bifida.

6.41 'Thumbprinting' in the Colon

Colitides
1. Ulcerative colitis*.
2. Crohn's disease*.
3. Ischaemic colitis — commonest at the splenic flexure, but anywhere possible. Air insufflation may obliterate the 'thumbprinting'.
4. Pseudomembranous colitis.
5. Amoebic colitis.
6. Schistosomiasis.

Neoplastic
1. Lymphoma*.
2. Metastases.

Differential Diagnosis
1. Pneumatosis coli — cysts may indent the mucosa, giving a similar appearance, but gas is seen in the wall.

6.42 Aphthoid Ulcers

Barium in a central ulcer
surrounded by a halo of
oedematous mucosa.

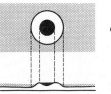

en face

Profile

In Colon
1. **Crohn's disease*** — the earliest sign in the terminal ileum
   and colon. Observed in 50% of patients.
2. **Yersinia enterocolitis.**
3. **Amoebic colitis.**
4. **Ischaemic colitis.**
5. **Behçet's disease** — mostly resembles Crohn's disease,
   but can occasionally simulate an idiopathic ulcerative
   proctocolitis.

In Small Bowel
1. **Crohn's disease*.**
2. **Yersinia enterocolitis.**
3. **Polyarteritis nodosa.**

Further Reading
Simpkins K.C. (1977) Aphthoid ulcers in Crohn's colitis. *Clin. Radiol.*, 28: 601–8.

6.43 Anterior Indentation of the Rectosigmoid Junction

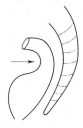

1. **Tumours**
   (a) Peritoneal metastases — common site. Particularly stomach, colon, pancreas and ovary.
   (b) Primary pelvic tumour.
2. **Abscess.**
3. **Haematoma.**
4. **Ascites** — if in erect position.
5. **Endometriosis** — common site.
6. **Hydatid** — metastatic cyst from rupture of a peripheral hepatic cyst.
7. **Surgical** — sling repair for rectal prolapse.

Further Reading

Schulman A. & Fataar S. (1979) Extrinsic stretching, narrowing, and anterior indentation of the rectosigmoid junction. *Clin. Radiol.* 30: 463–9.

6.44 Widening of the Retrorectal Space

The post-rectal soft-tissue space
at S3-S5 is greater than 1.5 cm.

Normal Variation
40% of cases and these are mostly large or obese individuals.

Inflammatory
1. **Ulcerative colitis*** — seen in 50% of these patients and
   the width increases as the disease progresses.
2. **Crohn's disease*** — the widening may diminish during the
   course of the disease.
3. **Radiotherapy.**
4. **Diverticulitis.**
5. **Abscess.**

Neoplastic
1. **Carcinoma of the rectum.**
2. **Metastases to the rectum** — especially from prostate,
   ovary and bladder.
3. **Sacral tumours** — metastases, plasmacytoma, chordoma
   and, in children, sacrococcygeal teratoma.

Others
1. **Anterior sacral meningocoele** — a sac containing CSF
   protudes through a round or oval defect in the anterior
   wall of the sacrum. The diagnosis is confirmed by
   myelography and/or C.T.
2. **Pelvic lipomatosis.**
3. **Enteric duplication cysts.**

Further Reading
Teplick S.K., Stark P., Clark R.E., Metz J.R and Shapiro J.H. (1978)
   The retrorectal space. *Clin. Radiol.*, 29: 177–84.

6.45   CT Retroperitoneal Cystic Mass

Pancreas
1. Pseudocyst.
2. Cystadenoma/carcinoma.
3. von Hippel–Lindau.

Kidney — see section 8.

Paraaortic Cystic Nodes
1. Testicular teratoma.
2. Carcinoma cervix.

Retroperitoneal Cystic Tumour
1. Lymphangioma.
2. Leiomyosarcoma.
3. Haemangiopericytoma.

N.B. Any tumour with a fatty content can appear cystic due to density averaging e.g. neurofibroma.

Others
1. Haematoma — late stage.
2. Abscess.
3. Lymphocoele.
4. Meningocoele.

Further Reading
Alpern M.B., Thorsen M.K., Kellman G.M., Pojunas K. & Lawson
    T.L. (1986) C.T. appearances of haemangiopericytoma. *J.
    Comput. Assist. Tomogr.*, 10 (2): 264–7.
Munechika H., Honda M., Kushihashi T., Koizumi K. & Gokan
    T. (1986) Computed tomography of retroperitoneal cystic
    lymphangiomas. *J. Comput. Assist. Tomogr.*, 11 (1): 116–19.

6.46   CT Mesenteric Cystic Lesion

Cyst
1. Pancreatic pseudocyst.
2. Enteric duplication cyst.
3. Mesothelial cyst.

Tumour
1. Teratoma.
2. Cystic leiomyoma/sarcoma.
3. Cystic mesothelioma.
4. Lymphangioma.

Further Reading
Ros P., Olmsted W., Moser R., Dachman A., Hjermstad B. & Sobin
   L. (1987) mesenteric and omental cysts: histologic classification
   with imaging correlation. *Radiology*, 164: 327–32.

Bibliography

General
Bartram C.I. & Kumar P. (1981) *Clinical Radiology in Gastroenterology*. Oxford: Blackwell Scientific Publications.
Laufer I. (1979) *Double Contrast Gastrointestinal Radiology*. Philadelphia: Saunders.
Margulis A.R. & Burhenne H.J. (1983) *Alimentary Tract Roentgenology*, 4th edn. St Louis: Mosby.
Sutton D. (1980) *A Textbook of Radiology and Imaging*. 3rd edn,
   chaps. 32–8. Edinburgh: Churchill Livingstone.

Abdomen
Fataar S. & Schulman A. (1981) Subphrenic abscess: the radiological
   approach. *Clin. Radiol.*, 32: 147–56.
Felson B. (ed.)(1973) The Acute Abdomen. Part I. Bowel obstruction.
   Semin. Roentgenol., 8 (3)
Felson B. (ed.)(1973) The Acute Abdomen. Part II. Inflammatory
   disease. *Semin. Roentgenol.*, 8 (4).
Meyers MA. (1981) Intraperitoneal spread of malignancies and its
   effects on the bowel. *Clin. Radiol.*, 32: 129–46.

Oesophagus
Donner M.W., Saba G.P. & Martinez C.R. (1981) Diffuse diseases
   of the esophagus: a practical approach *Semin. Roentgenol.*,
   16: 198–213.
Goldstein H.M., Zornoza J. & Hopens T. (1981) Intrinsic disease
   of the adult oesophagus: benign and malignant tumours.
   Semin. Roentgenol., 16: 183–97.
Zboralske F.F. & Dodds W.J. (1969) Roentgenographic diagnosis of
   primary disorders of oesophageal motility. *Radiol. Clin. North
   Am.*, 7: 147–62.

Stomach

Felson B. (ed.)(1971) Localised lesions of the stomach. *Semin. Roentgenol.*, 6 (2).

Ichikawa H. (1973) Differential diagnosis between benign and malignant ulcers of the stomach. *Clin. Gastroenterol.*, 2: 329–43.

Small Bowel

Eaton S.B. & Ferrucci J.T. (1973) *Radiology of the Pancreas and Duodenum*. Philadelphia: Saunders.

Marshak R.H. & Lindner A.E. (1976) *Radiology of the Small Intestine*, 2nd edn. Philadelphia: Saunders.

Sellink J.L. (1976) *Radiological Atlas of Common Diseases of the Small Bowel*. Massachusetts: Stenfert Kroese.

Theoni R.F. & Margulis A.R. (1979) Gastrointestinal tuberculosis. *Semin. Roentgenol.*, 14: 283–94.

Large Bowel

Felson B. (ed.)(1968) Inflammatory diseases of the colon. *Semin. Roentgenol.*, 3 (1).

Felson B. (ed.)(1976) Localised solitary lesions of the colon. *Semin. Roentgenol.*, 11 (2).

Gardiner R. & Stevenson G.W. (1982) The colitides. *Radiol. Clin. North Am.*, 20: 797–817.

Kolawole T.M. & Lewis E.A. (1974) Radiological observations on intestinal amoebiasis. *Am. J. Roentgenol.*, 122: 257–65.

Wittenberg J., Athanasoulis C.A., Williams L.F., Paredes S., O'Sullivan P. & Brown P. (1975) Ischaemic colitis. *Am. J. Roentgenol.*, 123: 287–300.

Young W.S. (1980) Further radiological observations in caecal volvulus. *Clin. Radiol.*, 31: 479–83.

Young W.S., Engelbrecht H.E. & Stoker A. (1978) Plain film analysis in sigmoid volvulus. *Clin. Radiol.*, 29: 553–60.

Computed Tomography

Haaga J.R. & Alfidi R.J. (1983) *Computed Tomography of the Whole Body*. Toronto. The C.V. Mosby Company.

Moss A.A., Gamsu G. & Gerant H.K. (1983) *Computed Tomography of the Body*. Philadelphia. W.B. Saunders Company.

Notes

Notes

Chapter 7
Gallbladder, Liver, Spleen, Pancreas and Adrenals

7.1 Non-visualization of the Gallbladder

During Oral Cholecystography
1. Technical failures
    (a) No fatty meal prior to taking of contrast medium.
    (b) Tablets not taken or taken at the wrong time.
    (c) Vomiting or diarrhoea.
    (d) Failure to fast after taking contrast medium.
    (e) Films taken too early or too late.
    (f) Bilirubin greater than 34 mmol.1^{-1}.
2. Previous cholecystectomy.
3. Ectopic gallbladder — confirmed by taking a film of the entire abdomen.
4. Cholecystitis.
5. Cystic duct obstruction.

During Intravenous Cholangiography
1. Technical failures
    (a) Contrast medium given too rapidly — renal excretion is seen.
    (b) Bilirubin greater than 50 mmol.1^{-1}.
2. Previous cholecystectomy.
3. Ectopic gallbladder.
4. Cystic duct obstruction.
5. Cholecystitis.

7.2 Filling Defect in the Gallbladder

Multiple

1. **Calculi** — 30% are radio-opaque. Freely mobile.
2. **Cholesterosis ('strawberry' gallbladder)** — characteristically multiple fixed mural filling defects.

Single and Small
1. **Calculus.**
2. **Adenomyomatosis** — three characteristic signs
   (a) Fundal nodular filling defect.
   (b) Stricture — anywhere in the gallbladder. Sharply localized or a diffuse narrowing. More prominent following contraction after a fatty meal.
   (c) Rokitansky-Aschoff sinuses — may only be visible after gallbladder contraction.

Single and Large
1. **Calculus.**
2. **Carcinoma** — difficult to diagnose as the radiological presentation is usually with a non-functioning gallbladder. Nearly always associated with gallstones and, therefore, if filling does occur it is indistinguishable from them.

7.3 Gas in the Biliary Tract

Irregularly branching gas shadows
which do not reach to the liver edge,
probably because of the direction of
bile flow. The gallbladder may also be
outlined.

Within the Bile Ducts
INCOMPETENCE OF THE SPHINCTER OF ODDI
1. Following sphincterotomy.
2. Following passage of a gallstone.
3. Patulous sphincter in the elderly.

POSTOPERATIVE
1. Cholecystoenterostomy.
2. Choledochoenterostomy.

SPONTANEOUS BILIARY FISTULA
1. **Passage of a gallstone directly from an inflamed gallbladder
   into the bowel** — 90% of spontaneous fistulae. 57%
   erode into the duodenum and 18% into the colon. May
   result in a gallstone ileus.
2. **Duodenal ulcer perforating into the common bile duct** —
   6% of spontaneous fistulae.
3. **Malignancy or trauma** — 4% of spontaneous fistulae.

Within the Gallbladder
1. **All of the above.**
2. **Emphysematous cholecystitis** — due to
   gas-forming organisms and associated
   with diabetes in 20% of cases. There
   is intramural and intraluminal gas but,
   because there is usually cystic duct
   obstruction, gas is present in the bile
   ducts in only 20%. The erect film may
   show an air/bile interface.

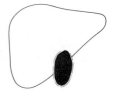

7.4 Gas in the Portal Veins

Gas shadows which extend to within 2 cm of the liver capsule because of the direction of blood flow in the portal veins. Gas may also be present in the portal and mesenteric veins and the bowel wall.

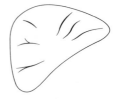

Children

1. **Necrotizing enterocolitis** — 10–20% develop gas in the portal vein. Necrotic bowel wall allows gas or gas-forming organisms into the portal circulation. The finding of portal vein gas is of serious significance.
2. **Umbilical vein catheterization** — with the inadvertent injection of air.
3. **Erythroblastosis fetalis.**

Adults

1. **Mesenteric infarction** — the majority of patients die soon after gas is seen in the portal veins.
2. **Air embolus during double contrast barium enema** — this has been observed during the examination of severely ulcerated colons and is not associated with a fatal outcome.
3. **Acute gastric dilatation** — in bedridden young people. May recover following decompression with a nasogastric tube.

Further Reading

Benson M.B. (1985) Adult survival with intrahepatic portal venous gas secondary to acute gastric dilatation, with a review of portal venous gas. *Clin Radiol.*, 36: 441–3.

Mindelzun R. & McCort J.J. (1980) Hepatic and perihepatic radiolucencies. *Radiol. Clin. North Am.*, 18: 221–38.

Radin D.R., Roson R.S. & Halls J.M. (1987) Acute gastric dilatation: a rare cause of portal venous gas. *Am. J. Roentgenol.*, 148: 279–80.

Sisk P.B. (1961) Gas in the portal venous system. *Radiology*, 77: 103–6.

Wiot J.F. & Felson B. (1961) Gas in the portal venous system *Am. J. Roentgenol.*, 86: 920–9.

7.5 Hepatomegaly

Neoplastic
1. Metastases.
2. Hepatoma.
3. Lymphoma*.

Raised Venous Pressure
1. Congestive cardiac failure.
2. Constrictive pericarditis.
3. Tricuspid stenosis.
4. Budd-Chiari syndrome.

Degenerative
1. Cirrhosis — especially alcoholic.
2. Fatty infiltration.

Myeloproliferative Disorders
1. Polycythaemia rubra vera.
2. Myelofibrosis.

Infective
1. **Viral** — infectious and serum hepatitis; infectious mononucleosis.
2. **Bacterial** — abscess; brucellosis.
3. **Protozoal** — amoebic abscess, malaria, trypanosomiasis and kala-azar.
4. **Parasitic** — hydatid.

Storage Disorders
1. Amyloid.
2. Haemochromatosis.
3. Gaucher's disease.
4. Niemann-Pick disease.

Congenital
1. Riedel's lobe.
2. Polycystic disease*.

7.6   Hepatic Calcification

Multiple and Small

1. **Healed granulomas** — tuberculosis, histoplasmosis and, less commonly, brucellosis and coccidioidomycosis.

Curvilinear

1. **Hydatid** — liver is the commonest site of hydatid disease. Most cysts are in the right lobe and are clinically silent but may cause pain, a palpable mass or a thrill. Calcification in 20–30% and although calcification does not necessarily indicate death of the parasite extensive calcification favours an inactive cyst. Calcification of daughter cysts produces several rings of calcification.
2. **Abscess** — especially amoebic abscess when the right lobe is most frequently affected.
3. **Calcified (porcelain) gall bladder** — strong association with gall bladder carcinoma.

Localized in Mass

1. **Metastases** — calcification is uncommon but colloid carcinoma of the rectum, colon or stomach calcify most frequently. It may be amorphous, flakey, stippled or granular and solitary or multiple. Calcification may follow radiotherapy or chemotherapy.
2. **Hepatoma** — rare. Calcifications are punctate, stippled or granular.

Sunray Spiculation

1. **Haemangioma** — phleboliths may also occur but are uncommon.
2. **Metastases** — infrequently in metastases from colloid carcinomas.
3. **Hepatoma.**

Diffuse Increased Density

1. **Haemochromatosis*.**
2. **Thorotrast** — lacy, bubbly increased density ± opacification of the liver capsule. Adjacent lymph nodes and spleen also show increased density, although the latter is more granular.

Further Reading

Ashur H., Siegal B., Oland Y. and Adam Y.G. (1978) Calcified gall bladder (porcelain gall bladder). *Arch. Surg.*, 113: 594–6.

Beggs I. (1985) The radiology of hydatid disease. *Am. J. Roentgenol.*, 145: 639–48.

Darlak J.J., Moskowitz M. & Katten K.R. (1980) Calcifications in the liver. *Radiol. Clin. North Am.*, 18: 209–19.

Gondos B. (1973) Late clinical roentgen observations following Thorotrast administration. *Clin. Radiol.*, 24: 195–203.

Levy D.W., Rindsberg S., Friedman A.C., Fishman E.K., Ros P.R., Radecki P.D., Siegelman S.S., Goodman Z.D., Pyatt R.S. & Grumbach K. (1986) Thorotrast-induced hepatosplenic neoplasia: CT identification. *Am. J. Roentgenol.*, 148: 997–1004.

7.7 Fetal or Neonatal Liver Calcification

Peritoneal

1. **Meconium peritonitis** — the commonest cause of neonatal abdominal calcification. US reveals intra-abdominal solid or cystic masses with calcified walls.
2. **Plastic peritonitis due to ruptured hydrometrocolpos** — similar appearance to meconium peritonitis but US may demonstrate a dilated, fluid-filled uterus and vagina.

Parenchymal

1. **Congenital infections** — TORCH complex (toxoplasmosis, rubella, cytomegalovirus, herpes simplex) and varicella. Randomly scattered nodular calcification. Often calcification elsewhere and other congenital abnormalities.
2. **Tumours** — haemangioma, hamartoma, hepatoblastoma, teratoma and metastatic neuroblastoma. Complex mass on US.

Vascular

1. **Portal vein thromboemboli** — subcapsular branching calcification.
2. **Ischaemic infarcts** — branching calcifications but distributed throughout the liver.

Further Reading

Brugman S.M., Bjelland J.J., Thomason J.E., Anderson S.F. & Giles H.R. (1979) Sonographic findings with radiologic correlation in meconium peritonitis. *J. Clin. Ultrasound*, 7: 305–6.

Friedman A.P., Haller J.O., Boyer B. & Cooper R. (1981) Calcified portal vein thromboemboli in infants: radiography and ultrasonography. *Radiology*, 140: 381–2.

Nguyen D.L. & Leonard J.C. (1986) Ischaemic hepatic necrosis: a cause of fetal liver calcification. *Am. J. Roentgenol.*, 147: 596–7.

Schackelford G.D. & Kirks D.R. (1977) Neonatal hepatic calcification secondary to transplacental infection. *Radiology*, 122: 753–7.

7.8 Ultrasound Liver — Generalized Hypoechoic

1. **Acute hepatitis** — mild hepatitis has normal echo pattern.
2. **Diffuse malignant infiltration.**

7.9 Ultrasound Liver — Generalized Hyperechoic (Bright Liver)

1. **Fatty infiltration.**
2. **Cirrhosis.**
3. **Hepatitis** — particularly chronic.
4. **Infiltration/deposition** — malignant, granulomata (e.g. TB, brucellosis, sarcoid), glycogen storage disease.

Further Reading

Barnett E. & Morley P. (eds) (1985) *Clinical Diagnostic Ultrasound.* D.O. Cosgrove, Liver and biliary tree. pp. 365–86. Chapter 22. Oxford: Blackwell Scientific Publications.

7.10 Ultrasound Liver — Focal Hyperechoic

1. **Metastases** — gastrointestinal tract, ovary, pancreas, urogenital tract.
2. **Capillary haemangioma.**
3. **Adenoma** — particularly if associated haemorrhage.
4. **Focal nodular hyperplasia** — may be hyperechoic.
5. **Focal fatty infiltration.**
6. **Debris within lesion** — e.g. abscess, haematoma.
7. **Hepatoma** — can be hyper or hypoechoic.

7.11 Ultrasound Liver — Focal Hypoechoic

1. **Metastasis** — including cystic metastases (e.g. ovary, pancreas, stomach, colon).
2. **Lymphoma.**
3. **Hepatoma** — can be hypo- or hyperechoic.
4. **Cysts** — benign, hydatid.
5. **Abscess** — ± hyperechoic wall due to fibrosis, ± surrounding hypoechoic rim due to oedema. Gas produces areas of very bright echoes.
6. **Haematoma** — acute stage.
7. **Cavernous haemangioma.**

7.12   Ultrasound Liver — Periportal Hyperechoic

1. Air in biliary tree.
2. Schistosomiasis.
3. Cholecystitis.
4. Recurrent pyogenic cholangitis (oriental).

Further Reading
Chau E.M.T., Leong L.L.Y. & Chan F.L. (1987) Recurrent pyogenic cholangitis: ultrasound evaluation compared with endoscopic retrograde cholangiopancreatography. *Clin Radiol.*, 38: 79–85.

7.13   CT Liver — Focal Hypodense Lesion Pre Intravenous Contrast

		Appearances post intravenous contrast
1.	Malignant tumours — e.g. hepatoma, metastases, lymphoma, haemangio-sarcoma intra hepatic cholangiocarcinoma.	± irregular patchy enhancement
2.	Benign tumours (a) Haemangioma — usually well defined, in right lobe of liver, ± multiple. Technetium 99^M labelled red blood cells may help make diagnosis.	75% peripheral enhancement 10% central enhancement 74% progressively isodense on delayed scan 24% partially isodense on delayed scan 2% remain hypodense on delayed scan
	(b) Adenoma — often young woman, related to use of oral contraceptive. Usually only slightly hypodense, and can be hyperdense due to predisposition to acute haemorrhage. Very rarely transforms to hepatoma.	85% hyperdense during arterial phase but rapidly (45 s – 1 min) becomes iso or hypodense.

3. **Cyst** — benign hepatic, polycystic, hydatid, von Hippel–Lindau. Water density if large enough. Small cysts can have higher density and apparently ill defined walls due to partial volume effect.

   margins more clearly demarcated

4. **Abscess**
   (a) Pyogenic

   ± peripheral enhancement

   (b) Fungal — immunosuppressed, multiple small lesions, can effect spleen.

   may not show any peripheral enhancement

   (c) Amoebic — ± crescent of low attenuation just peripheral to wall of abscess.

   ± peripheral enhancement

5. **Focal nodular hyperplasia** — usually only slightly hypodense. Often young female, asymptomatic unless large when pressure effects produce pain. Can contain sufficient functioning Kupfer cells to be normal or even increased in uptake on Technetium 99^M sulphur colloid scan which can help to discriminate it from other lesions, such as adenomas.

   most hyperdense during arterial phase but rapidly (45 s – 1 min) becomes iso or hypodense, ± stellate central low density due to scar, but this is not specific and occurs in adenomas, haemangiomas and fibrolamellar hepatomas.

6. **Focal fatty infiltration** — occasionally rounded in appearance, but usually diffuse or 'geographical' in distribution.

   no change

7. **Vascular** — infarction, laceration, old haematoma.

   no change

8. **Biliary tree dilatation** — no change
   Caroli's, choledochal.

Further Reading

Farman J., Javors B., Chao P., Fagelman D., Collins R. & Glanz S. (1987) C.T. demonstration of giant choledochal cysts in adults. *J. Comput. Assist. Tomogr.*, 11 (5): 771–4.

Freeny P.C. & Marks W.M. (1986) Hepatic haemangioma: dynamic bolus C.T. *Am. J. Roentgenol.*, 147: 711–19.

Mathieu D., Bruneton J.N., Drouillard J., Pointreau C.C. & Vasile N. (1986) Hepatic adenomas and focal nodular hyperplasia: dynamic C.T. study. *Radiology*, 160: 53–8.

Maxwell A.J. & Mamtora H. (1988) Fungal liver abscesses in acute leukaemia — a report of two cases. *Clin. Radiol.*, 39: 197–201.

Yates C.K. & Streight R.A. (1986) Focal fatty infiltration of the liver simulating metastatic disease. *Radiology*, 159: 83–4.

7.14 CT Liver — Focal Hyperdense Lesion

Pre Intravenous Contrast

1. Calcification in:
   - (a) Metastasis — usually colorectal, but ovary, stomach, islet cell pancreas also possible.
   - (b) Primary tumour — hepatoma, hepatoblastoma, haemangioendothelioma.
   - (c) Infective lesion — hydatid, tuberculous granuloma.
2. **Acute haemorrhage** — post traumatic or bleed into a vascular tumour e.g. adenoma.

Post Intravenous Contrast

1. Hypervascular masses
   - (a) Metastases — carcinoid, renal cell carcinoma, islet cell pancreas, and phaeochromocytoma.
   - (b) Adenoma ⎫

     enhancement only seen during arterial phase, i.e. within 1 minute of injection. After this they may appear hypodense.
   - (c) Focal nodular hyperplasia ⎭
2. **Vascular abnormalities** — e.g. arterio portal shunts which may occur in hepatoma.

Further Reading

Bressler E.L., Alpern M.B., Glazer G.M., Francis I.R. & Ensminger W.D. (1987) Hypervascular hepatic metastases: C.T. Evaluation. *Radiology*, 162: 49–51.

Scatarige J.C., Fishman E.K., Saksouk F.A. & Siegelman S.S. (1983) Computed tomography of calcified liver masses. *J. Comput. Assist. Tomogr.*, 7: 83–9.

7.15   CT Liver — Generalized Low Density Pre Intravenous Contrast

Assess by comparing liver with spleen. Also intrahepatic vessels stand out as 'high' density against low density background of liver, but aorta shows normal soft tissue density indicating the apparent high density of the intrahepatic vessels is not due to intravenous contrast.

1. **Fatty infiltration** — early cirrhosis, obesity, parenteral feeding, bypass surgery, malnourishment, cystic fibrosis, steroids, Cushing's, late pregnancy, carbon tetrachloride exposure, chemotherapy, high dose tetracycline, and glycogen storage disease.
2. **Malignant infiltration.**
3. **Budd–Chiari**
   (a) Acute — big low-density liver with ascites. After intravenous contrast there is patchy enhancement of the hilum of the liver due to multiple collaterals, and non visualisation of the hepatic veins and/or inferior vena cava.
   (b) Chronic — atrophied patchy low density liver with sparing and hypertrophy of caudate lobe. Post intravenous contrast scans show similar signs as the acute stage.
4. **Amyloid** — no change after intravenous contrast.

Further Reading

Halversen R.A., Korobkin M., Ram P.C. & Thomson W.M. (1982) C.T. appearance of focal fatty infiltration of the liver. *Am. J. Roentgenol.*, 139: 277–81.

Mathieu D., Vasile N., Menu Y., Van Beers B., Lorphelin J.M. & Pringot J. (1987) Budd Chiari syndrome: Dyamic C.T. *Radiology*, 165: 409–13.

Suzuki S., Takizawa K., Nakajima Y., Katayama M. & Sagawa F. (1986) C.T. findings in hepatic and splenic amyloidosis. *J. Comput. Assist. Tomogr.*, 10 (2): 332–4.

Vogelzang R.L., Anscheutz S.L. & Gore R.M. (1987) Budd Chiari syndrome: C.T. observations. *Radiology*, 163: 329–33.

Yates C.K. & Streight R.A. (1986) Focal fatty infiltration of the liver simulating metastatic disease. *Radiology*, 159: 83–4.

7.16 CT Liver — Generalized Increase in Density Pre Intravenous Contrast

Assess by comparing liver with spleen. Also intrahepatic vessels stand out as low density against high density background of liver.

1. **Haemochromatosis** — may be an associated hepatoma present.
2. **Haemosiderosis.**
3. **Iron overload** — e.g. from large number of blood transfusions.
4. **Glycogen storage disease** — liver may be increased or decreased in density.
5. **Amiodarone treatment** — contains iodine. Can also cause pulmonary interstitial and alveolar infiltrates.

Further Reading
Butler S. & Smathers R.L. (1985) Computed tomography of Amiodarone pulmonary toxicity. *J. Comput. Assist. Tomogr.*, 9 (2): 375–6.

7.17 CT Liver — Patchy Areas of Low Density Post Intravenous Contrast

1. Cirrhosis.
2. Hepatitis.
3. Portal vein thrombosis.
4. Budd–Chiari — chronic.
5. Lymphoma infiltration*.
6. Sarcoidosis*.

7.18   Splenomegaly

Huge Spleen
1. Chronic myeloid leukaemia.
2. Myelofibrosis.
3. Malaria.
4. Kala-azar.
5. Gaucher's disease.
6. Lymphoma*.

Moderately Large Spleen
1. All of the above.
2. Storage diseases.
3. Haemolytic anaemias.
4. Portal hypertension.
5. Leukaemias.

Slightly Large Spleen
1. All of the above.
2. Infections
   (a) Viral — infectious hepatitis, infectious mononucleosis.
   (b) Bacterial — septicaemia, brucellosis, typhoid and tuberculosis.
   (c) Rickettsial — typhus.
   (d) Fungal — histoplasmosis.
3. Sarcoidosis*.
4. Amyloidosis.
5. Rheumatoid arthritis (Felty's syndrome)*.
6. Systemic lupus erythematosus*.

7.19 Splenic Calcification

Curvilinear
1. Splenic artery atherosclerosis — including splenic artery aneurysm.
2. Cyst — hydatid or post-traumatic.

Multiple Small Nodular
1. Phleboliths — may have small central lucencies.
2. Haemangioma — phleboliths.
3. Tuberculosis.
4. Histoplasmosis.
5. Brucellosis.
6. Sickle-cell anaemia*.

Diffuse Homogeneous or Finely Granular
1. Sickle-cell anaemia*.
2. Thorotrast — densities also in the liver and upper abdominal lymph nodes.

Solitary Greater than 1 cm
1. Healed infarct or haematoma.
2. Healed abscess.
3. Tuberculosis.

Further Reading
McCall I.W., Vaidya S. & Serjeant G.R. (1981) Splenic opacification in homozygous sickle cell disease. *Clin. Radiol.*, 32: 611–15.

7.20   Pancreatic Calcification

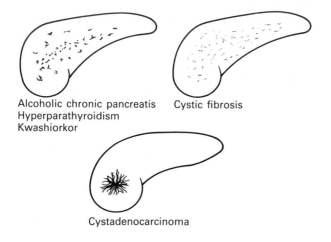

Alcoholic chronic pancreatis
Hyperparathyroidism
Kwashiorkor

Cystic fibrosis

Cystadenocarcinoma

1. **Alcoholic pancreatitis** — calcification, which is almost exclusively due to intraductal calculi is seen in 20–40% (compared with 2% of gallstone pancreatitis). Usually after 5–10 years of pain. Limited to head or tail in 25%. Rarely solitary. Calculi are numerous, irregular and generally small.
2. **Pseudocyst** — 12–20% exhibit calcification which is usually similar to that seen in chronic pancreatitis but may be curvilinear rim calcification.
3. **Carcinoma of the pancreas** — although for all practical purposes adenocarcinoma does not calcify there is an increased incidence of pancreatic cancer in chronic pancreatitis and the two will be found concurrently in about 2% of cases.
4. **Hyperparathyroidism*** — pancreatitis occurs as a complication of HPT in 10% of cases and 30% of these show calcification which is similar to that observed in chronic pancreatitis. 70% have nephrocalcinosis or urolithiasis and this should suggest the diagnosis.

5. **Cystic fibrosis*** — calcification occurs late in the disease when there is advanced pancreatic fibrosis associated with diabetes mellitus. Calcification is typically finely granular.

6. **Kwashiorkor** — pancreatic lithiasis is a frequent finding and appears before adulthood. Its pattern is similar to chronic alcoholic pancreatitis.

7. **Hereditary pancreatitis** — autosomal dominant. 60% show calcification which is typically rounded and often larger than in other pancreatic diseases. 20% die from pancreatic malignancy. The diagnosis should be considered in young, non-alcoholic patients.

8. **Tumours** — calcification is observed in 10% of cystadenomas and cystadenocarcinomas. It is non-specific but occasionally 'sunburst'. The rare cavernous lymphangioma contains phleboliths in and adjacent to it.

9. **Idiopathic.**

Further Reading

Ring E.J., Eaton S.B., Ferrucci J.T. & Short W.F. (1973) Differential diagnosis of pancreatic calcification. *Am. J. Roentgenol.*, 117: 446–52.

7.21   CT Focal Pancreatic Mass

1. **Adenocarcinoma** — 60% head, 10% body, 5% tail, 20% diffuse. 40% are isodense on pre-contrast scan, but most of these show reduced density on a post-contrast scan. Virtually never contain calcification. The presence of metastases (nodes, liver) or invasion around vascular structures (SMA, coeliac axis, portal and splenic vein) helps to distingiush this from focal pancreatitis.
2. **Focal pancreatitis** — usually in head of pancreas. Can contain calcification, but if not may be difficult to distingish from carcinoma.
3. **Metastasis** — e.g. breast, lung, stomach, kidney, thyroid.
4. **Islet cell tumour** — equal incidence in head, body and tail. 80% are functioning and so will present at a relatively small size. 20% are non-functioning and so are larger and more frequently contain calcification at presentation. In general functioning islet cell tumours, other than insulinomas, are often malignant, whereas 75% of non-functioning tumours are benign.
    (a) Beta cell:
        insulinoma — 90% benign, 10% multiple, 80% less than 2 cm in diameter. Usually isodense with marked contrast enhancement. Can calcify.
    (b) Non beta cell:
        gastrinoma — 60% malignant, 30% benign adenoma, 10% hyperplasia. 90% located in pancreas, 5% duodenum, occasionally stomach and splenic hilum. Shows marked contrast enhancement. Multiple adenomas seen as part of Multiple Endocrine Adenopathy I Syndrome (pituitary, parathyroid and pancreatic adenomas).
        glucagonoma —usually greater than 4 cm, since endocrine disturbance is often less marked.
5. **Mucinous cystadenoma** — multiple small (less than 2 cm) cysts usually in head. Frequently calcified. Usually female aged over 60.
6. **Mucinous cystadenocarcinoma** — multiple thick walled big (greater than 5 cm) cysts usually in body or tail. The thick walls may help to distinguish from pseudocysts. 15% calcify.

7. **Pancreatic abscess** — infected phlegmon/pseudocyst. Occurs in 3% of pancreatitis.

Further Reading

Breatnach E.S., Han S.Y., Rahatzad M.T. & Stanley R.J. (1985) C.T. evauation of glucagonomas. *J. Comput. Assist. Tomogr.*, 9 (1): 25–9.

Clark L.R., Jaffe M.H., Choyke P.L., Grant E.G. & Zaman R.K. (1985) Pancreatic Imaging. *Radiol. Clin. North Am.*, 23 (3): 489–501.

7.22   Adrenal Calcification

Child

1. **Cystic disease** — usually the result of haemorrhage which may be secondary to birth trauma, infection, haemorrhagic disorders of arterial or venous thromboses. Partial or complete ring-like calcification is observed initially but this later becomes compact as the cyst collapses. Frequently asymptomatic.

2. **Neuroblastoma** — in 30–50% of cases. Ill-defined, stippled and non-homogeneous. Lymph-node and liver metastases can also calcify.

3. **Ganglioneuroma** — similar appearance to neuroblastoma, but only 20% are within the adrenal.

4. **Wolman's disease** — a rare autosomal recessive lipoidosis. Hepatomegaly, splenomegaly and adrenomegaly with punctate cortical adrenal calcification is pathognomonic.

Adult

1. **Cystic disease** — similar to that seen in the child. Bilateral in 15% of cases.

2. **Carcinoma** — irregular punctate calcifications. Average size of tumour is 14 cm and there is frequently displacement of the ipsilateral kidney.

3. **Addison's disease** — now most commonly due to autoimmune disease or metastasis. In the past when tuberculosis was a frequent cause calcification was a common finding.

4. **Ganglioneuroma** — 40% occur over the age of 20 years. Slightly flocculent calcifications in a mass which is usually asymptomatic. If the tumour is large enough there will be displacement of the adjacent kidney and/or ureter.

5. **Inflammatory** — primary tuberculosis and histoplasmosis.

6. **Phaeochromocytoma** — calcification is rare but when present is usually an 'eggshell' pattern.

Further Reading

Queloz J.M., Capitanio M.A. & Kirkpatrick I.A. (1972) Wolman's disease. Roentgen observations in three siblings. *Radiology*, 104: 357–9.

Computed Tomography

Haaga J.R. & Alfidi R.J. (1983) *Computed Tomography of the Whole Body*. Toronto. The C.V. Mosby Company.

Moss A.A., Gamsu G. & Gerant H.K. (1983) *Computed Tomography of the Body*. Philadelphia. W.B. Saunders Company.

7.23 CT Adrenal Masses

Length of limbs is variable: can be up to 4 cm. Width of limb is normally less than 1 cm. The right adrenal lies behind inferior vena cava and above right kidney, i.e. not on same slice as the kidney. The left adrenal lies in front of upper pole of left kidney, i.e. on same slice as the kidney — do not mistake upper pole of left kidney for an adrenal mass.

Structures Mimicking Left Adrenal Mass

1. **Upper pole of left kidney.**
2. **Gastric diverticulum** — give oral contrast.
3. **Splenic lobulation/accessory spleen** — give intravenous contrast, should enhance to the same level as the body of the spleen.
4. **Large mass in tail of pancreas** — give intravenous contrast, pancreatic mass usually displaces splenic vein posteriorly whereas adrenal mass displaces it anteriorly.

Functioning Tumours

1. **Conn's adenoma** — accounts for 70% of Conn's syndrome. Usually small, 0.5 – 1.5 cm. Homogenous, relatively low density due to build up of cholesterol. 30% of Conn's syndrome due to hyperplasia which can occasionally be nodular and mimic an adenoma.
2. **Phaeochromocytoma** — usually large, 3 – 5 cm, with marked contrast enhancement (beware hypertensive crisis with intravenous contrast). 10% malignant, 10% bilateral, 10% ectopic (of these 50% are located around the kidney, particularly renal hilum. If CT does not detect, MIBG isotope scan may be helpful), 10% multiple (usually part of Multiple Endocrine Adenopathy II Syndrome). Associated with neurofibromatosis, von Hippel–Lindau, and MEA II.

3. **Cushing's adenoma** — accounts for 10% of Cushing's syndrome. Usually over 2 cm. 40% show slight reduction in density. 80% of Cushing's syndrome due to excess ACTH from pituitary tumour or ectopic source (oat cell carcinoma, pancreatic islet cell, carcinoid, medullary carcinoma thyroid, thymoma) which causes adrenal hyperplasia not visible on CT scan. Other 10% of Cushing's syndrome due to adrenal carcinoma. The possibilities for adrenal mass in Cushing's syndrome are:
   (a) Functioning adenoma/carcinoma.
   (b) Coincidental non-functioning adenoma.
   (c) Metastasis from oat cell primary.
   (d) Nodular hyperplasia, which occurs in 20% of Cushing's syndrome due to pituitary adenoma.
4. **Adrenal carcinoma** — 50% present as functioning tumours (Cushing's 35%, Cushing's with virilization 20%, virilization 20%, feminization 5%).

Malignant Tumours

1. **Metastases** — may be bilateral, usually greater than 2 – 3 cm, irregular outline with patchy contrast enhancement. Recent haemorrhage into a vascular metastasis (e.g. melanoma) can give a patchy high density on pre contrast scan.
2. **Carcinoma** — usually greater than 5 cm, mixed density, may calcify, and metastatic nodes or liver secondaries may be seen.
3. **Lymphoma** — 25% also involve kidneys at autopsy. Lymphadenopathy will be seen elsewhere.
4. **Neuroblastoma** — greater than 5 cm. Calcification in 70%. Extends across midline. Nodes commonly surround and displace the aorta and inferior vena cava.

Benign

1. **Non-functioning adenoma** — occurs in 5% at autopsy. Usually relatively small (50% less than 2 cm), homogenous, and well defined.
2. **Angiomyolipoma** — occurs in 0.2% at autopsy. Usually 1 – 2 cm. May contain fat density.
3. **Cyst** — well defined, water density.

4. **Post traumatic haemorrhage** — homogeneous, hyperdense. Occurs in 25% of severe trauma, 20% bilateral, 85% in right. Adrenal haemorrhage can also occur in vascular metastases, anticoagulant treatment, and severe stress (e.g. surgery, sepsis, burns, hypotension).

Further Reading

Falke T.H.M., te Strake L. & van Peters A.P. (1984) C.T. of the adrenal glands: adenoma or hyperplasia? *Radiology*, 153: 358.

Peretz G.S. & Lam A.H. (1985) Distinguishing neuroblastoma from Wilm's tumour by computed tomography. *J. Comput. Assist. Tomogr.*, 9 (5): 889–93.

Wilms, G., Marchal G., Baert A., Adisoejoso B. & Mangkuwerdojo (1987) C.T. and ultrasound features of post traumatic adrenal haemorrhage. *J. Comput. Assist. Tomogr.*, 11 (1): 112–15.

Notes

Notes

Chapter 8
Urinary Tract

8.1 Loss of a Renal Outline on the Plain Film

Not necessarily associated with a non-visualized kidney after intravenous contrast medium.

1. **Technical factors** — e.g. poor radiography, overlying faeces, etc.
2. **Congenital absence** — 1:1000 live births. Increased incidence of extrarenal abnormalities (ventricular septal defect, meningomyelocoele, intestinal tract strictures, imperforate anus, skeletal abnormalities and unicornuate uterus). The normal solitary kidney may approach twice normal size.
3. **Displaced or ectopic kidney** — presacral, crossed ectopia or intrathoracic.
4. **Perinephric haematoma** — obliteration of the perirenal fat. ± other signs of trauma, e.g. fractured transverse processes.
5. **Perinephric abscess** — scoliosis concave to the affected side. May be associated with gas in the perirenal tissues. ± localized ileus.
6. **Tumour** — when perinephric fat is replaced by tumour.
7. **Post-nephrectomy** — rare because residual perinephric fat preserves an apparent renal outline. Surgical resection of 12th rib is usually evident.

8.2   Renal Calcification

Calculi (q.v.)

Dystrophic Calcification Due to Localized Disease
Usually one kidney or part of one kidney.
1. **Infections**
    (a) Tuberculosis — variable appearance of nodular, curvilinear or amorphous calcification. Typically multifocal with calcification elsewhere in the urinary tract.
    (b) Hydatid — the cyst is usually polar and calcification is curvilinear or heterogeneous.
    (c) Xanthogranulomatous pyelonephritis.
    (d) Abscess.
2. **Carcinoma** — in 6% of carcinomas. Usually amorphous or irregular, but occasionally curvilinear.
3. **Aneurysm** — of the renal artery. Curvilinear.

Nephrocalcinosis
Parenchymal calcification associated with a diffuse renal lesion (i.e. dystrophic calcification) or metabolic abnormality, e.g. hypercalcaemia (metabolic or metastatic calcification). May be medullary or cortical.

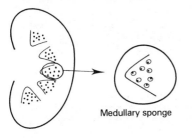

Medullary sponge

Medullary

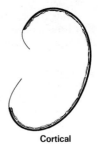

Cortical

MEDULLARY (PYRAMIDAL)
The first three causes account for 70% of cases.
1. **Hyperparathyroidism*.**
2. **Renal tubular acidosis** — may be associated with osteomalacia or rickets. Calcification tends to be more severe than that due to other causes. It is the commonest cause in children. Almost always a distal tubular defect.

3. **Medullary sponge kidney** — a variable portion of one of both kidneys contains numerous small medullary cysts which communicate with tubules and therefore opacify during excretion urography. The cysts contain small calculi giving a 'bunch of grapes' appearance. Big kidneys. ± multiple cysts or large medullary cystic cavities which may be > 2 cm diameter. (Although not strictly a cause of nephrocalcinosis, because it comprises calculi in ectatic ducts, it is included here because of the plain film findings which simulate nephrocalcinosis.)

4. **Renal papillary necrosis** — calcification of necrotic papillae. See section 8.19.

5. **Causes of hypercalcaemia or hypercalciuria**
   (a) Milk alkali syndrome.
   (b) Idiopathic hypercalciuria.
   (c) Sarcoidosis*.
   (d) Hypervitaminosis D.

6. **Primary hyperoxaluria** — rare. AR 65% present below 5 years of age (younger than the other causes). Radiologically — nephrocalcinosis (generally diffuse and homogeneous but may be patchy), recurrent nephrolithiasis, dense vascular calcification, osteopenia or renal osteodystrophy and abnormal metaphyses (dense and/or lucent bands).

CORTICAL

1. **Acute cortical necrosis** — classically 'tramline' calcification.
2. **Chronic glomerulonephritis** — rarely.
3. **Chronic transplant rejection.**

Further Reading

Daniel W.W., Hartman G.W., Witten D.M., Farrow G.M. & Kelalis P.P. (1972) Calcified renal masses. *Radiology*, 103: 503–8.

Day D.L., Scheinman J.I. & Mahan J. (1986) Radiological aspects of primary hyperoxaluria. *Am. J. Roentgenol.*, 146: 395–401.

Gedroyc W.M.W. & Saxton H.M. (1988) More medullary sponge variants. *Clin Radiol.*, 39: 423–5.

Lalli A.F. (1982) Renal parenchyma calcifications. *Semin. Roentgenol.*, 17 (2): 101–12.

Wrong O.M. & Feest T.G. (1976) Nephrocalcinosis. *Adv. Med.*, 12: 394–406.

8.3 Renal Calculi

Opaque
Calcium phosphate/calcium oxalate, calcium oxalate, calcium phosphate/magnesium ammonium phosphate and calcium phosphate. Calcium oxalate stones are more opaque than triple phosphate stones.

Poorly Opaque
Cystine (in cystinuria).

Non-opaque
Uric acid, xanthine and matrix (mucoprotein).

Calcium Containing
1. **With normocalcaemia** — obstruction, urinary tract infection, prolonged bedrest, 'horseshoe' kidney, vesical diverticulum, renal tubular acidosis, medullary sponge kidney and idiopathic hypercalciuria.
2. **With hypercalcaemia** — hyperparathyroidism, milk-alkali syndrome, excess vitamin D, idiopathic hypercalcaemia of infancy and sarcoidosis.

Pure Calcium Oxalate due to Hyperoxaluria
1. **Primary hyperoxaluria** — rare. AR 65% present below 5 years of age. Radiologically — nephrocalcinosis (generally diffuse and homogeneous but may be patchy), recurrent nephrolithiasis, dense vascular calcification, osteopenia or renal osteodystrophy and abnormal metaphyses (dense and/or lucent bands).
2. **Enteric hyperoxaluria** — due to a disturbance of bile acid metabolism. Mainly in patients with small bowel disease, either Crohn's disease or surgical resection.

Uric Acid
1. **With hyperuricaemia** — gout, myeloproliferative disorders and during the treatment of tumours with antimitotic agents.
2. **With normouricaemia** — idiopathic or associated with acid, concentrated urine (in hot climate and in ileostomy patients).

Xanthine
Due to a failure of normal oxidation of purines.

Matrix
Rare. In poorly functioning, infected urinary tracts.

Further Reading
Banner M.P. & Pollack H.M. (1982) Urolithiasis in the lower urinary tract. *Semin. Roentgenol.*, 17 (2): 140–8.
Day D.L., Scheinman J.I. & Mahan J. (1986) Radiological aspects of primary hyperoxaluria. *Am. J. Roentgenol.*, 146: 395–401.
Elkin M. (1983) Calcification in the urinary tract. In: Baker S.R. & Elkin M. *Plain Film Approach to Abdominal Calcifications.* pp. 39–46. Philadelphia: Saunders.
Singh, E.O. & Malek R.S. (1982) Calculus disease in the upper urinary tract. *Semin. Roentgenol.*, 17 (2): 113–32.
Thornbury J.R. & Parker T.W. (1982) Ureteral calculi. *Semin. Roentgenol.*, 17 (2): 133–9.

8.4 Gas in the Urinary Tract

Gas shadows which conform to the position and shape of the bladder, ureters or pelvicalyceal systems.

Gas Inside the Bladder
1. **Vesico-intestinal fistula** — diverticular disease, carcinoma of the colon or rectum and Crohn's disease.
2. **Cystitis** — due to gas-forming organisms and fermentation, especially in diabetics. Usually *Escherichia coli*. Clostridial infections are rare and usually secondary to septicaemia.
3. **Following instrumentation.**
4. **Penetrating wounds.**

Gas in the Bladder Wall
1. **Emphysematous cystitis** — usually in diabetics.

Gas in the Ureters and Pelvicalyceal Systems
1. **Any cause of gas in the bladder.**
2. **Ureteric diversion** — into the colon or bladder.
3. **Fistula** — Crohn's disease or perforated duodenal ulcer.
4. **Infection** — usually in diabetics. Gas may also be present in the renal parenchyma and retroperitoneal tissues.

8.5 Non-visualization of One Kidney During Excretion Urography

1. **Absent kidney** — congenital absence or post-nephrectomy.
2. **Ectopic kidney.**
3. **Chronic obstructive uropathy.**
4. **Infection** — pyonephrosis, xanthogranulomatous pyelonephritis or tuberculosis.
5. **Tumour** — an avascular tumour completely replacing the kidney or preventing normal function of residual renal tissue by occluding the renal vein or pelvis.
6. **Renal artery occlusion** — including trauma.
7. **Renal vein occlusion** — see section 8.21.
8. **Multicystic kidney** — see section 8.16.

8.6   Unilateral Scarred Kidney

NORMAL
Cortex parallel to
interpapillary line

FETAL LOBULATION
Normal size.
Cortical depressions between
papillae

DUPLEX KIDNEY
Renal size usually
larger than normal

SPLEEN IMPRESSION
Right kidney may
show hepatic
impression

OVERLYING BOWEL
Spurious
loss of cortex

REFLUX
NEPHROPATHY
Focal scars over
dilated calyces. Most
prominent at upper
and lower poles. May
be bilateral

LOBAR INFARCTION
Broad depression
over a normal calyx

Redrawn from Taylor C.M. & Chapman S. (1989) *Handbook
of Renal Investigations in Children*. London: Wright. By kind
permission of the publisher.

1. **Reflux nephropathy** — a focal scar over a dilated calyx. Usually multifocal and may be bilateral. Scarring is most prominent in the upper and lower poles. Minimal scarring, especially at a pole, may produce decreased cortical thickness with a normal papilla and is then indistinguishable from lobar infarction.
2. **Tuberculosis** — calcification differentiates it from the other members of this section.
3. **Lobar infarction** — a broad contour depression over a normal calyx. Normal interpapillary line.
4. **Renal dysplasia** — a forme fruste multicystic kidney. Dilated calyces. Indistinguishable from chronic pyelonephritis. Arteriography outlines a small thread-like renal artery.

Differential Diagnosis

1. **Persistent fetal lobulation** — lobules overlie calyces with interlobular septa between the calyces. **Normal-size kidney.**

Further Reading
Davidson, A.J. (1977) *Radiological Diagnosis of Renal Parenchymal Disease*. chap. 4, pp. 47–68. Philadelphia: Saunders.

8.7   Unilateral Small Smooth Kidney

In all these conditions chronic unilateral disease is associated with compensatory hypertrophy of the contralateral kidney.

With a Dilated Collecting System

1. **Post-obstructive atrophy** — ± thinning of the renal cortex and if there is impaired renal function this will be revealed by poor contrast medium density in the collecting system.

With a Small-volume Collecting System

This is a sign of diminished urinary volume and together with global cortical thinning, delayed opacification of the calyces, increased density of the opacified collecting system and delayed wash-out following oral fluids or diuretics, indicates ischaemia.

1. **Ischaemia due to renal artery stenosis** — ureteric notching is due to enlarged collateral vessels and differentiates this from the other causes in this group. See section 8.20.
2. **Radiation nephritis** — at least 23 Gy (2300 rad) over 5 weeks. The collecting system may be normal or small. Depending on the size of the radiation field both, one or just part of one kidney may be affected. There may be other sequelae of radiotherapy, e.g. scoliosis following radiotherapy in childhood.
3. **End result of renal infarction** — due to previous severe trauma involving the renal artery or renal vein thrombosis. The collecting system does not usually opacify during excretion urography.

With Five or Less Calyces

1. **Congenital hypoplasia** — the pelvicalyceal system is otherwise normal.

Further Reading

Davidson, A.J. (1977) *Radiological Diagnosis of Renal Parenchymal Disease*, chap. 5, pp. 69–95. Philadelphia: Saunders.

8.8 Bilateral Small Smooth Kidneys

1. **Generalized arteriosclerosis** — normal calyces.
2. **Chronic glomerulonephritis** — normal calyces. Reduced nephrogram density and poor calyceal opacification.
3. **Chronic papillary necrosis** (q.v.) — with other signs of necrotic papillae.
4. **Arterial hypotension** — distinguished by the time relationship to the contrast medium injection and its transient nature.
5. **Cause of unilateral small smooth kidneys occurring bilaterally** — e.g. obstructive uropathy or renal artery stenosis.

Further Reading

Davidson, A.J. (1977) *Radiological Diagnosis of Renal Parenchymal Disease*, chap. 6. pp. 96–131. Philadelphia: Saunders.

8.9 Unilateral Large Smooth Kidney

1. **Compensatory hypertrophy**
2. **Obstructed kidney** ⎫
3. **Pyonephrosis** ⎬ dilated calyces.
4. **Duplex kidney** — female:male, 2:1. Equal incidence on both sides and 20% are bilateral. Incomplete more common than complete. Only 50% are bigger than the contralateral kidney; 40% are the same size; 10% are smaller (Privett et al. 1976).
5. **Tumour** — see section 8.12.
6. **Crossed fused ectopia** — may be associated with anorectal anomalies and renal dysplasia. No kidney on the contralateral side and ureter crosses the midline.
7. **Multicystic kidney** — see section 8.16.
8. **Acute pyelonephritis** — impaired excretion of contrast medium. ± increasingly dense nephrogram. Attenuated calyces but may have non-obstructive pelvicalyceal or ureteric dilatation. Completely reversible within a few weeks of clinical recovery.
9. **Trauma** — haematoma or urinoma.
10. **Renal vein thrombosis** — see section 8.21.
11. **Acute arterial infarction.**
12. **Adult polycystic disease*** — asymmetrical bilateral enlargement, but 8% of cases are unilateral. Lobulated rather than completely smooth.

Further Reading

Davidson A.J. (1977) *Radiological Diagnosis of Renal Parenchymal Disease*, chap. 8, pp. 162–92. Philadelphia:Saunders.
Privett J.T.J., Jeans W.D. & Roylance J. (1976) The incidence and importance of renal duplication. *Clin. Radiol.*, 27: 521–30.

8.10 Bilateral Large Smooth Kidneys

It is often difficult to distinguish, radiologically, the members of this group from one another. The appearance of the nephrogram may be helpful — see section 8.18. Associated clinical and radiological abnormalities elsewhere are often more useful, e.g. in sickle-cell anaemia, Goodpasture's disease and acromegaly.

Proliferative and Necrotizing Disorders
1. Acute glomerulonephritis.
2. Polyarteritis nodosa.
3. Wegener's granulomatosis.
4. Goodpasture's disease.
5. Systemic lupus erythematosus*.

Deposition of Abnormal Proteins
1. Amyloid — renal involvement in 80% of secondary and 35% of primary amyloid. Chronic deposition results in small kidneys.
2. Multiple myeloma*.

Abnormal Fluid Accumulation
1. Acute tubular necrosis.
2. Acute cortical necrosis — may show an opacified medulla and outer rim with non-opacified cortex. Cortical calcification is a late finding.

Neoplastic Infiltration
1. Leukaemia and lymphoma.

Inflammatory Cell Infiltration
1. Acute interstitial nephritis.

Miscellaneous

1. **Renal vein thrombosis** (q.v.).
2. **Acute renal papillary necrosis** (q.v.).
3. **Polycystic disease*** — infantile form has smooth outlines.
4. **Acute urate nephropathy.**
5. **Sickle-cell anaemia***.
6. **Bilateral hydronephrosis.**
7. **Medullary sponge kidneys** — with 'bunch of grapes' calcification.
8. **Acromegaly*** **and gigantism** — as part of the generalized visceromegaly.

Further Reading

Davidson, A.J. (1977) *Radiological Diagnosis of Renal Parenchymal Disease*, chap. 7, pp. 132–61. Philadelphia: Saunders.

8.11 Localized Bulge of the Renal Outline

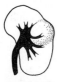

RENAL CYST
US confirms typical
echo-free cyst

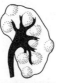

MULTIPLE RENAL
CYSTS
e.g. adult type
polycystic disease.
Spider leg deformity
of calyces

TUMOUR
Replacement of much
or all of normal renal
tissue

DROMEDARY HUMP
Left sided variant

PROMINENT SEPTUM
OF BERTIN
Increased activity on
Tc-DMSA scanning

HILAR LIP
Hyperplasia of
parenchyma adjacent
to the renal hilum.
Normal to Tc-DMSA scan

PSEUDOTUMOUR IN
REFLUX
NEPHROPATHY
Hypertrophy of
unscarred renal
parenchyma

DUPLEX KIDNEY WITH
HYDRONEPHROTIC
UPPER MOIETY
Drooping flower
appearance

DILATATION OF A
SINGLE CALYX
Most commonly due
to extrinsic
compression by an
intrarenal artery
(Fraley syndrome)

Redrawn from Taylor C.M. & Chapman S. (1989) *Handbook of Renal Investigations in Children*. London: Wright. By kind permission of the publisher.

1. **Cyst** — well defined nephrographic defect with a thin wall on the outer margin. Beak sign. Displacement and distortion of smooth-walled calyces without obliteration.
2. **Tumour** — mostly renal cell carcinoma in adults and Wilms' tumour in children. See section 8.12.
3. **Fetal lobulation** — the lobule directly overlies a normal calyx. Normal interpapillary line. See section 8.6.
4. **Dromedary hump** — on the mid portion of the lateral border of the kidney. The arc of the interpapillary line parallels the renal contour.
5. **Splenic impression** — on the left side only. This produces an apparent bulge inferiorly.
6. **Enlarged septum of Bertin** — overgrowth of renal cortex from two adjacent renal lobules. EU shows a pseudomass with calyceal splaying and associated short calyx ± attempted duplication. Tc-DMSA accumulates normally or in excess. On US echogenicity is usually similar to normal renal cortex but may be of increased echogenicity.
7. **Localized hypertrophy** — e.g. adjacent to an area of pyelonephritic scarring.
8. **Abscess** — loss of renal outline and psoas margin on the control film. Scoliosis concave to the involved side. Initially there is no nephrographic defect but following central necrosis there will be a central defect surrounded by a thick irregular wall. Adjacent calyces are displaced or effaced.
9. **Non-functioning moiety of a duplex** — usually a hydronephrotic upper moiety. Delayed films may show contrast medium in the upper moiety calyces. Lower moiety calyces have 'drooping flowers' appearance. See section 8.24.

Further Reading

Felson B. & Moskowitz M. (1969) Renal pseudotumours. The regenerated nodule and other lumps, bumps and dromedary humps. *Am. J. Roentgenol.*, 107: 720–9.

Hardwick D. & Hendry G.M.A. (1984) The ultrasonic appearances of the septa of Bertin in children. *Clin. Radiol.*, 34: 107–12.

Maklad N.F., Chuang V.P., Doust B.D., Cho K.T. & Curran J.E. (1977) Ultrasound characteristics of solid renal lesions. Echographic, urographic and pathological correlation. *Radiology*, 123: 733.

8.12 Renal Neoplasms

Malignant

1. **Renal cell carcinoma** — 90% of adult malignant tumours. Bilateral in 10% and an increased incidence of bilaterality in polycystic kidneys and von Hippel-Lindau disease. A mass lesion (showing irregular or amorphous calcification in 10% of cases). Calyces are obliterated, distorted and/or displaced. Half-shadow filling defect in a calyx or pelvis. Arteriography shows a typical pathological circulation in the majority.

2. **Transitional cell carcinoma** — usually papilliferous. May obstruct or obliterate a calyx or obstruct a whole kidney. Seeding may produce a second lesion further down the urinary tract. Bilateral tumours are rare. Calcification in 2%.

3. **Squamous cell carcinoma** — ulcerated plaque or stricture. 50% are associated with calculi. There is usually a large parenchymal mass before there is any sizeable intrapelvic mass. No calcification. Avascular at arteriography.

4. **Wilms' tumour** — 80% present in the first 3 years. Bilateral in 5%. The usual US appearance is that of a solid, usually hyperechoic mass with a rim of normal renal tissue. There may be necrotic and/or haemorrhagic areas within. On CT the tumour is usually of lower attenuation than kidney. Rarely the tumour may be multicystic.

   Mesoblastic nephroma is a rare congenital tumour which presents in the neonatal period. It may be solid or multicystic. It does not metastasize and complete excision results in cure. Indistinguishable from Wilms' tumour.

   Nephroblastomatosis is due to persistence of primitive blastema and may be a precursor of Wilms' tumour. It manifests as bilateral nephromegaly with relatively anechoic areas on US and nodules of decreased attenuation on CT seldom seen beyond 4 months of age.

   Multilocular cystic nephroma is also rare with two peaks of incidence — 3 months to 4 years and 40 to 60 years. Complete excision is curative in childhood but adult cases may metastasize.

5. **Leukaemia/lymphoma** — bilateral large smooth kidneys. Thickened parenchyma with compression of the pelvicalyceal systems.

6. **Metastases** — not uncommon. Usually multiple. Bronchus, breast and stomach.

Benign

1. **Hamartoma** — usually solitary but often multiple and bilateral in tuberous sclerosis. Diagnostic appearance on the plain film of radiolucent fat (but only observed in 9%). Other signs are of any mass lesion and angiography does not differentiate from renal call carcinoma.
2. **Adenoma** — usually small and frequently multiple. Majority are found at autopsy. Hypovascular at arteriography.
3. **Others** — myoma, lipoma, haemangioma and fibroma are all rare.

Further Reading

See end of chapter.

8.13   CT Kidney — Focal Hypodense Lesion

Tumours

1. **Malignant**
   (a) Renal cell carcinoma — usually inhomogenous and irregular if large.
   (b) Metastasis.
   (c) Lymphoma — usually late stage Non-Hodgkin's Lymphoma; only 5% at initial staging. 70% multiple and bilateral. Usually rounded in appearance.
   (d) Transitional cell carcinoma — can infiltrate and mimic renal cell carcinoma.
   (e) Wilms' — see section 8.12.
2. **Benign**
   (a) Oncocytoma — adenoma arising from proximal tubular cells. Round, well defined, homogenous (usually high density pre contrast, low density post contrast), ± central stellate low density scar if tumour bigger than 3 cm.
   (b) Angiomyolipoma — well defined containing fat densities. Association with tuberous sclerosis.

Inflammation

1. **Abscess** — thick irregular walls ± perirenal fascial thickening, but this can occur in malignancy.
2. **Xanthogranulomatous pyelonephritis** — obstructing calculus seen in 80% cases leading to chronic sepsis, perinephric fluid collections and fistula formation.
3. **Acute focal bacterial nephritis** — wedge shaped low density ± radiating striations after intravenous contrast.

Vascular

1. **Infarcts** — well defined, peripheral, wedge shaped.

Cyst — see 8.14 and 8.15.

Further Reading

Ishikawa I., Saito Y., Onouchi Z., Matsuura H., Saito T., Suzuki M. & Futyu Y. (1985) Delayed contrast enhancement in acute focal nephritis: C.T. features. *J. Comput. Assist. Tomogr.*, **9**(5): 894–7.

Neirius D., Braedel H.U., Schindler E., Hoene E. & Sch. Alloussi. (1988) Computed tomographic and angiographic findings in renal oncocytoma. *Br. J. Radiol.*, **61**: 1019–25.

Quinn M.J., Hartman D.S., Friedman A.C., Sherman J.L., Lautin E.M., Pyatt R.S., Ho C.K., Csere R. & Fromowitz F.B. (1984) Renal oncocytoma: new observations. *Radiology*, **153**:49–53.

8.14   Classification of Renal Cysts
(After Elkin & Bernstein, 1969).

Renal Dysplasia
1. Multicystic kidney — see section 8.16.
2. Focal and segmental cystic dysplasia.
3. Multiple cysts associated with lower urinary tract obstruction — usually posterior urethral valves in males.

Polycystic Disease*
1. Childhood polycystic disease — AR.
2. Adult polycystic disease — AD.

Cortical Cysts
1. Simple cyst — unilocular. Increase in size and number with age.
2. Multilocular cyst, multilocular cystic nephroma, cystic hamartoma or cystic Wilms' tumour — a tumour of multiple non-communicating cysts. Usually benign but may have more malignant elements (only diagnosable by histology). Most present below 2 years of age with an abdominal mass. Indistinguishable from a Wilms' tumour by urography but the multicystic nature with highly echogenic septae displacing normal kidney is typical on US.
3. Syndromes associated with cysts — Zellweger's syndrome, tuberous sclerosis, Turner's syndrome, von Hippel-Lindau disease, trisomy 13 and 18.
4. Haemodialysis.

Medullary Cysts
1. Calyceal cyst (diverticulum) — small, usually solitary cyst communicating via an isthmus with the fornix of a calyx.
2. Medullary sponge kidney — bilateral in 60–80%. Multiple, small, mainly pyramidal cysts which opacify during excretion urography and contain calculi.
3. Papillary necrosis — see 8.19.
4. Juvenile nephronophthisis (medullary cystic disease) — usually presents with polyuria and progressive renal failure. Positive family history. Normal or small kidneys. US shows a few medullary or corticomedullary cysts, loss of corticomedullary differentiation and increased parenchymal echogenicity.

Miscellaneous Intrarenal Cysts

1. **Inflammatory**
   (a) Tuberculosis.
   (b) Calculus disease.
   (c) Hydatid.
2. **Neoplastic** — cystic degeneration of a carcinoma.
3. **Traumatic** — intrarenal haematoma.

Extraparenchymal Renal Cysts

1. **Parapelvic cyst** — located in or near the hilum, but does not communicate with the renal pelvis and therefore does not opacify during urography. Simple or multilocular; single or multiple, unilateral or bilateral. It compresses the renal pelvis and may cause hydronephrosis.
2. **Perinephric cyst** — beneath the capsule or between the capsule and perinephric fat. Secondary to trauma, obstruction or replacement of haematoma. It may compress the kidney, pelvis or ureter, leading to hydronephrosis or causing displacement of the kidney.

Further Reading

Banner M.P., Pollack H.M., Chatten J. & Witzleben C. (1981) Multilocular renal cysts: radiologic pathologic correlation. *Am. J. Roentgenol.*, 136: 239–47.

Elkin M. & Bernstein J. (1969) Cystic diseases of the kidney — radiological and pathological considerations. *Clin. Radiol.*, 20: 65–82.

Madewell J.E., Hartman D.S. & Lichtenstein J.E. (1979) Radiologic-pathologic correlations in cystic disease of the kidney. *Radiol. Clin. North Am.*, 17: 261–79.

Hartmann D.S., Davies C.J., Sanders R.C., Johns T., Smirniotopoulos J. & Goldman S.M. (1984) The multiloculated renal mass: proposed classifications and differential features (Abstract). *Radiology*, 153: 18.

8.15 CT Renal Cysts — see section 8.14

1. **Simple** — thin walled, no enhancement. Occasionally haemorrhage can occur within one producing a round hyperdense lesion.
2. **Malignant** — 5% renal cell carcinomas are cystic. Suspect if thick walls or septations but this may just indicate previous infection/haemorrhage in cyst.
3. **Polycystic** — associated with hepatic cysts in approximately 60% of cases. Haemorrhage into cysts relatively common, so may be of varying density. Associated with increased incidence of renal cell carcinoma.
4. **Haemodialysis related cysts** — cysts develop in approximately 50% of long term haemodialysis, but can involute after a successful renal transplant. 7% incidence of associated renal cell carcinoma.
5. **von Hippel–Lindau** — associated pancreatic, hepatic cysts and renal cell carcinoma and phaeochromocytoma.
6. **Hydatid** — affected in 10% cases. ± curvilinear calcification in wall.
7. **Multicystic** — usually detected in infancy.
8. **Cystic hamartoma** — usually large with thick capsule and septations.

Further Reading

Beggs I. (1985) The radiology of hydatid disease. *Am. J. Roentgenol.*, 145: 639–48.

Cho C., Friedland G.W. & Swenson R.S. (1984) Acquired renal cystic disease and renal neoplasms in haemodialysis patients. *Urologic Radiology*, 6: 153–7.

Jennings C.M. & Gaines P.A. (1988) The abdominal manifestation of von Hippel–Lindau disease and a radiological screening protocol for an affected family. *Clin. Radiol.*, 39: 363–7.

8.16 Renal Mass in the Newborn and Young Infant

1. **Hydronephrosis** (q.v.) — uni- or bilateral.
2. **Multicystic kidney** — unilateral, but 30% have an abnormal contralateral kidney (mostly pelviureteric junction obstruction). Non-functioning, multilobulated kidney. Rarely, nephrographic crescents and late pooling of contrast medium in cysts is observed. Curvilinear calcification is characteristic but only seen occasionally. Ultrasound reveals multiple cysts of unequal size. The commonest renal mass in the first year of life.
3. **Polycystic kidneys** (see Polycystic disease*) — bilateral. Poor renal excretion. Striated nephrogram with no visualization of calyces. Highly echogenic on US.
4. **Renal vein thrombosis** (q.v.) — uni- or bilateral.
5. **Nephroblastomatosis or mesoblastic nephroma** — see section 8.12.
6. **Renal ectopia.**

Further Reading
Merten D.F. & Kirks D.R. (1985) Diagnostic imaging of paediatric abdominal masses. *Pediatr. Clin. North Am.*, 32: 1397–425.

8.17 Hydronephrosis in a Child

1. **Pelviureteric junction obstruction** — more common on the left side. 20% bilateral. Due to stricture, neuromuscular inco-ordination or aberrant vessels. Contralateral kidney is dysplastic in 25% of cases and absent in 12%.
2. **Bladder outflow obstruction** (q.v.) — bilateral upper tract dilatation.
3. **Ureterovesical obstruction** — more common in males and more common on the left side. May be bilateral.
4. **Reflux without obstruction.**
5. **Associated with urinary tract infection** — but no obstruction or reflux. ? represents atony.
6. **Neurogenic.**

Further Reading
Lebowitz R.L. & Griscom N.T. (1977) Neonatal hydronephrosis: 146 cases. *Radiol. Clin. North Am.*, 15: 49–59.

8.18   Nephrographic Patterns

Immediate Faint Persistent Nephrogram
1. Proliferative/necrotizing disorders — e.g. acute glomerulonephritis. See section 8.10.
2. Renal vein thrombosis.
3. Chronic severe ischaemia.

Immediate Distinct Persistent Nephrogram
1. Acute tubular necrosis — in 60% of cases.
2. Other causes of acute renal failure.
3. Acute-on-chronic renal failure.
4. Acute hypotension — uncommonly.

Increasingly Dense Nephrogram
1. Acute obstruction — including urate nephropathy.
2. Acute hypotension.
3. Acute tubular necrosis — in 30% of cases.
4. Acute pyelonephritis.
5. Multiple myeloma.
6. Renal vein thrombosis.
7. Acute glomerulonephritis.
8. Amyloid.
9. Acute papillary necrosis — and rarely chronic papillary necrosis.

Rim Nephrogram
1. Severe hydronephrosis — scalloped nephrogram with a negative pyelogram.
2. Acute complete arterial occlusion — smooth nephrogram from cortical perfusion by capsular arteries.

Striated Nephrogram
1. Acute ureteric obstruction.
2. Infantile polycystic disease — contrast medium in dilated tubules.
3. Medullary sponge kidney — in the medulla only. Parallel or fan-shaped streaks radiating from the papilla to the periphery of the kidney.
4. Acute pyelonephritis.

Further Reading
Newhouse, J.H. & Pfister, R.C. (1979) The nephrogram. *Radiol. Clin. North Am.*, 17: 213–26.

8.19   Renal Papillary Necrosis

1. Normal — small kidneys with smooth outlines.
2. Bilateral in 85% with multiple papillae affected.
3. Papillae may show
    (a) Enlargement (early).
    (b) Partial sloughing — a fissure forms and may communicate with a central irregular cavity.
    (c) Total sloughing — the sloughed papillary tissue may (i) fragment and be passed in the urine, (ii) cause ureteric obstruction, (iii) remain free in a calyx, or (iv) remain in the pelvis and form a ball calculus.
    (d) Necrosis-in-situ — the papilla is shrunken and necrotic but has not separated.
4. Calyces will appear dilated following total sloughing of a papilla.
5. Calcification and occasionally ossification of a shrunken, necrotic papilla. If marginal, it appears as a calculus with a radiolucent centre.

| Normal | Swollen | Partial papillary necrosis | Total papillary necrosis | Necrosis-in-situ |

A useful mnemonic is *ADIPOSE* —

A   Analgesics — phenacetin and aspirin
D   Diabetes
I   Infants in shock
P   Pyelonephritis
O   Obstruction
S   Sickle cell disease
E   Ethanol.

However, diabetes, analgesics and sickle-cell anaemia are the most important, with diabetes the most frequent cause.

Further Reading
Hare W.S.C. and Poynter J.D. (1974) The radiology of renal papillary necrosis as seen in analgesic nephropathy. *Clin. Radiol.*, 25: 423–43.

8.20 Renal Induced Hypertension

Signs of Unilateral Renal Artery Stenosis
1. Unilateral delay of 1 minute or more in the appearance of opacified calyces.
2. Small, smooth kidney
   — left more than 1.5 cm shorter than the right
   — right more than 2 cm shorter than the left.
3. Increased density of opacified calyces.
4. Ureteric notching by collateral vessels.

Renal Artery
1. **Arteriosclerosis** — 66% of renovascular causes. Stenosis of the proximal 2 cm of the renal artery; less frequently the distal artery or early branches at bifurcations. More common in males.
2. **Fibromuscular dysplasia** — 33% of renovascular causes. Stenoses ± dilatations which may give the characteristic 'string of beads' appearance. Mainly females less than 40 years. Bilateral in 60% of cases.
3. **Thrombosis/embolism.**
4. **Arteritis** — polyarteritis nodosa, thromboangiitis obliterans. Takayasu's disease, syphilis, congenital rubella or idiopathic.
5. **Neurofibromatosis*** — ± coarctation of the aorta. ± stenoses of other arteries. ± intrarenal arterial abnormalities.
6. **Trauma.**
7. **Aneurysm** — of the aorta or the renal artery.
8. **Arteriovenous fistula** — traumatic, congenital or a stump fistula following nephrectomy.
9. **Extrinsic compression** — neoplasm, aneurysm or lymph nodes.

Chronic Bilateral Parenchymal Disease
1. Chronic glomerulonephritis.
2. Chronic pyelonephritis.
3. Adult polycystic disease*.
4. Diabetic glomerulosclerosis.
5. Connective tissue disorders — systemic lupus erythematosus, scleroderma and polyarthritis nodosa.
6. Radiotherapy.
7. Hydronephrosis.

8. Analgesic nephropathy.
9. Renal vein thrombosis.

Unilateral Parenchymal Disease
Much less common as a cause of hypertension.
1. Chronic pyelonephritis.
2. Hydronephrosis.
3. **Tumours** — hypertension is more common with Wilms' tumour than with renal cell carcinoma. The rare juxta-glomerular cell tumour secretes renin.
4. Tuberculosis.
5. Xanthogranulomatous pyelonephritis.
6. Radiotherapy.
7. Renal vein thrombosis.

Further Reading
Webb J.A.W. & Talner L.B. (1979) The role of intravenous urography in hypertension. *Radio. Clin. North Am.*, **17**:187–95.

8.21   Renal Vein Thrombosis

Unilateral or bilateral.

Sudden —
1. Large non-functioning kidney which over a period of several months becomes small and atrophic.
2. Retrograde pyelography reveals thickened parenchyma (due to oedema) with elongation and compression of the major calyces.
3. Arteriography shows stretching and separation of arterial branches with decreased flow and a poor persistent nephrogram. No opacification of the renal vein.

Gradual —
1. Large kidney.
2. Nephrogram may be normal, poor persistent or increasingly dense.
3. Thickened parenchyma with elongation of major calyces.
4. Ureteric notching due to venous collaterals.

Children
1. **Dehydration and shock** — especially infants delivered of diabetic mothers.
2. **Nephrotic syndrome.**
3. **Cyanotic heart disease.**

Adults
1. **Extension of renal cell carcinoma into the renal vein.**
2. **Local compression by tumour or retroperitoneal nodes.**
3. **Extension of thrombus from the inferior vena cava.**
4. **Trauma.**
5. **Secondary to renal disease** — especially amyloid and chronic glomerulonephritis with nephrotic syndrome.

8.22 Non-visualization of a Calyx

1. **Technical factors** — incomplete filling during excretion urography.
2. **Tumour** — most commonly a renal cell carcinoma (adult) or Wilms' tumour (child).
3. **Obstructed infundibulum** — due to tumour, calculus or tuberculosis.
4. **Duplex kidney** — with a non-functioning upper or lower moiety. Signs suggesting a non-functioning upper moiety are
   (a) Fewer calyces than the contralateral kidney. This sign is only reliable in unilateral duplication (Calyceal distribution is symmetrical in 80% of normal individuals.)
   (b) A shortened upper calyx which does not reach into the upper pole.
   (c) The upper calyx of the lower moiety may be deformed by a dilated upper pole pelvis.
   (d) The kidney may be displaced downward by a dilated upper moiety pelvis. The appearances mimic a space occupying lesion in the upper pole.
   (e) The upper pole may be rotated laterally and downward by a dilated upper moiety pelvis and the lower pole calyces adopt a 'drooping flower' appearance.
   (f) Lateral displacement of the entire kidney by a dilated upper moiety ureter.
   (g) The lower moiety ureter may be displaced or compressed by the upper pole ureter, resulting in a series of scalloped curves.
   (h) The lower moiety renal pelvis may be displaced laterally and its ureter then takes a direct oblique course to the lumbosacral junction.
5. **Infection** — abscess or tuberculosis.
6. **Partial nephrectomy** — with a surgical defect in the 12th rib.

8.23   Radiolucent Filling Defect in the Renal Pelvis or a Calyx

Technical Factors
1. Incomplete filling during excretion urography.
2. Overlying gas shadows.

Extrinsic with a Smooth Margin
1. **Cyst** (q.v.).
2. **Vascular impression** — an intrarenal artery producing linear transverse or oblique compression lines and most commonly indenting an upper pole calyx, especially on the right side.
3. **Renal sinus lipomatosis** — most commonly in older patients with a wasting disease of the kidney. Fat in the renal hilum produces a relative lucency and narrows and elongates the major calyces.
4. **Collateral vessels** — most commonly ureteric artery collaterals in renal artery stenosis. Multiple small irregularities in the pelvic wall.

Inseparable from the Wall and with Smooth Margins
1. **Blood clot** — due to trauma, tumour or bleeding diathesis. May be adherent to the wall or free in the lumen. Change in size or shape over several days.
2. **Papilloma** — solitary or multiple.
3. **Pyeloureteritis cystica** — due to chronic infection. Multiple well-defined submucosal cysts project into the lumen of the pelvis and/or ureter.

Arising from the Wall with an Irregular Margin
1. **Transitional cell carcinoma**
2. **Squamous cell carcinoma** — } see section 8.12
3. **Renal cell carcinoma**
4. **Squamous metaplasia (cholesteatoma)** — occurs rarely in association with chronic irritation from a calculus. Indistinguishable from tumour and may be premalignant.

In the Lumen
1. Blood clot.
2. Lucent calculus (q.v.).
3. Sloughed papilla.
4. Air (q.v.).

Further Reading
Brown R.C., Jones M.C., Boldus R. & Flocks R.H. (1973) Lesions causing radiolucent defects in the renal pelvis. *Am. J. Roentgenol.*, 119: 770–8.

8.24   Dilated Calyx

With a Narrow Infundibulum
1. **Stricture** — tumour, calculus or tuberculosis.
2. **Extrinsic impression by an artery** — most commonly a right upper pole calyx (Fraley syndrome).
3. **Hydrocalycosis** — may be a congenital anomaly. Can only be safely diagnosed in childhood when calculus, tumour and tuberculosis are uncommon.

With a Wide Infundibulum
1. **Post-obstructive atrophy** — generally all the calyces are affected and associated with parenchymal thinning.
2. **Megacalyces** — dilated calyces ± a slightly dilated pelvis. ± stones. Increased number of calyces — 20–25 (normal 8–12). Because of the large volume collecting system full visualization during urography is delayed. Normal cortical thickness and good renal function differentiate it from post obstructive atrophy.
3. **Polycalycosis** — rare. ± ureteric abnormalities.

Further Reading
Talner L.B. & Gittes R.F. (1974) Megacalyces, further observations and differentiation from obstructive renal disease. *Am. J. Roentgenol.*, 121: 473–86.

8.25   Dilated Ureter

Obstruction

WITHIN THE LUMEN
1. Calculus (q.v.).
2. Blood clot.
3. Sloughed papilla.

IN THE WALL
1. **Oedema or stricture due to calculus.**
2. **Tumour** — carcinoma or papilloma.
3. **Tuberculous stricture** — a particular hazard during the early weeks of treatment.
4. **Schistosomiasis** — especially the distal ureter. ± calcification in the ureter or bladder.
5. **Post surgical trauma** — e.g. a misplaced ligature.
6. **Ureterocoele.**
7. **Megaureter** — symmetrical tapered narrowing above the uretero-vesical junction.

OUTSIDE THE WALL
1. **Retroperitoneal fibrosis** (q.v.).
2. **Carcinoma of cervix, bladder or prostate.**
3. **Retrocaval ureter** — right side only. Distal ureter lies medial to the dilated proximal portion.

Vesico-ureteric Reflux.

No Obstruction or Reflux
1. **Post partum** — more common on the right side.
2. **Following relief of obstruction** — most commonly calculus of prostatectomy.
3. **Urinary tract infection** — due to the effect of P fimbriated *E. coli* on the urothelium.
4. **Primary non-obstructive megaureter** — children > adults. The juxtavesical segment of ureter is of normal calibre but fails to transmit an effective peristaltic wave.

Further Reading
Hamilton S. & Fitzpatrick J.M. (1987) Primary non-obstructive megaureter in adults. *Clin. Radiol.*, 38: 181–5.

8.26 Retroperitoneal Fibrosis

1. Ureteric obstruction of variable severity. 75% bilateral.
2. Tapering lumen or complete obstruction — usually at L4–5 level and never the extreme lower end.
3. Medial deviation of the ureters — more significant if there is a right-angled step in the course of the ureter rather than a gentle drift. The position of the ureters is frequently normal.
4. Easy retrograde catheterization of ureter(s);
5. Retroperitoneal, periaortic mass — demonstrable by CT or US.
6. Clinically — back pain, high ESR and elevated creatinine.

1. **Retroperitoneal malignancy** — lymphoma and metastases from colon and breast especially. The tumour initiates a fibrotic reaction around itself.
2. **Inflammatory conditions** — Crohn's disease, diverticular disease, actinomycosis, pancreatitis and extravasation of urine from the pelvicalyceal system.
3. **Aortic aneurysm** ⎫ fibrosis occurs secondary to
4. **Trauma** ⎬ blood in the retroperitoneal
5. **Surgery** ⎭ tissues.
6. **Drugs** — methysergide.
7. **Idiopathic** — > 50% all cases. May be due to an immune reaction to atheromatous material in the aorta.

Differential Diagnosis of Medially Placed Ureters
1. **Normal variant** — 15% of individuals. Commoner in blacks, in whom bilateral displacement is also commoner.
2. **Pelvic lipomatosis** — other signs suggesting the diagnosis are (a) elevation and elongation of the bladder, (b) elongation of the rectum and sigmoid with widening of the retrorectal space, and (c) increased lucency of the pelvic wall.
3. **Following abdomino-perineal resection** — the ureters are medially placed inferiorly.
4. **Retrocaval ureter** — the right ureter passes behind the inferior vena cava at the level of LV4. The distal ureter lies medial to the dilated proximal portion.

Further Reading

Brooks A.P., Reznek R.H., Webb J.A.W. & Baker R.I. (1987)
    Computed tomography in the follow-up of retroperitoneal
    fibrosis. *Clin. Radiol.*, 38: 597–601.

Dixon A.K., Mitchinson M.J. & Sherwood T. (1984) Computed
    tomographic observations in peri-aortitis: a hypothesis. *Clin.
    Radiol.*, 35: 39–42.

Minford J.E. & Davies P. (1984) The urographic appearances in
    acute and chronic retroperitoneal fibrosis. *Clin. Radiol.*, 35:
    51–7.

8.27 Filling Defect in the Bladder (in the Wall or in the Lumen)

1. **Prostate.**
2. **Neoplasm** — especially transitional cell carcinoma in an adult and rhabdomyosarcoma in a child.
3. **Blood clot.**
4. **Instrument** — urethral or suprapubic catheter.
5. **Calculus.**
6. **Ureterocoele.**
7. **Schistosomiasis.**
8. **Endometriosis.**

8.28 Bladder Calcification

In the Lumen
1. **Calculus.**
2. **Foreign body** — encrustation of the balloon of a Foley catheter.

In the Wall
1. **Transitional and squamous cell carcinoma** — radiographic incidence about 0.5%. Usually surface calcification which may be linear, curvilinear or stippled. Punctate calcification of a villous tumour may suggest chronicity. No extravesical calcification.
2. **Schistosomiasis** — an infrequent cause in the Western hemisphere but the commonest cause of mural calcification worldwide. Thin curvilinear calcification outlines a bladder of normal size and shape. Calcification spreads proximally to involve the distal ureters (appearing as two parallel lines) in 15%.
3. **Tuberculosis** — rare and usually accompanied by calcification elsewhere in the urogenital tract. Unlike schistosomiasis the disease begins in the kidney and spreads distally. Contracted bladder.
4. **Cyclophosphamide-induced cystitis.**

Further Reading
Pollack H.M., Banner M.P., Martinez L.O. & Hodson C.J. (1986) Diagnostic considerations in urinary bladder wall calcification. *Am. J. Roentgenol.*, 136: 791–7.

8.29   Bladder Fistula

Congenital
1. Ectopia vesicae.
2. Imperforate anus — high type.
3. Patent urachus.

Inflammatory
1. Diverticular disease.
2. Crohn's disease*.
3. Appendix abscess — and other pelvic sepsis.

Neoplastic
1. Carcinoma of the colon, bladder or reproductive organs.
2. Radiotherapy.

Trauma
1. Accidental.
2. Iatrogenic — particularly in obstetrics and gynaecology.

8.30 Bladder Outflow Obstruction in a Child

1. Distended bladder with incomplete emptying.
2. ± bilateral upper tract dilatation.
3. ± upper tract cystic disease.

Causes (from proximal to distal)
1. **Vesical diverticulum** — posteriorly behind the bladder base. It fills during micturition and compresses the bladder neck and proximal urethra. More common in males.
2. (**Bladder neck obstruction** — probably not a distinct entity and only occurs as part of other problems such as ectopic ureterocoele and rhabdomyosarcoma.)
3. **Ectopic ureterocoele** — 80% are associated with the upper moiety of a duplex kidney. 15% are bilateral. More common in females. Opens into the urethra, bladder neck or vestibule. May be largely outside the bladder and the bladder base may be elevated. 'Drooping flower' appearance of lower moiety. May prolapse into the urethra.
4. **Posterior urethral valves** — posterior urethra is dilated and the distal urethra is small. Almost exclusively males.
5. **Urethral stricture** — post-traumatic strictures are most commonly at the peno-scrotal junction and follow previous instrumentation or catheterization.
6. **Anterior urethral diverticulum** — a saccular wide-necked, ventral expansion of the anterior urethra, usually at the peno-scrotal junction. The proximal lip of the diverticulum may show as an arcuate filling defect and during micturition the diverticulum expands with urine and obstructs the urethra.
7. **Prune-belly syndrome** — almost exclusively males. High mortality. Bilateral hydronephrosis and hydroureters with a distended bladder are associated with undescended testes, hypoplasia of the anterior abdominal wall and urethral obstruction.
8. **Calculus or foreign body.**
9. **Meatal stenosis** ⎫ clinical diagnosis.
10. **Phimosis** ⎭

N.B. The commonest cause in males is posterior urethral valves and in females is ectopic uretercoele.

8.31   Calcification of the Seminal Vesicles or Vas Deferens

1. **Diabetes mellitus** — the cause in the vast majority of cases.
2. **Chronic infection** — tuberculosis, schistosomiasis, chronic urinary tract infection and syphilis.
3. **Idiopathic.**

Further Reading
King J.C. & Rosenbaum H.D. (1971) Calcification of the vasa deferentia in non-diabetes. *Radiology*, 100: 603–6.

Bibliography

General
Chrispin A.R., Gordon I., Hall C. & Metreweli C. (1980) *Diagnostic Imaging of the Kidney and Urinary Tract in Children*. Berlin: Springer International.
Davidson A.J. (1977) *Radiological Diagnosis of Renal Parenchymal Disease*. Philadelphia: Saunders.
Davidson A.J. (ed.) (1979) Advances in uroradiology. *Radiol. Clin. North Am.*, 17 (2).
Sherwood T. (1980) *Uroradiology*. Oxford: Blackwell.
Sutton D. (ed.)(1980) *Textbook of Radiology and Imaging*. 3rd edn, chaps. 39–46. Edinburgh: Churchill Livingstone.
Witten D.M., Myers G.H. & Utz D.C. (1977) *Clinical Urography*. 4th edn. Philadelphia: Saunders

Infections
Felson B. (ed.)(1971) Infections of the urinary tract. *Semin. Roentgenol.*, 6 (3).
Gingell J.C., Roylance J., Davies E.R. & Penry J.B. 1973) Xanthogranulomatous pyelonephritis, *Br. J. Radiol.*, 46: 99–109.
Kirkland K. (1966) Urological aspects of hydatid disease, *Br. J. Urol.*, 38: 241–54.
Roylance J., Penry J.B., Davies E.R. & Roberts M. (1970) The radiology of tuberculosis of the urinary tract. *Clin. Radiol.*, 21: 163–70.
Silver T.M., Kass E.J., Thornbury J.R., Konnack J.W. & Wolfman M.G. (1976) The radiological spectrum of acute pyelonephritis in adults and adolescents. *Radiology*, 118: 65–71.
Tonkin A.K. & Whitten D.M. (1979) Genitourinary tuberculosis, *Semin. Roentgenol.*, 14: 305–18.
Watt I. & Roylance J. (1975) Pyonephrosis. *Clin. Radiol.*, 27: 513–19.

Neoplasms

Bruneton J.N., Ballanger P., Ballanger R., & Delorme G. (1979) Renal adenomas. *Clin. Radiol.*, 30: 343–52.

Cope J.R., Roylance J. & Gordon I.R.S. (1972) The radiological features of Wilms' tumours. *Clin. Radiol.*, 23: 331–9.

Lowe P.P. & Roylance J. (1976) Transitional cell carcinoma of the kidney. *Clin. Radiol.*, 27: 503–12.

Martinez-Maldonado M. & Ramirez de Arellano G.A. (1966) Renal involvement in malignant lymphomas. *J. Urol.*, 95: 485–8.

McCallum R.W. (1975) The preoperative diagnosis of renal hamartoma. *Clin. Radiol.*, 26: 257–60.

Thomas J.L., Barnes P.A., Bernardino M.E. & Lewis E. (1982) Diagnostic approaches to adrenal and renal metastases. *Radiol. Clin. North Am.*, 20: 531–44.

Notes

Notes

Chapter 9
Soft Tissues

9.1 Gynaecomastia

Physiological
1. **Neonatal** — due to high placental oestrogens.
2. **Pubertal** — due to an excess of oestradiol over testosterone.
3. **Senile** — due to falling androgen and rising oestrogen levels with age.

Pharmacological
1. **Oestrogen** — especially in the treatment of carcinoma of the prostate.
2. **Digitalis** — binds to oestrogen receptors.
3. **Anti-cancer drugs** — producing testicular damage.
4. **Anti-androgens** — spironolactone.
5. **Reserpine.**
6. **Phenothiazines.**
7. **Tricyclic antidepressants.**
8. **Methyldopa.**

Pathological
1. **Carcinoma of the bronchus** ⎫ secreting human chorionic gonadotrophin.
2. **Teratoma of the testis** ⎭
3. **Cirrhosis** — due to increased conversion of androgens to oestrogens.
4. **Hypogonadism** — e.g. Klinefelter's syndrome and castration.
5. **Hypopituitarism** — including acromegaly.
6. **Testicular feminization** — androgen insensitivity.
7. **Adrenal tumours** ⎫ secreting oestrogens
8. **Leydig cell tumours** ⎭

9.2 Linear and Curvilinear Calcification in Soft Tissues

Arterial
1. Atheroma/aneurysm.
2. Diabetes.
3. **Hyperparathyroidism*** — more common in secondary than primary.
4. **Werner's syndrome** — premature ageing in a Jewish diabetic (male or female).

Nerve
1. Leprosy.
2. Neurofibromatosis*.

Ligament
1. **Tendinitis** — Pellegrini–Stieda syndrome, supraspinatus.
2. **Ankylosing spondylitis***.
3. **Fluorosis**.
4. **Diabetes**.
5. **Alkaptonuria**.

Bismuth Injection — in the buttocks. ± neuropathic joints.

Parasites

1. Cysticerci	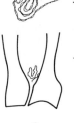	— oval with lucent centre. Often arranged in the direction of muscle fibres.
2. Guinea worm		— irregular coiled appearance.
3. Loa loa		— thread-like coil. Particularly in the web spaces of the hand.
4. Armillifer		— 'comma' shaped. Only in trunk muscles.

See also section 9.4.

9.3   Conglomerate Calcification in Soft Tissues

Collagenoses
1. Scleroderma* — acrolysis and flexion contractures in the hands.
2. Dermatomyositis.
3. Ehlers–Danlos syndrome.

Metabolic
1. Hyperparathyroidism* — more common in secondary hyperparathyroidism. Vascular calcification is common.
2. Gout* — calcified tophus.

Traumatic
1. Haematoma.
2. Burns.
3. Myositis ossificans — outer part is more densely calcified than the centre.

Infective
1. Tuberculous abscess/node.

Neoplastic
1. Benign
   (a) Parosteal lipoma — lucent. ± pressure erosion of adjacent bone.
   (b) Haemangioma — Suspect if phleboliths present in an unusual site. ± soft-tissue mass with adjacent bone destruction.
2. Malignant
   (a) Parosteal osteosarcoma — age 20–40. Lobulated calcification around a metaphysis. Inner part is more densely calcified than the periphery. Early – a thin lucent line may separate it from underlying bone.
   (b) Juxta-cortical chondrosarcoma — particularly pelvis.
   (c) Liposarcoma.

9.4 'Sheets' of Calcification/Ossification in Soft Tissues

1. Congenital myositis ossificans progressiva — manifest in childhood. Initially neck and trunk muscles involved. Short first metacarpal and metatarsal.
2. Dermatomyositis.

9.5 Periarticular Soft-tissue Calcification

Inflammatory
1. Scleroderma* — ± acro-osteolysis.
2. Dermatomyositis.
3. Gout* — calcified tophi. Punched-out erosions.
4. Bursitis — can be dense and lobulated.

Degenerative
1. Calcific periarthritis (calcium hydroxyapatite deposition disease).
2. Calcium pyrophosphate deposition disease*.

Renal Failure
1. Secondary hyperaparathyroidism — ± vascular calcification.
2. Treatment with 1-α-OHD$_3$ — particularly shoulder, hip and metacarpophalangeal joints.

Hypercalcaemia
1. Sarcoidosis* — rare. Affects hands and feet. ± lace-like trabecular pattern in tubular bones.
2. Hypervitaminosis D.
3. Milk–alkali syndrome.

Neoplastic
1. Synovial osteochondromatosis — age 20–50 years. Most commonly affects a large joint. Multiple calcified loose bodies. ± secondary degenerative changes or pressure erosion of bone.
2. Synovioma — age 20–50 years. Soft-tissue mass with amorphous calcification, irregular bone destruction and osteoporosis.

Idiopathic
1. Tumoral calcinosis — age 20–30 years. Adjacent to a major joint. Firm, non-tender, moveable mass which is well defined, lobulated and calcified on X-ray. Osseous involvement is rare. ± calcium fluid level.

9.6 Soft-tissue Ossification

Traumatic
1. Myositis ossificans.
2. Burns
3. **Paraplegia** — ossification adjacent to the ischium — may be related to pressure sores.

Neoplastic
1. Parosteal osteosarcoma.
2. Liposarcoma.

Congenital Myositis Ossificans Progressiva

9.7 Increased Heel Pad Thickness

males: if 'x' is greater than 23 mm.
females: if 'x' is greater than 21.5 mm.
1. Acromegaly*.
2. Obesity.
3. Peripheral oedema.
4. Infection/injury.
5. Myxoedema.
6. Epanutin therapy.

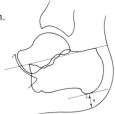

Further Reading
Kattan K.R. (1975) Thickening of the heel pad associated with long-term Dilantin therapy. *Am. J. Roentgenol.*, 124: 52–6.
Kho K.M., Wright A.D. & Doyle F.H. (1970) Heel pad thickness in acromegaly. *Br. J. Radiol.*, 43: 119–22.

Bibliography

Cockshott P. & Middlemiss J.H. (1979) *Clinical Radiology in the Tropics*. Edinburgh: Churchill Livingstone.
Griffiths H.J. (1976) *Radiology of Renal Failure*. Philadelphia: Saunders.
Palmer P.E.S. (1966) Tumoral calcinosis. *Br. J. Radiol.*, 39: 518–23.

Notes

Notes

Chapter 10
Mammography

Michael Collins

Introduction

Modern mammography demands meticulously high standards in all its aspects. This includes X-ray equipment, radiographic technique, film-screen combinations, processing, viewing conditions and interpretation. Shortcomings in any of these factors will lead to serious errors. Other factors that lead to difficulty include dense parenchymal background that may obscure tumours; benign conditions that mimic malignancy; and malignant tumours with benign appearances on mammography. Close co-operation between radiologists, radiographers, surgeons and pathologists is essential.

10.1	Benign vs	Malignant
1. Opacity	Smooth margin	Ill defined margin — stellate, spiculated, comet tail. May only involve part of margin.
	Low/mixed density	High density
	Homogenous	Inhomogenous
	Thin 'halo'	Wide 'halo'
2. Calcification	see below	
3. **Surrounding parenchyma**	Normal	Disrupted
4. **Nipple**	± Retracted	± Retracted
5. **Skin**	Normal	Thickened, retracted

6. Cooper ligaments	Normal	Thickened, increased number
7. Ducts	Normal	Focal dilatation
8. Subcutaneous/ retromammary space	Normal	± Obliterated

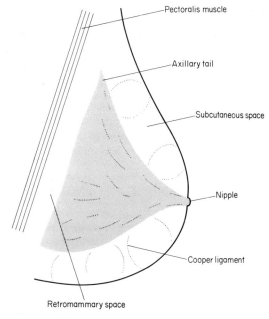

Typical normal

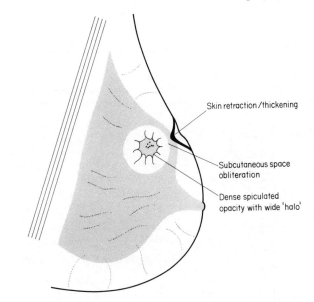

Skin retraction /thickening

Subcutaneous space
obliteration

Dense spiculated
opacity with wide 'halo'

Typical carcinoma

10.2 Calcification

1. Microcalcification not as specific an indication of malignancy as once thought.
2. Seen in 30–40% of carcinomas.
3. Macrocalcification is defined as > 0.5 mm diameter.
4. Microcalcification is defined as < 0.5 mm diameter.

Definitely Benign

1. 'Arterial'

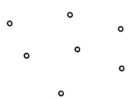

2. Widespread punctuate ± lucent centre

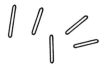

3. Thick linear ± lucent centre

4. 'Eggshell'

5. 'Popcorn'-in fibroadenoma

6. Large calcific density

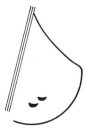

7. 'Floating' calcification

Microcalcification and/or mixture of shapes

1. Arterial — tortuous, tramline.
2. Smooth, widely separated, some with radiolucent centre.
3. Thick linear, widespread, some with radiolucent centre.
4. 'Egg-shell' curvilinear margin of cyst or papilloma.
5. 'Pop-corn' in fibroadenoma.
6. Large individual calcific opacity > 2 mm.
7. 'Floating' calcification — seen as calcific/fluid level on erect film.

Probably Benign
1. Widespread — all one/both breasts.
2. Macrocalcification of uniform size.
3. Symmetrical distribution.
4. Well separated opacities.
5. Superficial distribution.

Possibly malignant — biopsy indicated — see figure showing microcalcification and mixture of shapes
1. Microcalcification — particularly segmental, cluster distribution (five particles each measuring < 0.5 mm in 1.0 cm^3 space. Of these, 30% of cases will be malignant).
2. Mixture of shapes and sizes — linear, branching, punctate.
3. Associated soft tissue opacity of suspicious shape and density.
4. Suspicious calcification (see above) eccentric to soft tissue opacity.
5. Increased number of calcific opacities visible on magnification.
6. Deterioration on serial mammography

Further Reading
Sickles E.A. (1986) Breast calcification: mammographic evaluation. *Radiology*, 160: 289–93.

10.3 Benign Conditions that Mimic Malignancy

1. **Microcalcification**
   (a) Sclerosing adenosis — irregular opacity.
   (b) Recent surgery — parenchymal distortion and skin thickening.
2. **Suspicious soft tissue opacity**
   (a) Fibroadenoma — occasionally part of margin is irregular or ill defined.
   (b) Fat necrosis — ill defined opacity, occasionally with a radiolucent centre.
   (c) Post biopsy — ill defined opacity.
   (d) Radial scar — spiculated margin.
   (e) Haematoma — ± ill defined.

10.4 Benign Lesions with Typical Appearances

1. **Lipoma** — rounded often large, radiolucent with compression of adjacent parenchyma.
2. **Fibroadenoma** — rounded, lobulated with eccentrically sited 'pop-corn' calcification.
3. **Intramammary lymph nodes** — well defined, usually < 1.0 cm, eccentric radiolucency.

N.B. Any well-defined opacity > 1.0 cm in diameter that is solid on ultrasound should be subjected to biopsy, particularly if any of the margins are ill-defined or if a 'comet-tail' is evident. A small group of carcinomas look 'benign' on mammography, i.e. medullary, mucoid, encephaloid, papillary.

10.5 Single Well-defined Soft Tissue Opacity

1. **Benign**
   (a) Cyst (herimenopausal) (haemenopausal).
   (b) Fibroadenoma.
   (c) Intramammary lymph node.
   (d) Skin lesion, e.g. sebaceous cyst.
   (e) Intraductal papilloma (usually small).
   (f) Nipple not in profile.
   (g) Cystosarcoma phylloides — can have malignant potential.
2. **Malignant**
   (a) Carcinoma — in particular medullary, mucoid, encephaloid, intracystic, papillary and carcinoma in fibroadenoma

10.6 Multiple Well-defined Soft Tissue Opacities

1. **Cysts.**
2. **Fibroadenomata** — 10–20% are multiple.
3. **Skin lesions** (e.g. neurofibromata).
4. **Silicone injections** — usually quite dense.
5. **Papillomatosis** — often localized.
6. **Intramammary lymph nodes.**
7. **Metastases** — lymphoma and melanoma are the commonest primary lesions.

10.7 Large (> 5 cm) Well-defined Opacity

1. **Giant cyst.**
2. **Giant fibroadenoma.**
3. **Lipoma** (radiolucent).
4. **Sebaceous cyst.**
5. **Cystosarcoma phylloides.**

10.8 Mixed Density Well-defined Single Opacity

1. Intramammary lymph node.
2. Fibroadenoma lipoma — usually large.
3. Galactocele — seen during lactation.
4. Haematoma — history of trauma.

10.9 Causes of Disappearance of Calcification

1. Recent surgery.
2. Radiotherapy.
3. Chemotherapy.
4. Spontaneous.

Further Reading

Buckley J.H. & Roebuck E.J. (1986) Mammographic changes following radiotherapy. *Br. J. Radiol.*, 59: 337–44.
Fewins H.E., Whitehouse G.H. & Leinster S.J. (1988) The spontaneous disappearance of breast calcification. *Clin. Radiol.*, 39: 257–261.

10.10 Oedematous Breast

Signs on Mammography:
1. Diffuse increased density.
2. Skin thickening (> 1.5 mm).
3. Coarse reticular pattern.
4. Prominent Cooper ligaments.

Causes:
1. Diffuse carcinoma.
2. Lymphatic obstruction (usually due to tumour).
3. Venous obstruction.
4. Recent surgery.
5. Radiotherapy.
6. Breast abscess.
7. Heart/renal failure.

10.11 Ultrasound in Breast Disease

Uses and indications:
1. Dense parenchyma.
2. During pregnancy, lactation.
3. Breast tenderness (compression for mammography not possible).
4. Breast prosthesis.
5. Non-palpable opacity seen on mammography.
6. Palpable lump with negative mammography.
7. Biopsy guidance.

Typical appearances of carcinoma:
1. Hypoechoic mass.
2. Heterogeneous internal echoes.
3. Ill-defined margin.
4. Surrounding hyperechoic 'halo'.
5. Absent far wall echoes.
6. Distant acoustic shadowing.

10.12 Breast Cancer Screening — Forrest Report

Summary
1. Screening by mammography alone.
2. 50–64 year age group.
3. Screening at 3 yearly intervals.
4. Single projection (lateral oblique).
5. Leads to 33% reduction in mortality.

Other points
1. Basic screening unit — population of 41 150 women.
2. Expected acceptance rate (attendance) — 70%.
3. Expected referral to assessment clinic — 10% of screening attendances.
4. Expected biopsy rate — 1.5% of screening attendances.
5. Incidence of carcinoma in screened population — 0.55%.

Further Reading
Forrest Report (1986) Breast Cancer Screening. HMSO.

10.13   Radiation Risk from Mammography

Modern mammography: typical mammary gland dose: 0.15 cGy (single view each breast).
Xeromammography: dose 5–6 times greater than X-ray mammography.

One excess cancer per year (after latent period of 10 years) in two million women screened. This is contrasted with an incidence of new cases of breast cancer of 1800/10 000 000/ year at age 50.

Further Reading

Fieg S.A. (1986) *Diagnostic Radiology: A Textbook of Organ Imaging. The Breast*, pp. 1631–68. Edinburgh: Churchill Livingstone.
Forrest Report (1986) Breast Cancer Screening. HMSO.

Bibliography

Fieg S.A. (1986) *Diagnostic Radiology: A Textbook of Organ Imaging. The Breast*, pp. 1631–68. Edinburgh: Churchill Livingstone.
Forrest Report (1986) Breast Cancer Screening. HMSO.
Gravelle I.H. (1987) *Textbook of Radiology and Imaging*, 4th edn, pp. 1396–410. Edinburgh: Churchill Livingstone.
Sickles E.A. (ed.) (1987) *Breast Imaging. Radiol. Clin. North Am.*, 25 (1).
Tabar L. & Dean P. (1985) *Teaching Atlas on Mammography*, 2nd edn, Stuttgart, New York: George Thieme Verlag.
Wolfe, J.N. (ed.) (1983) *Mammography. Radiol. Clin. North Am.*, 21 (1).

Notes

Notes

Chapter 11
Face and Neck

11.1 Unilateral Exophthalmos

Dysthyroid
This is the commonest cause, most cases being diagnosed clinically.

Orbital Lesions
1. **Primary neoplasms in a child**
    (a) Rhabdomyosarcoma — rapidly progressive proptosis compared with the reduction in visual acuity. Arises from extraocular muscles. Commonest site is the superonasal quadrant. Commonly fills the adjacent nasal cavity and sinuses.
    (b) Haemangioma — presents during the first 6 months during its period of active growth. Majority have skin stigmata.
    (c) Optic nerve glioma — rapid reduction of vision compared with the degree of proptosis.
2. **Secondary neoplasms in a child**
    (a) Neuroblastoma — usually in the presence of well advanced abdominal disease. High CT attenuation, probably due to calcification and haemorrhage. Rarely → preseptal extension compared with rhabdomysarcoma.
    (b) Leukaemia — excluded by blood and marrow examination. Most likely diagnosis if the tumour is confined to the conal muscles only.
3. **Neoplasms in an adult**
    (a) Haemangioma.
    (b) Lymphoma*.
    (c) Optic nerve glioma — age usually less than 35 years. Optic canal enlarged in 90%.
    (d) Orbital meningioma — age usually over 35 years. Optic canal enlarged in 10%.

    (e) Neurofibromatosis* — 'bare' orbit and widened superior orbital fissure.
    (f) Metastases — often show lytic bone changes.
    (g) Dermoid.
    (h) Lacrimal gland tumour.
4. **Trauma** — haematoma and/or fracture.
5. **Orbital pseudotumour.**

Intracranial Lesions

1. **Meningioma** — ± hyperostosis of the apex of the orbit, or lesser wing of sphenoid.
2. **Glioma.**
3. **Infraclinoid aneurysm.**
4. **Cavernous sinus thrombosis.**

Sinus/bone Lesions

1. **Fibrous dysplasia*** — leontiasis ossea of the antrum.
2. **Neoplasms**
    (a) Carcinoma of paranasal sinus.
    (b) Osteoma.
    (c) Dermoid — typical expansion of the superolateral part of the orbital roof.
3. **Mucocele** — extending inferiorly from the frontal sinus.
4. **Craniostenosis** (q.v.).

Further Reading

Price H & Danziger A. (1979) The computerised tomographic findings in paediatric orbital tumours. *Clin. Radiol.*, 30: 435–40.
Vade E. & Armstrong D. (1987) Orbital rhabdomyosarcoma in childhood. *Radiol. Clin. North Am.*, 25: 701–14.

11.2 CT Characteristics of Orbital Masses in Children (see facing table)

Further Reading

Lallemand D.P., Brasch R.C., Char D.H. & Norman D. (1984) Orbital tumours in children. Characterisation by computed tomography. *Radiology*, 151: 85–8.

CT Characteristics of Orbital Masses in Children (modified from Lallemand et al.)

	Location				Orbital expansion	Bone destruction	Calcification	Extension		Attenuation		Enhancement
	Preseptal	Extraconal	Intraconal	Muscle only				Intracranial	Facial	High	Low	
Optic nerve glioma	+/-		+		+			+				+
Rhabdomyosarcoma	+/-	+				+	−		+			+
2° Neuroblastoma	+	+				+	+	+	+	+		+/-
Lymphangioma	+	+	+		+						mixed	
Haemangioma	+	+	+		+		+				mixed	++ irregular
Histiocytosis X	+/-	+				+		+	+			
Infection	+	+				+			+			
Leukaemia	+	+		+		+				+		
Lymphoma	+								+			+
Dermoid	+	+	+		+				+		mixed	
Pseudotumour	with dacryo adenitis	+	+	+								+

11.3   Optic Nerve Enlargement

1. **Optic nerve glioma** } see list.
2. **Meningioma**
3. **Extension of 1° ocular tumours** — retinoblastoma or melanoma.
4. **Optic neuritis** — diffuse, smooth expansion of the optic nerve. Contrast enhanced CT may show the tram-track sign typical of meningioma. Usually idiopathic but CT or MRI may reveal periventricular plaques suggesting multiple sclerosis.
5. **Raised intracranial pressure** — produces widening of the subarachnoid space around the optic nerve. Clinical and/ or radiological evidence of intracranial disease.
6. **Pseudotumour** — painful proptosis with an early decrease in visual acuity. CT shows thickening and enhancement of the sclera extending along the optic nerve. Striking response to steroids.
7. **Secondary to systemic diseases** — lymphoma, toxoplasmosis, tuberculosis and syphilis.

Further Reading

Azar-Kia B., Naheedy, M.H., Elias D.A., Mafee M.F. & Fine M. (1987) Optic nerve tumours: role of magnetic resonance imaging and computed tomography. *Radiol. Clin. North Am.*, 25 (3): 561–81.

Curtin H.D. (1987) Pseudotumour. *Radiol. Clin. North Am.*, 25 (3): 583–99.

Flanders A.E., Espinosa G.A., Markiewicz D.A. & Howell D.D. (1987) Orbital lymphoma. Role of CT and MRI. *Radiol. Clin. North Am.*, 25 (3): 601–13.

11.4 Optic Nerve Glioma *vs* Orbital Meningioma Clinical and CT Differentiation

Optic nerve glioma	Meningioma
50% less than 5 years of age	Usually middle-aged women
+/− bilateral	+/− bilateral
Well defined margins	More infiltrative Tubular thickening in 66% Fusiform enlargement in 25%
Calcification rare without prior radiotherapy	Calcification more common
No orbital hyperostosis	Hyperostosis
Enhancement, but with mottled lucencies due to extensive mucin deposition	Diffuse homogeneous enhancement
Kinking and buckling of the optic nerve is common	Straight optic nerve Negative image of optic nerve within tumour (tram-track sign)
Widened optic canal in 90%	Widened optic canal in 10%
25% have neurofibromatosis (NFT); 15% of NFT have optic nerve glioma; bilateral disease strongly suggests neurofibromatosis	Less frequently associated with neurofibromatosis

Further Reading

Azar-Kia B., Naheedy M.H., Elias D.A., Mafee M.F. & Fine M. (1987) Optic nerve tumours: role of magnetic resonance imaging and computed tomography. *Radiol. Clin. North Am.*, 25 (3): 561–81.

Linder B., Campos M. & Schafer M. (1987) CT and MRI of orbital abnormalities in neurofibromatosis and selected craniofacial anomalies. *Radiol. Clin. North Am.*, 25 (4): 787–802.

11.5 Enlarged Orbit

Exclude small contralateral orbit, e.g. enucleation as a child.

1. **Neurofibromatosis*** — ± 'bare' orbit due to elevation of the lesser wing of the sphenoid and associated dysplasia.
2. **Congenital glaucoma (buphthalmos)** — asymmetrical enlargement.
3. **Any space occupying lesion** — if present long enough. The enlargement in children occurs much faster. (See section 11.1.)

11.6 'Bare' Orbit

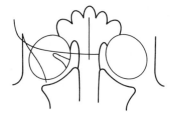

1. **Neurofibromatosis*** — dysplasia of the sphenoid.
2. **Metastasis** — bone destruction.
3. **Meningioma** — adjacent bone sclerosis.

Further Reading

Burrows E.H. (1963) Bone changes in orbital neurofibromatosis. *Br. J. Radiol.*, 36: 549–61.

11.7 Enlarged Optic Foramen

Diameter greater than 7 mm (normal range of 4.4–6 mm is reached by the age of four). However, the final arbiter is always comparison with the asymptomatic side. A difference in diameter of 1 mm is abnormal.

Concentric Enlargement
1. **Optic nerve glioma** — child/young adult. 25% associated with neurofibromatosis. Bone margins intact.
2. **Neurofibroma** — may occur without any associated glioma.
3. **Extension of retinoblastoma.**
4. **Vascular** — ophthalmic artery aneurysm, arterovenous malformation.
5. **Granuloma** — very rarely in sarcoid or pseudotumour.

Local Defect
ROOF
1. **Adjacent neoplasm** — meningioma, metastases, glioma.
2. **Raised intracranial pressure** (q.v.) — due to thinning of the floor of the anterior cranial fossa.

MEDIAL WALL
1. **Adjacent neoplasm** — carcinoma of the ethmoid/sphenoid.
2. **Sphenoid mucocele.**

INFEROLATERAL WALL
1. Same conditions as cause **enlargement of superior orbital fissure** (q.v.).

Further Reading
Lloyd G.A.S. (1975) *Radiology of the Orbit*, pp. 26–9. Philadelphia: Saunders.

11.8   Enlarged Superior Orbital Fissure

1. Normal variant.
2. Neurofibromatosis*.
3. Extension of intracranial lesion
   (a) Meningioma — adjacent sclerosis.
   (b) Infraclinoid aneurysm — occurs in 75%. Usually accompanied by erosion of the inferior surface of the anterior clinoid.
   (c) Parasellar chordoma.
4. Metastasis to wing of sphenoid.
5. Extension of orbital lesion (anterior clinoids not eroded)
   (a) Arteriovenous malformation.
   (b) Haemangioma.
   (c) Orbital meningioma.
   (d) Lymphoma.

11.9   Intraorbital Calcification

In the Globe
1. Cataract.
2. Retinoblastoma — young children. Very fine, stippled calcification. 30% are bilateral. ± proptosis. Siblings may also be affected.
3. Old trauma/infection — of the vitreous humour.

Outside the Globe
1. Phleboliths
   (a) Arteriovenous malformation — enlarged orbit and proptosis. ± prominent vascular markings. Can also occur in an arterovenous shunt (e.g. secondary to a traumatic carotico-cavernous fistula).
   (b) Haemangioma — only rarely have calcified phleboliths.
2. Orbital meningioma — 12% calcify (more common in extradural location). 10% show enlargement of the optic foramen. Sclerosis of the orbital apex may be present if extradural in location.
3. Others — rarely in neurofibroma, intraorbital dermoid and adenocarcinoma of the lacrimal gland.

11.10   Hyperostosis in the Orbit

1. **Meningioma.**
2. **Sclerotic metastases.**
3. **Fibrous dysplasia*** — bone expansion may cause some reduction in size of the orbit.
4. **Paget's disease*** — usually widespread changes in the calvarium.
5. **Osteopetrosis*** — and other sclerosing bone dysplasias, see 12.6.
6. **Chronic osteomyelitis** — adjacent to a chronically infected frontal sinus.
7. **Lacrimal gland malignancy.**
8. **Histiocytosis X*.**
9. **Radiotherapy.**

11.11   Small or Absent Sinuses

Congenital
1. **Congenital absence** — absence of the frontal sinuses occur in 5% of the normal population.
2. **Cretinism*.**
3. **Down's syndrome*** — 90% have absent frontal sinuses.
4. **Kartagener's syndrome** — dextrocardia, bronchiectasis and absent frontal sinuses.

Overgrowth of Bony Wall
1. **Paget's disease*.**
2. **Fibrous dysplasia*.**
3. **Haemolytic anaemia*.**
4. **Post Caldwell–Luc operation.**

11.12 Opaque Maxillary Antrum

Traumatic
1. **Fracture** — blood in the antrum.
2. **Overlying soft-tissue swelling** — gives apparent opacification of the antrum.
3. **Postoperative** — washout/Caldwell-Luc.
4. **Epistaxis.**
5. **Barotrauma.**

Inflammatory/Infective
1. Infection.
2. Allergy.
3. Pyocele — infected mucocele (rare in the antrum). Severe systemic symptoms.

Neoplastic
1. Carcinoma — ± bone destruction and extension of the soft-tissue mass.
2. Lymphoma*.

Others
1. Fibrous dysplasia* — ± bone expansion.
2. Cysts — dentigerous and mucous retention cysts may be large enough to fill the antrum.
3. Wegener's granulomatosis.
4. Technical — overtilted view.
5. Anatomical — thick skull vault, sloping antral wall.

11.13   Mass in the Maxillary Antrum

1. Cysts
    (a) Mucous retention cyst — complication of sinusitis. Maxillary antrum is a common site, and it often arises from the floor. Commoner than a polyp, but hard to differentiate between them.
    (b) Dentigerous cyst — expands upwards into the floor of the antrum. The involved tooth may be displaced into the antrum.
2. Trauma — due to 'tear-drop' of prolapsed muscle through the roof of the antrum in an orbital blow-out fracture.
3. Neoplasms
    (a) Polyp — complication of sinusitis.
    (b) Carcinoma — ± bone destruction and soft-tissue mass extending beyond the boundary of the antrum.
4. Wegener's granulomatosis — age usually 40–50. Early mucosal thickening progresses to a mass with bone destruction.

11.14 Cystic Lesion in the Mandible

Dental

1. **Periodontal cyst** — periapical rounded lucency with a sclerotic margin. Due to chronic infection.
2. **Dentigerous cyst** — adjacent to the crown of an unerupted tooth (usually a wisdom tooth or canine). Multiple cysts occur in children with Gorlin's syndrome — multiple basal cell naevi which may become malignant. Autosomal dominant inheritance.

Non-dental

1. **Hyperparathyroidism** — common site for a brown tumour.
2. **Neoplasms**
   (a) Cystic adamantinoma — multilocular. Usually at the angle of the mandible.
   (b) Aneurysmal bone cyst*.
   (c) Giant cell tumour*.
   (d) Haemangioma.
   (e) Histiocytosis X*.
   (f) Metastases.
3. **Fibrous dysplasia*** — rare site.
4. **Bone cyst.**

11.15 'Floating' Teeth

No obvious supporting bone for the teeth.

1. **Severe periodontal disease.**
2. **Histiocytosis X*.**
3. **Hyperparathyroidism*.**
4. **Metastes.**
5. **Multiple myeloma*.**

11.16 Loss of Lamina Dura of Teeth

Generalized
1. Endocrine/metabolic
   (a) Osteoporosis (q.v.).
   (b) Hyperparathyroidism*.
   (c) Cushing's syndrome*.
   (d) Osteomalacia (q.v.).
2. Paget's disease*.
3. Scleroderma* — thickened periodontal membrane.

Localized
1. Infection.
2. Neoplasms — leukaemia, multiple myeloma, metastases, Burkitt's lymphoma, Histiocytosis X.

11.17 Mass in the Nasopharynx

1. Adenoids — enlargement is normal between 1–7 years of age.
2. Trauma — fracture of the base of the skull or upper cervical spine with associated haematoma.
3. Infection — abscess may be confined above C2 by strong attachment of the prevertebral fascia. ± speckled gas in the mass.
4. Neoplasms, benign
   (a) Adolescent angiofibroma — very vascular. Young male — ± spontaneous regression after adolescence. Can cause pressure erosion of the sphenoid and opacification of the antra.
   (b) Antro-choanal polyp.
5. Neoplasms, malignant
   (a) Nasopharyngeal carcinoma.
   (b) Lymphoma*.
   (c) Rhabdomyosarcoma.
   (d) Plasmacytoma*.
   (e) Extension — carcinoma of the sphenoid/ethmoid, and chordoma.
6. Encephalocele — midline defect in the base of the skull.

11.18 Prevertebral Soft-tissue Mass in the Cervical Region

Child
N.B. Anterior buckling of the trachea, which may occur in expiration, flexion or oblique views, can simulate a prevertebral mass. An ear lobe may also mimic a prevertebral mass.
1. **Trauma/haematoma** — ± an associated fracture.
2. **Abscess** — gas lucencies within it.
3. **Neoplasms**
    (a) Neuroblastoma.
    (b) Teratoma.
    (c) Lymphoma*.
    (d) Cystic hygroma.

Adult
1. **Trauma.**
2. **Abscess.**
3. **Neoplasms**
    (a) Post-cricoid carcinoma.
    (b) Lymphoma*.
    (c) Chordoma.
4. **Pharyngeal pouch** — ± air/fluid level within it.
5. **Retropharyngeal goitre.**

See also section 11.17.

Notes

Notes

Chapter 12
Skull and Brain

12.1 Lucency in the Skull Vault, with No Surrounding Sclerosis — Adult

Neoplastic
1. **Multiple myeloma*** — involves cancellous and cortical bone, hence punched out appearance. It can affect the mandible (metastases rarely do) and paranasal sinuses. Lesions are cold on radioisotope bone-scan. The skull may be normal even with widespread lesions elsewhere.
2. **Metastases** — usually irregular and ill defined. Especially breast, kidney, thyroid.
3. **Haemangioma** — may have 'soap bubble' appearance, and can cause 'hair-on-end' appearance (q.v.).
4. **Neurofibroma** — may cause a lucent defect in the occipital bone (usually adjacent to the left lambdoid suture).
5. **Adjacent malignancy** — e.g. rodent ulcer, carcinoma of the ear.
6. **Paget's sarcoma.**

Traumatic
1. **Burr hole** — very well defined.

Idiopathic
1. **Osteoporosis circumscripta** — occurs in the active lytic phase of Paget's disease*. It starts in the lower part of the frontal and occipital regions (i.e. rare in the vertex) and can cross suture lines to involve large areas of the calvarium. Basilar invagination and loss of the lamina dura around the teeth may occur.
2. **Sarcoidosis*** — can occur without other bony lesions in the hands. Usually small and multiple with no sclerotic margin. Can affect inner and outer tables.

Metabolic

1. **Hyperparathyroidism*** — 'pepper pot skull'. Rarely severe enough to cause overt lytic lesions. The calvarium is affected in approximately 20% of primary hyperparathyroidism causing 'pepper pot' appearance. The mandible is a common site for 'brown' tumours and there may be loss of the lamina dura around the teeth. Basilar invagination may occur.

Infective

1. **Tuberculosis** — tuberculous osteomyelitis is much less common than tuberculous arthritis and the skull is a rare site (the spine being the most common). It can produce a punched out lytic lesion.
2. **Hydatid**.
3. **Syphilis** — 'moth-eaten' appearance.

12.2 Lucency in the Skull Vault, with no Surrounding Sclerosis — Child

Neoplastic

1. **Metastases** — especially neuroblastoma and leukaemia. ± wide sutures.
2. **Histiocytosis X*** — eosinophilic granuloma usually produces a solitary lesion which only causes local pain. It can have bevelled edges, due to differential destruction of the inner and outer tables, and can grow several centimetres in size in a few weeks. There is no sclerosis unless the lesion is healing.

   Hand–Schüller–Christian syndrome produces the 'geographical' skull, with associated systemic symptoms. Exophthalmos and diabetes insipidus accompany it in less than 10% of cases. Chronic otitis media, and loose teeth due to surrounding lucencies ('floating' teeth), commonly occur. 'Honeycomb lung' occurs in 10% of cases and worsens the prognosis.

Traumatic

1. **Leptomeningeal cyst** — if the dura is torn, the arachnoid membrane can prolapse, and the pulsations of the CSF can cause progressive widening and scalloping of the fracture line. The bone changes take several weeks to appear and may persist into adult life.

2. **Burr hole.**

N.B. Normal variants such as parietal foramina and venous lakes, apart from having characteristic configurations, will also be 'cold' on a radioisotope bone-scan.

12.3 Lucency in the Skull vault, with Surrounding Sclerosis

Fibrous Dysplasia*

Developmental

1. **Epidermoid** — scalloped appearance with thin sclerotic margins. It is intramedullary in origin and so can expand both inner and outer tables. Although any site is possible, it is commonly in the squamous portion of the occipital or temporal bones.
2. **Meningocele** — this is a mid-line defect and has a smooth sclerotic margin with an overlying soft-tissue mass. It usually occurs in the occipital bone, but may occur in the frontal, parietal or basal bones.

Neoplastic

1. **Haemangioma** — only rarely has a sclerotic margin. Radiating spicules of bone within it are a helpful discriminatory sign.
2. **Histiocytosis X*** — only has a sclerotic margin if it is in the healing phase.

Infective

1. **Chronic osteomyelitis** — sclerosis dominates, with only a few lytic areas.
2. **Frontal sinus mucocoele** — secondary to sinusitis.

Further Reading

Lane B. (1974) Erosions of the Skull. *Radiol. Clin. North Am.*, 12: 257–82.

12.4   Multiple Lucent Lesions in the Skull Vault

1. **Neoplasms**
   (a) Metastases.
   (b) Multiple myeloma*.
   (c) Histiocytosis X*.
2. **Osteomyelitis.**
   (a) Acute — multiple small ill-defined lucencies associated with frontal sinusitis mastoiditis, scalp wound or infected bone flap. There is no surrounding sclerosis or periosteal reaction.
   (b) Chronic — sclerosis becomes a feature.
3. **Avascular necrosis** — of bone flap is identical in appearance to acute osteomyelitis, but it is slower in progression and there is no clinical evidence of an infection.
4. **Radiotherapy** — can cause multiple small lucencies.
5. **Hyperparathyroidism*** — rarely produces overt lytic lesions.
6. **Sarcoidosis*** — can occur without bony lesions in hands. Usually small and multiple with no sclerotic reaction.

12.5   Generalized Thickening of the Skull Vault in Children

With Homogeneous Increased Density
1. **Normal variant.**
2. **Sclerosing bone dysplasias** — see list 12.6.
3. **Chronic decreased intracranial pressure** — in cerebral atrophy or following successful shunting of hydrocephalus.

With Non-homogeneous Sclerosis or No Sclerosis
1. **Chronic haemolytic anaemias.**
2. **Renal osteodystrophy.**
3. **Fibrous dysplasia*.**

Further Reading
Anderson R., Kieffer S.A., Wolfson J.J. & Peterson H.O. (1970) Thickening of the skull in surgically treated hydrocephalus. *Am. J. Roentgenol.*, **110**: 96–101.

Griscom N.T. & Kook Sang O. (1970) The contracting skull; inward growth of the inner table as a physiologic response to diminution of intracranial content in children. *Am. J. Roentgenol.*, **110**: 106–10.

12.6 Bone Dysplasias with Increased Density of the Skull

With Normal Modelling of Long Bones
1. Normal newborn.
2. Osteopetrosis*.
3. Pycnodysostosis.

With Abnormal Modelling of Long Bones
1. Metaphyseal dysplasia (Pyle's disease).
2. Craniometaphyseal dysplasia.
3. Craniodiaphyseal dysplasia.
4. Frontometaphyseal dysplasia.
5. Osteodysplasty (Melnick–Needles syndrome).

With Overgrowth of Long Bones
1. Endosteal hyperostosis — types van Buchem and Worth.
2. Sclerosteosis.
3. Diaphyseal dysplasia (Camurati–Engelmann disease).
4. Hyperphosphatasia.

Further Reading
Kozlowski K. & Beighton P. (1984) *Gamut Index of Skeletal Dysplasias*. Berlin: Springer-Verlag.

12.7 Generalized Increase in Density of the Skull Vault

1. **Paget's disease*** — multiple islands of dense bone. Later the differentiation between the inner and outer tables is lost and the skull vault is thickened (2–5 times normal). Basilar invagination may occur. The sinuses may be involved giving an appearance similar to leontiasis ossea. Loss of lamina dura may occur.

2. **Sclerotic metastases** (q.v.).

3. **Fibrous dysplasia*** — if the lesions are widespread throughout the skeleton, then the skull always has a lesion. However, if only the facial bones and base of skull are involved (leontiasis ossea), the rest of the skeleton is rarely affected. Younger age group than Paget's disease.

4. **Myelosclerosis** — there is endosteal thickening which causes narrowing of the diploë. The spleen is greatly enlarged.

5. **Renal osteodystrophy*** — osteosclerosis occurs in 25%. The skull and spine are commonly involved and can look similar to Paget's disease. ± vascular calcification.

6. **Fluorisis** — mottling of the tooth enamel is a pronounced feature. The calvarium is a rare site for changes to be seen, the axial skeleton being the most frequent. Calcification or muscle attachments.

7. **Acromegaly*** — enlarged frontal sinuses, prognathism, enlarged sella, thick vault.

8. **Phenytoin therapy**.

9. **Chronic haemolytic anaemias**.

10. **Congenital** — see 12.6 and 1.8.

    (a) Osteopetrosis — 'bone in bone' appearance in the spine. The mandible is not affected. Flask-shaped femora.

    (b) Pyknodysostosis — particularly involves the skull base. Wormian bones. Wide sutures.

    (c) Pyle's disease — associated with metaphyseal splaying of the long bones.

12.8 Localized Increase in Density of the Skull Vault

In Bone

1. **Neoplasms**
   (a) Sclerotic metastases (q.v.).
   (b) Osteoma — rare in vault. More common in frontal sinus (ivory osteoma).
   (c) Treated lytic metastases — especially breast primary.
   (d) Treated 'brown' tumour.
2. **Paget's disease***.
3. **Fibrous dysplasia***.
4. **Depressed fracture** — due to overlapping bone fragments.
5. **Benign hyperostosis** — commonly seen in post menopausal females (rare in men). Mainly involves the frontal region, and is characteristically bilateral and symmetrical. Thickening of inner table — 'choppy sea' appearance.

Adjacent to Bone

1. **Meningioma** — mainly involves the inner table, but if it breaks through the outer table it may cause a 'hair-on-end' appearance. About 15% show calcification in the tumour itself. There may be an abnormal increase in the vascular channels and also signs of raised intracranial pressure. The characteristic sites are parasagittal, olfactory groove, sphenoid ridge and tentorium.
2. **Calcified sebaceous cyst.**
3. **Old cephalhaematoma** — it is usually in the parietal region, and may be bilateral.
4. **Soft-tissue tumours** — e.g. neurofibroma, sebaceous cyst.
5. **Hair bunch.**

12.9 Increase in Density of the Skull Base

Localized

1. Fibrous dysplasia*.
2. Meningioma.
3. Sclerotic metastases (q.v.).
4. Chronic suppurative otitis media.

Generalized

1. Paget's disease*.
2. Fibrous dysplasia*.
3. Other causes of generalized increase in bone density (q.v.).

12.10   Destruction of Petrous Bone — Apex

1. **Acoustic neuroma** — eighth nerve. Increase in size of IAM (greater than 1 cm in diameter or more than 2 mm asymmetry between the sides). Erosion of the crista transversalis and apparent 'shortening' of the IAM may occur. Bilateral in neurofibromatosis.
2. **Congenital cholesteatoma** — lytic defect with no sclerosis. Petrous ridge may be elevated. Seventh nerve may be involved (this is rare in acoustic neuroma).
3. **Meningioma.**
4. **Metastases** — particularly breast, kidney and lung. Irregular lytic defect. Pain, bleeding and nerve palsy are common.
5. **Fifth nerve neuroma.**
6. **Nasopharyngeal carcinoma** — usually large area of destruction in the floor of the middle cranial fossa also.
7. **Chordoma.**
8. **Apical petrositis.**

Further Reading
Livingstone P.A. (1974) Differential diagnosis of radiolucent lesions of the temporal bone. *Radiol. Clin. North Am.*, 12: 571–83.

12.11   Destruction of Petrous Bone — Middle Ear

Adult
1. **Acquired cholesteatoma** — usually diagnosed by auroscopy. Bony destruction extending from the epitympanic recess, with clear cut but not sclerotic margins. Earliest sign is destruction of the spur (80%). Ossicles may be destroyed. The mastoid antrum is often sclerotic due to the associated chronic infection.
2. **Carcinoma of the middle ear** — 30% associated with chronic otitis media. Pain and bleeding are late. 12% show bone destruction (particularly of the articular fossa of the temporomandibular joint).
3. **Metastases.**
4. **Glomus jugulare** — the jugular foramen is enlarged and destroyed, with minimal or no sclerosis. Very vascular — can look like an aneurysm.
5. **Tuberculosis** — rare. Destruction with no sclerosis. May be no evidence of TB elsewhere.

Child
1. **Rhabdomyosarcoma** — commonest primary malignancy of ear in childhood. Pain is rare.

Further Reading
Phelps P.D. & Lloyd G.A.S. (1981) The radiology of carcinoma of the ear. *Br. J. Radiol.* 54: 103–9.
Phelps P.D. & Lloyd G.A.S. (1980) The radiology of cholesteatoma. *Clin. Radiol.* 31: 501–12.
Livingstone P.A. (1974) Differential diagnosis of radiolucent lesions of the temporal bone. *Radiol. Clin. North Am.*, 12: 571–83.

12.12   Metastases in the Skull Base

1. **Breast**
2. **Bronchus** } metastatic disease is best shown by CT.
3. **Prostate**

Patients may present with one of four clinical syndromes:
   Orbital syndrome — pain, diplopia, proptosis and external ophthalmoplegia.
   Parasellar and middle fossa syndrome — headache, ocular paresis without proptosis and facial numbness caused by invasion of the maxillary and mandibular divisions of the fifth cranial nerve. Radiographic changes occur late.
   Jugular foramen syndrome — hoarseness and dysphagia. Radiography is often normal.
   Occipital condyle syndrome — stiffness and pain in the neck, worse on flexion.

The differential diagnosis of these clinical syndromes includes:
1. **Carotid or vertebrobasilar aneurysm.**
2. **Tolosa Hunt syndrome.**
3. **Primary neoplasms of the skull base.**

Further Reading
Kagan R.A., Steckel R.J., Bassett L.W. & Gold R.H. (1986) Radiologic contributions to cancer management. Bone metastases. *Am. J. Roentgenol.*, 147: 305–12.

12.13   Basilar Invagination

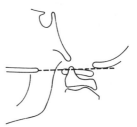

McGregor's line (tip of hard
palate to the base of the occiput).
The tip of the odontoid peg is
normally less than 0.5 cm above
this line. If basilar invagination is
severe obstructive hydrocephalus
may occur.

Primary Anomalies of the Occiput, Atlas and Axis

Generalized Bone Disease
1. Rickets*/osteomalacia (q.v.).
2. Paget's disease*.
3. Fibrous dysplasia*.

Delayed or Defective Cranial Ossification
1. Osteogenesis imperfecta*.
2. Achondroplasia*.
3. Cleidocranial dysplasia*.
4. Cranial thinning in hydrocephalus.
N.B.
1. Platybasia — does not
   always accompany basi-
   lar invagination, but
   occurs in similar circum-
   stances. The index of this
   is the basal angle, normal
   < 140°. By itself it is
   symptomless, but if
   associated with basilar
   invagination, then
   obstructive hydrocephalus may occur.

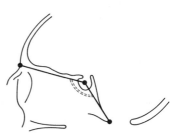

Basal angle

2. **Basilar invagination** — elevation of the floor of the
   posterior cranial fossa. This may be associated with
   anomalies of the cervical spine such as atlanto-occipital
   fusion or Klippel–Feil syndrome.

Further Reading
Dolan K.D. (1977) Cervicobasilar relationships. *Radiol. Clin. North
    Am.*, 15: 155–66.

12.14 'Hair-on-end' Skull Vault

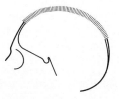

Haemolytic Anaemias

1. **Sickle-cell anaemia*** — occurs in 5%. Begins in the frontal region and can affect all the calvarium except that which is below the internal occipital protuberance, since there is no marrow in this area. The diploic space is widened due to marrow hyperplasia.

2. **Thalassaemia*** — marrow hyperplasia in thalassaemia major is more marked than in any other anaemia. May be severe enough to cause marrow hyperplasia of the facial bones, resulting in obliteration of the maxillary antra. (This does not occur in sickle-cell anaemia.)

3. **Others** — hereditary spherocytosis, elliptocytosis and pyruvate kinase deficiency.

Neoplastic

1. **Haemangioma.**

2. **Meningioma** — only rarely, when it breaks through the outer table.

3. **Neuroblastoma metastases** — may involve the sutures (particularly coronal suture) also, causing widening and irregularity. Orbital deposits causing proptosis are common.

4. **Osteosarcoma** — very rare.

5. **Plasmacytoma*** — spiculation may occur with the expansion of the diploë (usually parietal or occipital).

Others

1. **Cyanotic heart disease** — due to erythroid hyperplasia. Hypertrophic pulmonary osteoarthropathy may occur.

2. **Iron-deficiency anaemia** — severe childhood cases.

12.15 Craniostenosis

Simple Primary

1. **Scaphocephaly** — long, narrow, 'boat-shaped' skull. Commonest type. Premature fusion of the sagittal suture. Usually uncomplicated and relatively benign but may be part of a complex craniofacial malformation.
2. **Trigonocephaly** — premature fusion of the metopic suture. Wedge-shaped frontal region with a narrow forehead and hypotelorism.
3. **Turricephaly, oxycephaly and acrocephaly** — high forehead with a 'tower-' or 'turret-shaped' head. Premature fusion of the coronal and sphenofrontal sutures. This type of skull deformity is present in the acrocephalosyndactyly syndromes (Apert, Carpenter, Pfeiffer and Saethre–Chotzen).
4. **Plagiocephaly** — asymmetry of the skull due to asymmetrical sutural fusion.
5. **Triphyllocephaly** — 'cloverleaf skull' or *Kleeblattschädel* Trilobular skull with temporal and frontal bulges.

Complex Primary

1. **Apert syndrome (acrocephalosyndactyly, type 1)**
   (a) Acrocephaly with shallow orbits.
   (b) Mental retardation.
   (c) Severe osseous and cutaneous syndactyly (mitten hands and feet).
   (d) Abnormal thumb and hallux.
2. **Carpenter syndrome (acrocephalopolysyndactyly)** — similar to Apert syndrome but distinguished from it by
   (a) Duplication of the proximal phalanx of the thumb and hallux.
   (b) Cardiac abnormalities, obesity and hypogonadism may also be present.
3. **Crouzon syndrome (craniofacial dysostosis)**
   (a) Craniostenosis of the sagittal, coronal and lambdoid sutures.
   (b) Midface hypoplasia with relative mandibular prognathism.
   (c) Hypertelorism and proptosis.
   (d) Normal intelligence.
   (e) Normal hands.

Secondary
1. **Microcephaly** — failure of brain growth in the first few years of life.
2. **Treatment of severe hydrocephalus** — by low pressure ventricular shunting.

Metabolic Disorders Sometimes Complicated by Craniostenosis
1. **Rickets.**
2. **Hyperthyroidism.**
3. **Polycythaemia.**
4. **Thalassaemia*.**

Further Reading
David D.J., Poswillo D. & Simpson D. (1982) *The Craniosynostoses.* Berlin: Springer-Verlag.

12.16 Wormian Bones

A few wormian bones may be considered as normal; only when multiple should they be considered significant.
1. **Osteogenesis imperfecta***
2. **Cleidocranial dysplasia*** — autosomal dominant. Brachycephaly with open sutures and anterior fontanelle. The teeth are always poorly formed/delayed and multiple supernumerary teeth may be present. Small facial bones.
3. **Pyknodysostosis** — autosomal recessive. Short-limbed dwarf, with some features of osteopetrosis and cleidocranial dysplasia.
4. **Hypophosphatasia*** — autosomal recessive. Low alkaline phosphatase, and excessive phosphoethanolamine in the urine. Premature fusion of the sutures.
5. **Cretinism*** — delayed, fragmented epiphyses. There is usually a hypoplastic 'bullet-shaped' vertebra at L1 or L2 level.
6. **Acro-osteolysis** — particularly Hajdu-Cheney syndrome.
7. **Chromosomal disorders** — particularly trisomy 21.
8. **Pachydermoperiostosis.**
9. **Menkes kinky hair syndrome.**
10. **Increased frequency in mentally retarded individuals.**

Further Reading
Pryles C.V. Khan A.J. (1979) Wormian bones. *Am. J. Dis. Child.,* 133: 380–2.

12.17 Defective Ossification of the Skull Vault

1. Retarded ossification of the calvarium.
2. Wormian bones.
3. Large fontanelles.
4. Wide sutures.

Bone Dysplasias

1. **Osteogenesis imperfecta***.
2. **Cleidocranial dysplasia***.
3. **Cretinism***.
4. **Hypophosphatasia***.
5. **Pycnodysostosis** — dense bones, hypoplastic outer ends of clavicles and short terminal phalanges.
6. **Osteodysplasty (Melnick–Needles syndrome).**

12.18 Raised Intracranial Pressure

Child

1. **Suture diastasis** — occurs easily up to the age of 8 years and may take only a few days to appear. Particularly noticeable in coronal and sagittal sutures. If chronic, excess interdigitations may be seen.
2. **Increased head size.**
3. **Craniolacunia** — oval/finger-shaped pits on inner table, with bony ridges between. Seen in the neonate and gradually fade by 6 months. Associated with myelomeningocoele, encephalocoele, aqueduct stenosis and Arnold–Chiari malformation.
4. **Erosion of the dorsum sellae** — late sign (takes several weeks to develop). Only seen in 30%. If no associated suture diastasis, then look for parasellar pathology.
5. **Increased convolutional markings** — unreliable. Normal variant age 4–10 years.

Adult

1. Erosion of the dorsum sellae — occurs earliest at the base of the dorsum sellae.
2. Pineal displacement — if the raised intracranial pressure is due to a space occupying lesion.
3. Calcification — may occur in space occupying lesion.

N.B. If symptoms have been present for longer than 5 weeks, then 30% have signs on SXR. Headache and papilloedema may be absent even in the presence of signs on the SXR.

1. **Space-occupying lesion**
   (a) Tumour.
   (b) Abscess.
   (c) Haematoma — intracerebral, extra/subdural.
2. **Obstructive hydrocephalus**
   (a) Communicating — e.g. post-meningitis/subarachnoid haemorrhage, superior sagittal sinus thrombosis.
   (b) Non-communicating — e.g. congenital stenosis, SOL causing obstruction to ventricular pathway.
3. **Craniostenosis.**
4. **Cerebral oedema.**
5. **Toxic** — e.g. lead.

12.19   Large Head in Infancy

1. **Hydrocephalus** — this may be congenital or acquired. Commonest congenital causes are aqueduct stenosis, stenosis of the foramen of Monroe (producing unilateral ventricular enlargement), Dandy–Walker cyst and Arnold–Chiari malformation. Acquired hydrocephalus most commonly follows meningitis or an intracranial haemorrhage.
2. **Hydranencephaly.**
3. **Benign external hydrocephalus** — onset at about 9 months of age with a self limiting course. Prominent forehead clinically. Large ventricles with wide sulci.
4. **Subdural haematoma.**
5. **Congenital syndromes** — chondrodystrophies i.e. achondroplasia, achondrogenesis, thanatophoric dwarfism and metatropic dwarfism, cleidocranial dysplasia, Soto's syndrome, Beckwith–Wiedmann syndrome.
6. **Megalencephaly.**
7. **Storage diseases** — MPS etc.
8. **Neurofibromatosis***.

Further Reading
DeMeyer W. (1972) Megalencephaly in children. *Neurology*, 22: 634–43.
Harwood-Nash D.C. & Fitz C.R. (1975) Large heads and ventricles in infants. *Radiol. Clin. North Am.*, 13: 119–224.
Holt J.F. & Kuhns L.R. (1976) Macrocranium and macrocephaly in neurofibromatosis. *Skeletal Radiol.*, 1: 25–8.

12.20   Wide Sutures

1. Birth to 1 month — suture width greater than 1 cm.
2. Over 3 months — suture width greater than 3 mm.
Beware the normal prominent coronal suture in infancy. If the saggital suture is normal the appearance of the coronal suture is probably physiological.

Raised Intracranial Pressure (q.v.)
Suture diastasis only if onset before 10 years of age.
1. **Space-occupying lesion.**
2. **Hydrocephalus.**
3. **Deprivational dwarfism** — when children are removed from their deprived environment rebound growth of brain and skull occurs. Rapid brain growth results in raised intracranial pressure and separation of sutures.

Infiltration of the Sutures
1. **Neuroblastoma** — ± lucencies in skull vault and 'sunray' spiculation (a reaction to subpericranial deposits).
2. **Leukaemia** ⎱
3. **Lymphoma*** ⎰ — in children.

Defective Ossification
1. **Rickets*.**
2. **Renal osteodystrophy*.**
3. **Bone dysplasias with defective skull mineralization** — see list 12.17.

Further Reading
Capitanio M.A. & Kirkpatrick J.A. (1969) Widening of the cranial sutures, a roentgen observation during periods of accelerated growth in patients treated for deprivation dwarfism. *Radiology*, 92: 53–9.

Swischuk L.E. (1974) The growing skull. *Semin. Roentgenol.*, 9: 115–24.

Swischuk L.E. (1984) *Differential Diagnosis in Paediatric Radiology*, pp. 347–9. Baltimore: Williams and Wilkins.

12.21 Pneumocephalus

1. **Trauma** — fracture of the ethmoid or frontal sinuses is commonest. Fluid levels in sinus. Dural tear permits CSF rhinorrea (positive for glucose).
2. **Iatrogenic** — postoperative/air encephalogram.
3. **Abscess.**
4. **Osteoma** — if erodes cribriform plate.
5. **Nasopharyngeal/ethmoid carcinoma.**

12.22 Small Pituitary Fossa

1. **Normal variant.**
2. **Dystrophia myotonica** — hereditary. Usually starts in early adult life. Cataracts, frontal baldness, testicular atrophy, thick skull and large frontal sinus.
3. **Radiotherapy as child.**
4. **Hypopituitarism.**

12.23 Expanded Pituitary Fossa

1. Size — normal range is: height 6.5–11 mm
   length 9–16 mm
   breadth 9–19 mm
2. **Double floor** — can be a normal variant (asymmetrical development), but a tumour should be suspected.
3. **Elevation/destruction of clinoid processes.**
4. **Loss of lamina dura.**

1. **Para/intrasellar mass.**
   (a) Pituitary adenoma
      (i) Chromophobe (non-functioning); commonest cause of expansion and commonest adenoma to produce suprasellar extension. 10% do not expand the sella.
      (ii) eosinophilic (acromegaly); only slight expansion.
      (iii) basophilic (Cushing's syndrome); virtually never expands.
   (b) Craniopharyngioma — 50% cause expansion — usually slight.
   (c) Prolactinoma — typically a blister on the antero-inferior wall. SXR abnormal in 20%. Tomography detects abnormality in 50%. CT useful for detecting suprasellar extension.
      N.B. Other causes of hyperprolactinaemia are:
      (i) Physiological — pregnancy.
      (ii) Drugs — phenothiazines, tricyclics, methyldopa, metoclopramide and oral contraceptives.
      (iii) Hypothalamic and stalk lesions — encephalitis, tumours, trauma and histiocytosis X.
      (iv) Severe hypothyroidism.
      (v) Renal failure.
   (d) Meningioma — usually produces sclerosis, but may cause erosion and expansion of the sella.
   (e) Aneurysm — well-defined pressure resorption of bone ± curvilinear calcification.
2. **Raised intracranial pressure** (q.v.) — due to dilated third ventricle.

3. **Empty sella**
   (a) Primary — defect in diaphragma sellae allows pulsating CSF to expand the sella. Typically obese with hypertension. Headache common. Visual and endocrine defects uncommon. Associated with benign intracranial hypertension. SXR abnormal in 85% — symmetrical expansion with no erosion.
   (b) Secondary — pituitary tumour or treatment of a pituitary lesion may distort the diaphragma sellae.
4. **Nelson's syndrome** — post adrenalectomy for Cushing's syndrome.

Further Reading

Doyle F.H. (1979) Radiology of the pituitary fossa. In: Lodge T. & Steiner R.E. (eds) *Recent Advances in Radiology*, Vol. 6, pp. 121–43. Edinburgh, Churchill Livingstone.

Sage M.R., Chan E.S.H. & Reilly P.L. (1980) The clinical and radiological features of the empty sella syndrome. *Clin. Radiol.*, 31: 513–19.

Teasdale E., Macpherson P. & Teasdale G. (1981) The reliability of radiology in detecting prolactin-secreting pituitary microadenomas. *Brit. J. Radiol.*, 54: 556–71.

12.24 J-shaped Sella

Flattened tuberculum sellae with a prominent sulcus chiasmaticus. Rare in adults.

1. **Normal variant** — 5% of normal children.
2. **Optic chiasm glioma** — if the chiasmatic sulcus is markedly depressed (W- or omega-shaped sella), the tumour may be bilateral.
3. **Chronic hydrocephalus** — due to downward pressure of an enlarged third ventricle.
4. **Mucopolysaccharidoses.**
5. **Achondroplasia***.
6. **Neurofibromatosis*** — sphenoid dysplasia.

12.25   Erosion and Osteoporosis of the Sella, with no Expansion

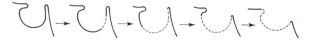

1. **Erosion** — the earliest sign is interruption of the lamina dura at the base of the dorsum sellae. The line of the lamina dura should normally be complete, even in the elderly, and any defect is significant.
2. **Osteoporosis** (q.v.) — the cortex may become blurred.

Raised Intracranial Pressure (q.v.) — commonest cause of erosion. (In children, suture diastasis is a more prominent sign.) 30% show this if raised ICP has been present more than 5–6 weeks. In 20% of those with X-ray changes papilloedema is not present.

Parasellar Masses
1. Craniopharyngioma.
2. Meningioma.
3. Pituitary adenoma.
4. Aneurysm.
5. Chordoma.
6. Metastases — kidney, bronchus, breast, prostate, malignant melanoma.
7. Local invasion — (e.g. carcinoma of the sphenoid or nasopharynx).

Generalized Decrease in Bone Density
1. Osteoporosis (q.v.).
2. Osteomalacia (q.v.).
3. Hyperparathyroidism*.

Malignant Hypertension

12.26 Unifocal Intracranial Calcification

Physiological — pineal, choroid plexus, etc.

Neoplastic
1. **Glioma** — overall 5–10% calcify, especially if slow growing. About 20% of astrocytomas and 50% of oligodendrogliomas calcify (the latter being typically serpiginous in form), but astrocytomas are much more common.
2. **Meningioma** — 15% calcify (characteristically homogeneous and rounded) in psammoma bodies. Hyperostosis and an increase in the vascular channels may be seen.
3. **Metastases** — may occasionally calcify, particularly from colon, breast and osteosarcoma.
4. **Craniopharyngioma** — 90% calcify in children and 40% in adults. Two types — solid (walnut sized) and cystic (may be very large). The sella is abnormal (expanded or eroded) in 50%.
5. **Chordoma** — 50% show dense calcification adjacent to the clivus. 50% erode the clivus and reactive bone sclerosis may occur at the margins. 30% may have a nasopharyngeal mass. Skeletal metastases may occur.
6. **Others**
   (a) Pituitary adenoma (chromophobe) — 1–6% calcify.
   (b) Pinealoma — suspect if pineal calcification is greater than 1 cm in diameter or occurs below the age of ten.
   (c) Lipoma — characteristically two curvilinear bands of calcification, one on each side of the corpus callosum.
   (d) Hamartoma — usually in temporal lobe.
   (e) Teratoma — 50% occur in the pineal region and usually present in the first decade of life.
   (f) Dermoid — majority in the midline of the posterior cranial fossa (cerebellar vermis, fourth ventricle, and base of skull). Usually presents in adolescence.
   (g) Epidermoid — majority not in the midline. Cerebellopontine angle is the commonest site. These inclusions can also occur in the skull vault.
   (h) Choroid plexus papilloma — the commonest site is the fourth ventricle in children, and the temporal horn of the lateral ventricle in adults.

Vascular

1. **Atherosclerosis** — usually carotid siphon.
2. **Aneurysm** — 1% calcify. (Most patients present with subarachnoid haemorrhage and these aneurysms virtually never show calcification.) However, 'giant' aneurysms greater than 2.5 cm in diameter show curvilinear calcification in 50% of cases and are large enough to cause erosion of the sella in 20%.
3. **Arteriovenous malformations** — 15% calcify. Vascular grooves may be prominent.
4. **Chronic subdural haematoma** — 1–5% calcify. 15% bilateral. Usually parietal region.
5. **Old infarct.**
6. **Sturge–Weber syndrome** — capillary and venous agiomas associated with ipsilateral cutaneous 'port wine' naevus. The calcification is gyriform and occurs in the occipital/parietal region. The hemicranium is smaller on the affected side. Association with coarctation of the aorta.

Infective

1. **Abscess** — calcification occurs late. Usually frontal/temporal regions.
2. **Tuberculoma** — 1–5% calcify. Usually multiple but can be solitary.
3. **Tuberculous meningitis** — 50% of those children who recover show calcification which is usually in the thickened basal meninges. It takes 15 months–3 years to develop. Obstructive hydrocephalus is common.

Extracerebral (i.e. mimics intracranial calcification)

1. Calcified sebaceous cyst.
2. Osteoma of the calvarium.
3. Foreign body.

12.27 Multifocal Intracranial Calcification

Infective

1. **Toxoplasmosis** — transplacental infection of the fetus. 80% show nodular calcification in infancy (cortical, basal ganglia, periventricular). Microcephaly, dilated ventricles and bilateral choroidoretinitis are usually present.
2. **Cytomegalovirus/rubella** — may be indistinguishable from toxoplasmosis, but tends to be more periventricular in distribution.
3. **Cysticercosis** — calcification occurs in the dead cysts of *Taenia solium*, and takes 1–10 years to develop. It is always supratentorial and is about 0.5 cm in size. Only 5% of infections produce cysts in the brain.
4. **Hydatid** — only 2% of infections produce cysts in the brain and these rarely calcify.
5. **Others** — tuberculomata, histoplasmosis, coccidiomycosis, cryptococcosis, torulosis, paragonimiasis.

Metabolic

1. **Hypo-, pseudohypo- and pseudopseudohypoparathyroidism*** — characteristically basal ganglia.
2. **Chronic renal failure.**
3. **Excess vitamin D.**

Toxic

1. **Lead** — subcortical, basal ganglia and cerebellar.
2. **Carbon monoxide.**

Tuberous Sclerosis*

Scattered nodular calcification (mm's – 1 cm in size). Cortical and periventricular. The nodules may bulge into the ventricle. Calcification not visible until 2 years old. 15% develop glioma (characteristically at the foramen of Munro) in adolescence. Multiple hamartomas occur in other organs, particularly kidney. Periosteal thickening may be seen in the phalanges.

Further Reading

Reyes P.F., Gonzalez C.F., Zalewska M.K. & Besarab A. (1986) Intracranial calcification in adults with chronic lead exposure. *Am. J. Roentgenol.*, 146: 267–70.

12.28 Parasellar Calcification

Neoplastic
1. Craniopharyngioma.
2. Meningioma.
3. Pituitary adenoma (chromophobe).
4. Chordoma.
5. Optic chiasm glioma.
6. Cholesteatoma.

Vascular
1. **Aneurysm** — circle of Willis or basilar artery.
2. **Atheroma** — carotid siphon.

Infective
1. **Tuberculous meningitis** — calcification in the basal meninges.

12.29 Basal Ganglia Calcification

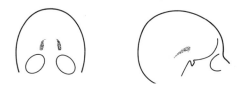

Idiopathic
Accounts for over 50% of cases and can be familial.

Metabolic
1. **Hypoparathyroidism*** — commonest pathological cause. Low serum calcium.
2. **Pseudohypoparathyroidism*** — short 4th and 5th metacarpals. End organ unresponsiveness to parathormone.
3. **Pseudopseudohypoparathyroidism***.
4. **Hyperparathyroidism***.

Infective
1. Congenital cytomegalovirus.
2. Congenital toxoplasmosis.

Toxic
1. Lead — subcortical, basal ganglia and cerebellar.
2. Carbon monoxide.

Others
1. Tuberous sclerosis*.
2. Fahr's disease — presents in childhood with choreoathetoid movements and progressive mental deterioration.
3. Cockayne's syndrome — microcephaly and truncal dwarfism. Progeria. Also has cortical calcification.

Further Reading
Reyes P.F., Gonzalez C.F., Zalewska M.K. & Besarab A. (1986) Intracranial calcification in adults with chronic lead exposure. *Am. J. Roentgenol.*, 146: 267–70.

12.30 Curvilinear Calcification

Vascular
1. Aneurysm.
2. Atheroma.
3. Angioma.
4. Haematoma.

Neoplastic
1. Cystic glioma (astrocytoma).
2. Cystic craniopharyngioma.
3. Teratoma.
4. Lipoma of corpus callosum.

12.31 Surface Enhancement of the Brain

Rim or Linear Enhancement

Indicates the presence of an abnormal fluid collection over the surface of the brain. The enhancing rim is either a segment of normal dura displaced by an extradural collection or arachnoid membrane displaced by a subdural collection.

1. **Haematoma.**
2. **Empyema** — a thick and/or serpiginous outline differentiates a subdural empyema from an uninfected subdural haematoma.

Gyriform Enhancement

WIDESPREAD i.e. DISSEMINATED MENINGEAL DISEASE no mass effect; no accompanying oedema.

1. **Infection** — viral, bacterial or tuberculous.
2. **Tumour** — primary or secondary.
3. **Sarcoidosis***.
4. **Lymphoma***.

FOCAL

1. **Arteriovenous malformation.**
2. **Infarction**
3. **Encephalitis**   } parenchymal lesions infiltrating the
4. **Glioma**   cortex and obliterating the sulci.

Basal Cistern Enhancement

1. **Tuberculous meningitis** — often accompanied by hydrocephalus and infarction which are bad prognostic indicators.
2. **Meningeal neoplasms.**
3. **Torulosis.**

Further Reading

Burrows E.H. (1985) Surface enhancement of the brain. *Clin. Radiol.*, 36: 233–9.

12.32 Posterior Fossa Neoplasms in Childhood

50–60% of paediatric cerebral tumours. Majority arise within the 4th ventricle and cerebellum. Cerebellar astrocytomas, medulloblastomas and ependymomas present with symptoms of raised intracranial pressure and ataxia. Brain stem gliomas involve the cranial nerve nuclei and long tracts at an early stage.

1. **Cerebellar astrocytoma** — 20–25% of posterior fossa tumours. Vermis (50%) or hemispheres (20%) or both sites (30%) ± extension into the cavity of 4th ventricle. Calcification in 20%.

   CT
   Large lesion displacing 4th ventricle → obstructive hydrocephalus. Cystic type (80%) — well defined cyst > CSF attenuation. 50% have a mural nodule (usually iso-dense) which shows enhancement or a multicystic mass with enhancement of the main bulk of the tumour, cyst walls and cerebellum beyond the cysts. Larger tumour at diagnosis than the solid type. Solid type (20%) — low density lesion with less well-defined margins; more inhomogeneous. Homogeneous, ring or no enhancement. May only be detected by the surrounding oedema.

   CT will detect recurrence long before onset of symptoms. Attenuation of recurrent cystic tumour 2x CSF.

2. **Medulloblastoma** — 50% occur in first decade; second peak in adults. 20–40% of all posterior fossa tumours. In childhood — 85% are midline; adults — more laterally in the cerebellar hemispheres. Increased incidence in Basal Cell Naevus Syndrome.

   CT
   Moderately well defined, ovoid or spherical mass; slightly > surrounding cerebellum; rim of oedema. Usually uniform enhancement; non-enhancement rarely. Calcification (in 10%) is usually small, homogeneous and eccentric. Dystrophic calcification occurs after radiotherapy. Small cystic or necrotic areas are unusual.

   Dissemination by (1) seeding of the subarachnoid space, (2) retrograde ventricular extension or (3) extracranial metastases bone, lymph nodes or soft tissues.

Recurrence of tumour is demonstrated by (1) enhancement at the site of the lesion, (2) enhancement of the subarachnoid space (basal cisterns, Sylvian, fissures, sulci and ependymal surfaces of ventricles, or (3) progressive ventricular enlargement.

3. **Ependymoma** — most commonly in the floor of the 4th ventricle. Usually solitary but may be multiple in neurofibromatosis.

CT

Variable features. 80% isodense; non-homogeneous or homogeneous enhancement. Calcification in 50% — small round calculi. Calcification within a 4th ventricular mass or adjacent to the 4th ventricle ≡ ependymoma. Small lucencies in 50%.

4. **Brainstem glioma** — insidious onset because of the location and tendency to infiltrate cranial nerve nuclei and long tracts without producing CSF obstruction until late. Pons > midbrain. They frequently extend down into medulla and cervical cord, up into thalamus or posterolaterally along the cerebellar peduncle into the hemisphere.

CT

Usually low density, either same as or lower than adjacent tissue. Non-homogeneous contrast enhancement minimum θ moderate. Calcification is extremely uncommon. May be cystic.

5. **Choroid plexus papilloma** — commonest in the lateral ventricle but may be in 4th.

Further Reading

Faerber E.N. (1986) *Cranial Computed Tomography In Infants and Children*. Chapter 9, pp. 171–204. London: Spastics International Medical Publications.

12.33 CT Attenuation of Cerebral masses
(relative to normal brain)

Hyperdense
1. Neoplasms
   - (a) Meningioma 95%.
   - (b) Microglioma (primary lymphoma).
   - (c) Metastases 30%.
   - (d) Glioma 10% (most glioblastomas show mixed attenuation).
   - (e) Ependymoma.
   - (f) Papilloma.
   - (g) Medulloblastoma 80%.
   - (h) Pituitary adenoma 25%.
   - (i) Craniopharyngioma (if solid).
   - (j) Acoustic neuroma 5%.
2. Haematoma — if ≤ 2 weeks old.
3. Giant aneurysm.
4. Colloid cyst — 50%.

Isodense
1. Neoplasms
   - (a) Acoustic neuroma 95%.
   - (b) Pituitary adenoma 65%.
   - (c) Glioma 10%.
   - (d) Metastases 10%.
   - (e) Chordoma.
   - (f) Pinealoma.
2. Haematoma — if 2–4 weeks old.
3. Tuberculoma.
4. Colloid cyst — 50%.

Hypodense
1. Tumours
   - (a) Craniopharyngioma.
   - (b) Glioma (95% of astrocytomas).
   - (c) Metastases.
   - (d) Prolactinoma.
   - (e) Haemangioblastoma.
   - (f) Lipoma.
   - (g) Epidermoid.
   - (h) Dermoid.

2. **Haematoma** — ± if >4 weeks old.
3. **Abscess** — pyogenic.
4. **Tuberculoma.**
5. **Cyst**
    (a) Arachnoid.
    (b) Porencephalic.
    (c) Hydatid.

12.34 CT Appearances of Cerebral Masses

A.

Tumours	Attenuation (μ)	Surrounding oedema	Contrast enhancement
Glioma	Increased or decreased (if cystic/necrotic)	Yes	95% if high grade; relatively infrequent in low grade; often *irregular ring*, but may be homogeneous or patchy
Metastases	Increased or decreased; often multifocal	Yes, extensive	Marked; may be *irregular ring*, homogeneous or patchy
Meningioma	Increased; multifocal in 5%	Minimal, perifocal (moderate in 20%)	Marked, homogeneous
Microglioma (i.e. primary lymphoma)	Increased (occasionally decreased, infiltrating); multifocal 50%	Yes	Marked, homogeneous
Pituitary adenoma	Isodense 65%; increased 25%	No	Marked, homogeneous
Prolactinoma	Hypodense	No	No
Craniopharyngioma	Decreased if cystic; increased if solid	No	± moderate homogeneous (solid), or *ring* (cystic)
Pinealoma	Isodense	No	Marked, homogeneous
Acoustic neuroma	Isodense 95%; increased 5%	No	Marked, homogeneous
Epidermoid (cholesteatoma)	Decreased	No	No
Medulloblastoma	Increased	Minimal, perifocal	Moderate, homogeneous
Haemangioblastoma	Decreased	Minimal	Moderate, homogeneous

Dermoid	Decreased	No	No
Chordoma	Isodense, poorly defined	No	Variable

Lipoma	Decreased	No	No
Papilloma	Increased	No	Marked, homogeneous
Ependymoma	Increased	May occur	± patchy
Glomus jugulare	Isodense	No	Moderate

B.

Infections	Attenuation (μ)	Surrounding oedema	Contrast enhancement
Pyogenic abscess	Decreased	Yes	*Regular-ring* (thin walled)
Tuberculoma	Decreased or isodense; often multifocal	Yes	*Regular or irregular ring*; ± central ('target') enhancement characteristic
Hydatid	Decreased	No	No

C.

Vascular	Attenuation (μ)	Surrounding oedema	Contrast enhancement
Giant aneurysm	Increased	No	*Ring* or homogeneous
Arteriovenous malformation	± patchy increased	± patchy low attenuation due to surrounding infarcts	± marked, sinuous
Haematoma	Increased if fresh (isodense at 2 weeks; ± decreased at 4 weeks)	No	No (some peripheral enhancement may occur during the resorption phase)

D.

Cysts	Attenuation (μ)	Surrounding oedema	Contrast enhancement
Colloid	Increased 50%; isodense 50%	No	No
Arachnoid	Decreased (CSF)	No	No
Porencephalic	Decreased (CSF)	No	No

Further Reading

Lange S., Grumme T. & Meese W. (1980) *Computerized Tomography of the Brain*. Berlin: Schering A.G. Medico-scientific book series.

Bibliography

duBoulay G.H. (1980) *Principles of X-Ray Diagnosis of the Skull*, 2nd edn. London: Butterworths.

Chase N.E. & Kricheff I.I. (eds) (1974) The skull and brain. *Radiol. Clin. North Am.*, 12 (2).

Felson B. (ed.) (1974) The normal skull and its variations. *Semin. Roetgenol.*, 9 (2).

Leeds N.E. (ed.) (1982) Neuroradiology. *Radiol. Clin. North Am.*, 20 (1).

Sutton D. (ed.) (1980) *Textbook of Radiology and Imaging*, 3rd edn., chaps. 56–8, 63–4. Edinburgh: Churchill Livingstone.

Notes

Chapter 13
Nuclear Medicine

Keith Harding

13.1 Increased Uptake on Bone Scans

1. **Metastatic disease** — multiple, randomly scattered lesions especially in the axial skeleton.
2. **Joint disease** — commonly degenerative in the cervical spine, hips, hands, knees. Also inflammatory joint disease.
3. **Traumatic fractures**
   (a) Aligned fractures in ribs are traumatic.
   (b) Single lesions elsewhere — always ask if history of trauma.
   (c) Stress fractures.
4. **Post surgery** — after joint replacement. Increased uptake lasts 1 year.
5. **Paget's disease*** — diffuse involvement with much increased uptake. Commonly affects the pelvis, skull, femur, and spine. Involvement of the whole of the vertebra is typical.
6. **Super scan** — high uptake throughout the skeleton often due to disseminated secondary disease with poor or absent renal images but often with bladder activity. Look carefully at the skull and ribs where the inhomogeneity may be apparent.
7. **Metabolic bone disease** — high uptake in the axial skeleton, proximal long bones, with prominent calvarium and mandible. Faint or absent kidney images.
8. **See 'increased uptake on bone scans not due to skeletal abnormalities'.**

13.2 Increased Uptake on Bone Scans Not Due to Skeletal Abnormality

Artefacts
These are common.
1. **Patient**
   (a) Beware spots of urine in the pelvic area and urine on handkerchiefs.
   (b) Sweat — axillae.
   (c) Injection site.
   (d) Scars of recent operations.
   (e) Breast — accentuation of ribs at the lower border of the breast due to small angle scatter.
2. **Equipment**
   (a) Edge effect — increase in intensity at the edge of the field of view, especially in vertebrae.
   (b) Contamination of the collimator or crystal — check using a uniformity source.

Physiological Variants
1. **Epiphyses in children.**
2. **Inferior angle of the scapula.**
3. **Calcification of cartilages** — especially those in the ribs and anterior neck.
4. **Bladder diverticulum.**
5. **Nipples** especially confusing if at different heights.

Soft Tissue Uptake
1. Calcification
   (a) Myositis ossificans.
   (b) Soft tissue osseous metaplasia.
   (c) Soft tissue tumours with calcification.
   (d) Vascular calcification.
   (e) Calcific tendinitis.
   (f) Abscess.
2. Others
   (a) Acute infarction of the myocardium, cerebrum, skeletal muscle.
   (b) Malignant pleural effusion.
   (c) Inflammatory carcinoma of the breast.
   (d) Hepatic necrosis.
   (e) Hepatic metastases — colon, breast, oat cell carcinoma.
   (f) Tumour uptake.

Visualization of Normal Organs
1. **Free pertechnetate** — thyroid, stomach, salivary glands.
2. **Colloid formation** — liver, spleen and sometimes lung.
3. **Study on the previous day.**

13.3   Photopenic Areas (Defects) on Bone Scans

1. **Artefacts** — the commonest cause.
    (a) external — metal objects — coins, belts, lockets, buckles.
    (b) internal — joint prosthesis, pace makers.
2. **Avascular lesions** — for example cysts.
3. **Multiple myeloma*** — may show increased uptake.
4. **Leukaemia** — may show increased uptake.
5. **Haemangiomas of the spine** — occasionally slightly increased uptake.
6. **Radiotherapy fields** — usually oblong in shape.
7. **Advanced cancer** — especially breast. Possibly related to chemotherapy.
8. **Spina bifida.**

Further Reading
Fogelman I. (ed.) (1987) *Bone Scanning in Clinical Practice*. London: Springer-Verlag.

13.4 Abnormal Bone Scan with Normal or Minimal Radiographic Changes

1. Early disease
   (a) Metastatic.
   (b) Paget's.
   (c) Osteomyelitis.
   (d) Asceptic necrosis.
   (e) Arthritides.
2. Fractures
   (a) Ribs.
   (b) Hands or feet.
3. Lymphoma*.
4. Myelofibrosis.
5. Primary hyperparathyroidism*.
6. Osteodystrophy
   (a) Renal.
   (b) Pulmonary.

Further Reading

Silberstein E.B. & McAfee J.G. (eds) (1984) *Differential Diagnosis in Nuclear Medicine*. New York: McGraw-Hill.

13.5 Positive Radiograph with Normal Bone Scan

1. Benign conditions
   (a) Bone cyst.
   (b) Bone island.
   (c) Exostoses.
2. Recent fractures — within 48 h.
3. Multiple myeloma*.
4. Osteoporosis — q.v.
5. Metastases — very rare but occurs if there is no osteoblastic reaction.

Further Reading

Silberstein E.B. & McAfee J.G. (eds) (1984) *Differential Diagnosis in Nuclear Medicine*. New York: McGraw-Hill.

13.6 Localization of Infection

Technique: ^{111}In leucocytes or ^{99m}Tc HMPAO leucocytes
 1. **Collection of pus.**
 2. **False positive**
     (a) Surgical scars.
     (b) Drip sites and drainage tubes.
     (c) i/v injection sites.
     (d) Lung accumulation in early images.
     (e) Gastro intestinal bleeding (q.v.).
     (f) Sites of bone marrow aspiration.
     (g) Swallowed WBC from lung, sinuses, mouth.
     (h) Fractures within the first 2 weeks.
     (i) Inflammatory arthritis.
     (j) Biliary and renal tract (HMPAO only).
 3. **False negative**
     (a) Walled off avascular pus.
     (b) Chronic inflammatory (lymphocytic) reaction.
     (c) Steroid therapy.
     (d) Immunosuppression.
     (e) Effective antibiotic therapy.
 4. **Inflammatory bowel disease** — uptake at 2 h and reduces by 24 h.
     (a) Crohn's disease.
     (b) Ulcerative colitis.
     (c) Infective colitis.
 5. **Infected prosthesis.**
 6. **Sinusitis.**
 7. **Acute infarcts** — including bowel, myocardial, cerebral.
 8. **Myocarditis.**
 9. **Rejected transplant** — kidney.
10. **Pancreatitis.**
11. **Infected tumour** — especially bronchial.

13.7 Gallium Uptake

Technique: Imaging 24 h after ^{67}Ga injection for inflammatory lesions; up to 72 h for tumour.

Inflammatory
1. Inflammation or abscess.
2. **Sarcoidosis** — lacrimal and salivary gland uptake are typical.
3. **Diffuse lung disease** — interstitial fibrosis, scleroderma, asbestosis.
4. **Heart** — myocarditis, pericarditis, systemic lupus erythematosis.

Tumours
1. **Lymphoma** — positive in 90% of patients and 80% of affected sites.
2. **Bronchial carcinoma** — (90%). Used for staging.
3. **Gastrointestinal tumours** — (20%).
4. **Phaeochromocytoma.**
5. **Hypernephroma.**
6. **Hepatoma.**

Normal Variants
1. **Nasopharynx.**
2. **Bowel** — diffuse or outlining the colon.
3. **Breast** — often due to antiemetics. Intense uptake if recent breast feeding.

13.8 Whole Body Iodine Scan for Localizing Metastases

Technique: The test is usually undertaken when there is a rising level of Thyroglobulin. Transfer patient to T3 one month and stop the T3 for 4 days before imaging.

1. **Metastases** — visualization depends on the amount of ^{131}I given. A low dose gives false negative results.
2. **Thyroid bed** — a small amount of uptake is normal.
3. **Normal thyroid tissue**
   (a) Ectopic, retrosternal, sublingual.
   (b) Aberrant — liver, thyroid lymph nodes (unless an ablative dose of iodine has already been given).
4. **Normal uptake** — genito urinary tract, nasopharynx, salivary glands, stomach, breasts.

Further Reading
Wu S., Brown T., Milne N., Egbert R., Kebok A., Lyons K.P. & Hickey J. (1986) Iodine 131 Total Body Scan — extrathyroidal uptake of radioiodine. *Sem. Nucl. Med.*, 16: 82–4.

13.9 Photopenic (Cold) Areas in Thyroid Imaging

Localized
1. **Colloid cyst.**
2. **Adenoma** — non functioning.
3. **Carcinoma** — medullary may be bilateral.
4. **Multinodular goitre.**
5. **Local thyroiditis** — may be increased uptake also
   (a) Acute.
   (b) De Quervain's.
   (c) Hashimito's.
   (d) Riedel's.
6. **Vascular** — haemorrhage or infarct.
7. **Artefacts.**
8. **Abscesses.**

Generalized reduction in uptake

1. **Medication** — thyroxine, glucocorticoids, phenylbutazone sulphonylureas.
2. **Hypothyroidism** — primary or secondary.
3. **Ectopic hormone production.**
4. **De Quervain's thyroiditis.**
5. **Ectopic thyroid** — lingual or retrosternal.

Further Reading

Fogelman I. & Maisey M. (1988) *An Atlas of Clinical Nuclear Medicine*, pp. 160–216. London: Martin Dunitz.

13.10 Parathyroid Imaging

Technique: ^{201}Tl, ^{99}Tc^m subtraction.

The technique should be limited to localizing adenomas, diagnosis is made using clinical information, serum calcium and parathyroid hormone levels.

1. **Parathyroid adenomas** — approximately two-thirds are demonstrated — related to size.
2. **Thyroid nodules** — adenoma or carcinoma.
3. **Hyperplasia** — several areas of uptake evident. More difficult to demonstrate than adenomas.
4. **Parathyroid carcinoma.**
5. **False positive results** — may occur in patients on thyroxine, or with thyroiditis.
6. **Other disease**
   (a) Lymphoma*.
   (b) Metastases.
   (c) Sarcoidosis*.

Further Reading

Winzelberg G.G. (1987) Thallium 201/^{99m}Tc parathyroid subtraction scintigraphy of the neck: single area of increased thallium uptake. *Sem. Nucl. Med.*, 17: 273–5.
Winzelberg G.G. (1987) Thallium 201/^{99m}Tc parathyroid subtraction scintigraphy of the neck: multiple areas of increased thallium uptake. *Sem. Nucl. Med.*, 17: 276–7.
Winzelberg G.G. (1987) Thallium 201/^{99m}Tc parathyroid subtraction scintigraphy of the mediastinum. *Sem. Nucl. Med.*, 17: 278–9.

13.11 Brain Isotope Angiogram

Technique: Dynamic injection of $^{99}Tc^m$.

Increased Vascularity

1. **Tumours** — glioblastoma multiforme, meningioma, astrocytoma.
2. **Metastases** — thyroid, kidney, lung, breast, melanoma.
3. **Lesions of skin or scalp** — Paget's disease, fibrous dysplasia, metastases, primary tumours, myeloma, sinusitis.
4. **Arteriovenous malformations.**
5. **Jugular reflux** — reflux up the jugular vein if the patient holds their breath at the time of injection.

Vascularity — Localized Decreased Vascularity

1. **Cerebro vascular occlusion.**
2. **Carotid stenosis or occlusion.**
3. **Subdural haematoma.**
4. **Avascular brain masses**
   (a) Tumour.
   (b) Cysts.
   (c) Haematoma.
   (d) Abscess.
   (e) Gliomas (occasionally).
5. **Ventricular enlargement.**
6. **Cortical atrophy** — if marked.

Bilaterally Decreased Vascularity

1. **Poor bolus.**
2. **Low cardiac output.**
3. **Venous return** — obstruction of venous return to the heart.
4. **Raised intracranial pressure** — marked increase.
5. **Brain death.**

Further Reading

Lin D.S. (1986) Hypervascularity on cerebral radionuclide angiogram. *Sem. Nucl. Med.*, 16: 74–6.
Lin D.S. (1986) Hypovascularity on cerebral radionuclide angiogram. *Sem. Nucl. Med.*, 16: 77–9.

13.12   Ventilation Perfusion Mismatch

Mismatched Perfusion Defects
Perfusion defect greater than ventilation defect.
1. **Pulmonary embolus** — especially if multiple and segmental.
2. **Bronchial carcinoma** — but more commonly matched.
3. **Tuberculosis** — typically affecting an apical segment.
4. **Vasculitis** — polyarteritis nodosa, systemic lupus erythematosis etc.
5. **Tumour embolus.**
6. **Fat embolus.**
7. **Post radiotherapy.**

Mismatched Ventilation Defects
Bronchial obstruction with normal blood supply. Ventilation defect greater than perfusion defect.
1. **Chronic obstructive airways disease.**
2. **Pneumonia.**
3. **Carcinoma** — the rarest appearance with bronchial carcinoma.
4. **Lung collapse** — of any cause.
5. **Pleural effusion.**

Further Reading
Carvandho P. & Lavender J.P. (1988) Incidence and aetiology of the reverse (V/Q) mismatch defect. *Nucl. Med. Commun.*, 9: 167.

13.13 Myocardial Perfusion Imaging

Technique: ²⁰¹Tl (thallium).

Focal defect on exercise but not on reperfusion
1. Exercise induced ischaemia.
2. Hypertrophic cardiomyopathy.
3. Aortic stenosis.
4. Mitral valve prolapse.
5. Myocarditis.

Focal defect on exercise and reperfusion images
1. Myocardial infarct — old or recent.
2. Peri-infarct ischaemia.
3. Angina pectoris — during pain (also reported when free of pain).
4. Sarcoidosis*.
5. Mitral valve prolapse.
6. Congestive cardiomyopathy.
7. Artefact — breast, diaphragm.

Further Reading
Gerson M.C. & Gelford M.J. (1984) ²⁰¹Tl-thallium myocardial perfusion imaging. In: Silbertstein E.B. & McAfee J.G. (eds), *Differential Diagnosis in Nuclear Medicine*, pp. 17–22. New York: McGraw-Hill.

13.14 Gated Blood Pool Imaging

Technique: ⁹⁹Tcᵐ labelled red blood cells.

Dyskinesia Focal
1. Myocardial infarct.
2. Ischaemic cardiomyopathy.
3. Unstable angina pectoris.
4. Aneurysm — paradoxical movement.

13.15 Photopenic (Cold) Areas in Colloid Liver Scans

Single
1. Single metastasis.
2. Cyst.
3. Abscess.
4. **Primary tumour** — haemangioma, adenoma. Hepatoma may be multiple.
5. Subphrenic abscess.
6. **Adjacent organs** — kidney, stomach, pancreas, especially if involved by tumour.
7. **Non pathological**
   (a) Contrast media — in the bowel.
   (b) Breast — on anterior view and less apparent on the right lateral view.
   (c) Gallbladder fossa.
   (d) Costal margin indentation.
   (e) Porta hepatis.

Multiple
1. **Metastases** — commonly from the bowel.
2. **Hepatoma** — see above.
3. **Dilated intrahepatic ducts** — obstructive jaundice.
4. **Non uniformity of the gamma camera** — producing hexagonal defects.

Diffuse
1. **Cirrhosis** — with increased bone marrow and spleen uptake, and a large left lobe of liver.
2. **Metastases** — if extensive.
3. **Acute hepatitis.**
4. **Fatty liver.**
5. **Amyloid infiltration.**
6. **Budd–Chiari** — especially over the right lobe with an enlarged caudate lobe.

13.16 Non Visualization of the Gallbladder with HIDA

Technique: Deithyl HIDA satisfactory, but di-isopropyl or iodo HIDA are excreted at higher bilirubin levels.

No Bowel Activity
1. **Common bile duct obstruction** — of any cause.
2. **Severe hepatitis.**
3. **Opiates** — because of their effect on the sphincter of Oddi.

With Bowel Activity
1. **Acute cholecystitis.**
2. **Chronic cholecystitis** — usually fills after 1 h.
3. **Cholecystectomy.**
4. **Inadequate fasting** — including i/v feeding.
5. **Biliary pancreatitis.**
6. **Severe diffuse hepatocellular disease.**

Further Reading
Lecklitner M.L. & Growcock G. (1984) Hepatobiliary scintigraphy: non visualization of activity in the area of the gallbladder associated with intestinal activity. *Sem. Nucl. Med.*, 14: 345–6.

13.17   Spleen Imaging

Technique: For almost all purposes a colloid image of the liver and spleen provides perfectly satisfactory spleen images. However $^{99}Tc^m$ heat damaged red blood cells required after splenectomy or with equivocal colloid images.

Splenunculus
Post splenectomy — more uptake than in the liver. Note that the liver may fall into the splenic bed. There is normally some activity in the renal tract.

Photopenic Areas (Defects) in the Spleen
1. **Trauma** — leak of the radiopharmaceutical into the abdomen proves that bleeding is currently taking place.
2. **Infarct**
   (a) Infective endocarditis.
   (b) Vasculitis.
   (c) Tumour invasion.
   (d) Pancreatitis.
3. **Involvement by other disease**
   (a) Lymphoma*.
   (b) Melanoma.
   (c) Secondaries, usually from lung or breast.
4. **Artefact** — breast, barium, metal objects.

Absent or Much Reduced Splenic Uptake
Using heat damaged red blood cells or $^{99}Tc^m$ colloid
1. **Splenectomy.**
2. **Vascular occlusion.**
3. **Haemoglobinopathies.**
4. **Polycythaemia rubra vera.**
5. **Infiltrative** — tumour, amyloid.
6. **Coeliac disease.**
7. **Chronic active hepatitis.**

13.18 Meta iodo benzyl guanidine (MIBG) Imaging

Technique: Images at 4 and 24 h after ^{123}I MIBG; 1–3 days after ^{131}I MIBG.

Normal
1. Myocardium.
2. Liver.
3. Bladder.
4. Adrenal glands — more marked with ^{123}I MIBG.

Abnormal
1. Phaeochromocytoma.
2. Neuroblastoma.
3. Carcinoid tumour.

Further Reading
McEwan A.H., Shapiro B., Sisson J.C., Beierwaltes W.H. & Ackery D.M. (1985). Radioiodobenzylguanidine for the scintigraphic localisation and therapy of adrenergic tumours. *Sem. Nucl. Med.*, **15**: 132–53.

13.19 Unilateral Adrenal Visualization

Technique: Images at 3–10 days after injection of ^{75}Se selenocholesterol.

1. Adenoma — suppressing the other adrenal.
2. Metastases — breast or lung commonly.
3. Aldosteronism — after dexamethasone suppression.
4. Carcinoma.
5. Adrenalectomy — unilateral.
6. Infarct.

Further Reading
Standalik R.C. (1981) Unilateral visualisation of the adrenal gland. *Sem. Nucl. Med.*, **11**: 224–5.

13.20 Cortical Defects in Renal Images

Technique: $^{99}Tc^m$ DMSA but may be apparent with other renal imaging agents.

1. **Scars** — note that apparent scars present during infection may resolve later. Oblique views are required.
2. **Hydronephrosis.**
3. **Trauma** — subcapsular or intra-renal.
4. **Renal cysts.**
5. **Carcinoma.**
6. **Infarct or ischaemia.**
7. **Abscesses.**
8. **Metastases.**
9. **Wilm's tumour.**

Further Reading
Fogelman I. & Maisey M. (1988) *An Atlas of Clinical Nuclear Medicine*, pp. 217–373. London: Martin Dunitz.

13.21 Localization of Gastrointestinal Bleeding

Technique: For acute or continuous bleeding image for 30 min using $^{99}Tc^m$ colloid (or DTPA) which can detect a blood loss of 0.1 ml/min. If this is negative or the blood loss is known to be intermittent use $^{99}Tc^m$ labelled red blood cells and image for up to 24 h. This is sensitive to 0.5 ml/min blood loss.

1. **Ulcers** — benign or malignant.
2. **Vascular lesions** — telangiectasia, haematoma, fistula, angiodysplasia.
3. **Tumours** — leiomyoma, adenoma.
4. **Inflammatory lesions** — gastritis, duodenitis.
5. **Varices** — oesophageal or stomach.
6. **Surgical anastomosis.**
7. **Meckel's diverticulum** (q.v.).
8. **Intusussception.**
9. **Metastatic disease.**
10. **Diverticula.**
11. **False positive**
    (a) Renal tract, liver, spleen, small bowel vascularity.
    (b) Uterus.
    (c) Accessory spleen.
    (d) Marrow uptake of colloid, especially if irregular.

Further Reading
Silberstein E.B. & McAfee J.G. (eds) (1984) *Differential Diagnosis in Nuclear Medicine*, pp. 191–3. New York: McGraw-Hill.

13.22 Meckel's Diverticulum.

Technique: $^{99}Tc^m$ pertechnetate (perchlorate must not be given).

Meckels's Diverticulum
Appears at the same time as the stomach and the activity increases in intensity with the stomach. May change in position during the study and may empty its contents into the bowel.

Gastrointestinal Bleeding
Any blood leaking into the bowel would be apparent, although it would not show the rounded appearance of a Meckel's diverticulum.

False Positive Results
1. Physiological
   (a) Gastric emptying.
   (b) Renal tract — pelvis, ureter, bladder diverticulum.
   (c) Iliac vessels.
   (d) Uterus.
2. Pathological
   (a) Ectopic gastric mucosa in the small bowel.
   (b) Infection — for example acute appendicitis.
   (c) Intussusception.
   (d) Haemangioma of the bowel — gradual reduction in activity.

False Negative
1. No ectopic gastric mucosa in the diverticulum.
2. Hidden by bladder or stomach.

Further Reading
Merrick M.V. (1986) In: P.J.A. Robinson (ed.) *Nuclear Gastroenterology*, pp. 163–8. Edinburgh: Churchill Livingstone.

Notes

Notes

Chapter 14

Obstetric and Gynaecological Ultrasonography

Josephine McHugo

Obstetric ultrasound can broadly be divided into four sections:

1. Normality/abnormality of the first trimester.
2. Assessment of gestational age and fetal number.
3. Structural abnormalities.
4. Growth and fetal well being throughout pregnancy.

For simplicity these will be dealt with separately but an accurate knowledge of gestational age is essential before abnormal growth can be implied and gestational age is often vital in assessing structural abnormalities.

14.1 Measurements for Dating (in weeks post LMP)

		range
Sac volume	5 wks	+/–1.5 wks
Crown–rump length	$6\frac{1}{2}$ wks	+/–0.7 wks
Biparietal diameter	12 wks–term	+/–1 wk < 20 wks
		+/–1.5 wks at 20–26 wks
		+/–2–3 wks at 26–30 wks
		3–4 wks after 30 wks
Femur length	12 wks–term	+/–22 day > 34 wks
Cerebellar width	15–16–term	

From the above it can be seen that gestational age measurements are less variable in early pregnancy. To accurately date a fetus with an uncertain LMP serial scans are essential.

14.2 Ultrasound Features of a Normal Intrauterine Pregnancy (Using Abdominal Scanning)

The earliest ultrasound sign of pregnancy is fundal endometrial thickening.

At 5 weeks
1. Gestational sac should be visible.
2. The gestational sac is surrounded by an echo dense ring.
3. Asymmetry of this ring is apparent.

At 6 weeks
Embryonic structures apparent (the yolk sac and developing amniotic sac).

At $6\frac{1}{2}$ weeks
Cardiac movement identifiable in the fetus
Crown rump length approximately 5 mm.

These dates will not always apply in obese patients where ultrasound images are not ideal. In these cases ultrasound evidence of a normal pregnancy will not be seen so readily. The above appearances are easily seen using transvaginal scanning.

Normal sac growth
A normal gestational sac grows at a rate of 0.7–1.75 mm/day (mean = 1.33) from 5–11 weeks.

Using transvaginal ultrasound

Gestational sac — seen as early as 32 days and present in all normal pregnancies with HCG level of 1000 mIU ml^{-1}.

Yolk sac — seen in 100% of normal pregnancies with HCG level of 7200 mIU ml^{-1}. Yolk sac first seen in every pregnancy between 36 and 40 days and when the gestational sac is between 6 and 9 mm.

Embryo with a heart beat — in all pregnancies greater than 40 days and when the gestational sac diameter is greater than 9 mm.

Further Reading
Bree R.L., Edwards M., Böhm-Vélez M., Beyler S., Roberts J. & Mendelson E.B. (1989) Transvaginal sonography in the evaluation of normal early pregnancy: correlation with HCG level. *Am. J. Roentgenol.*, 153: 75–9.

14.3 Indications for Ultrasound Scanning in the First Trimester

Common
1. Threatened abortion.
2. Suspected ectopic pregnancy.
3. Uncertain dates (LMP); size discrepancy.
4. Evaluation of retained products post spontaneous abortion.

Less common
1. Assessment of success of ovulation induction.
2. Assessment of multiple pregnancies.
3. Guidance for chorionic villus sampling.
4. Retained intrauterine contraceptive device.
5. Adjunct for therapeutic abortion.
6. Evaluation for pelvic masses in early pregnancy.

It should be noted that ultrasound should not be simply used to diagnose an uncomplicated pregnancy.

14.4 Threatened Abortion

Definition (clinical)
Blood loss PV with a closed cervical os.

Incidence
25% pregnancies (clinically apparent)
50% of these go on to abort.

Demonstration of a living fetus
90–97% favourable outcome.

Ultrasound findings in threatened abortion
1. Intact pregnancy approx 50%. Fetal viability depends on imaging a fetal heart beat or fetal movements.
2. Blighted ovum 20–25%.
3. Missed abortion 25–30%.
4. Incomplete abortion 2–5%.
5. Ectopic pregnancy 1–3%.
6. Hydatidiform mole < 1%.

14.5 Blighted Ovum (Anembryonic Pregnancy)

Definition
A fertilized ovum in which development has been arrested. The majority have chromosomal abnormalities.

Ultrasound signs of an 'empty' sac
1. No fetal parts seen with a sac diameter > 30 mm.
2. No yolk sac seen with a sac > 20 mm.
3. Irregular sac contour.

14.6 Ectopic Pregnancy

Risk factors
1. Previous ectopic.
2. IUCD *in situ*.
3. History of pelvic inflammatory disease.
4. Previous tubal surgery.
5. *In vitro* fertilization.

Ultrasound findings
1. Ultrasound evidence of an intrauterine pregnancy excludes the diagnosis if there are no risk factors. (1:30 000 approx. rate of concomitant intra and extrauterine pregnancy. This increases to 1:7000 following ovulation induction.)
2. Endometrial thickening (decidual cast/pseudogestational sac).
3. Adnexal mass (complex).
4. Fluid in the Pouch of Douglas.
5. Demonstration of a living fetus outside the uterus (demonstrated in approx. 10% of cases of ectopic pregnancy).
6. Absence of any ultrasound abnormality does not exclude the diagnosis (approx. 20% of proven cases have no ultrasound abnormalities).
7. hCG level > 1800 mIU/ml with no evidence of an intrauterine pregnancy strongly suggests an ectopic.
   Sensitivity 44%.
   Specificity 100%.

14.7   Absent Intrauterine Pregnancy with Positive Pregnancy Test

1. Ectopic.
2. Early intrauterine pregnancy < 5 weeks.
3. Recent complete/incomplete abortion.

14.8   Liquor Volume

The liquor volume increases in normal pregnancy until approx. 34/40 and then decreases towards term (approx 400 ml at 20 weeks).

Assessment of liquor volume is usually subjective; (accurate and reproducible with experienced observers). <2 cm pools in any direction indicates a reduction.

Differential diagnosis of abnormal liquor volume

1. **Severe oligohydramnios**
   (a)   Renal agenesis/bilaterally nonfunctioning kidneys.
   (b)   Premature rupture of membranes.
   (c)   Severe growth retardation.
2. **Moderate oligohydramnios**
   (a)   Renal anomalies (bilateral).
   (b)   Premature rupture of membranes.
   (c)   Growth retardation.
3. **Polyhydramnios**
   (a)   Diabetes (maternal).
   (b)   Fetal anomaly (30% cases) — fetus may be hydropic. See 14.9.
        Cardiovascular decompensation.
        Obstructive malformations of the GI tract, e.g. TOF, duodenal stenosis/atresia.
        Diaphragmatic hernia.
        Anencephaly/other severe cranial anomalies.
   (c)   Rarer causes e.g. bone dysplasis, neuromuscular abnormalities.

14.9   Fetal Hydrops

Defined as excessive fluid accumulation in the extravascular compartment = subcutaneous oedema, plus at least one of the following — ascites, pleural or pericardial effusions.
In the fetus ascites and pericardial effusions occur earlier than pleural fluid in cardiac failure.

Immune hydrops
1. Rhesus incompatibility
2. Other blood group incompatibility

Nonimmune Hydrops (late manifestations of many severe diseases)
1. **Cardiovascular**
   (a) Arrhythmias.
   (b) Anatomic defects.
   (c) Cardiomyopathies.
2. **Chromosomal**
   (a) Trisomies.
   (b) Turners syndrome.
   (c) Triploidy
3. **Infections**
   (a) CMV (Cytomegalic virus).
   (b) Toxoplasmosis.
   (c) Rubella.
   (d) Syphilis.
   (e) Other congenital infections.
4. **Twin pregnancies**
   (a) Twin to twin transfusion.
5. **Haematological**
   (a) Alpha–thalassaemia.
   (b) A–V shunts (large).
6. **Thoracic mass lesions e.g.**
   (a) Diaphragmatic hernia.
   (b) Cystic adenoma of the lung.
   (c) Pulmonary lymphangiectasia.
7. **Gastrointestinal**
   (a) Atresias.
   (b) Volvulus.
   (c) Perforation.

8. **Umbilicus/placenta**
   (a) Chorioangioma.
   (b) Fetomaternal transfusion.
9. **Urinary**
   (a) Congenital nephrosis.
   (b) Bladder outlet obstruction with perforation.
10. **Miscellaneous**
    (a) Skeletal dysplasias.
    (b) Sacrococcyageal teratoma etc.

14.10 Raised Serum Alphafeto Protein (AFP)

(This protein is produced by the fetus and crosses the placenta to enter the maternal blood. The level rises during normal pregnancy. Discrimination between normal and abnormal is best between 16–18 weeks when termination for lethal abnormalities can be offered.)

1. **Wrong dates** — (a normal pregnancy which is more advanced).
2. **Twins.**
3. **Missed abortion.**
4. **CNS abnormalities**
   (a) Anencephaly.
   (b) Spina bifida (open).
   (c) Encephalocoele.
   (d) Hydrocephalus.
5. **Renal anomalies**
   (a) Renal agenesis.
   (b) Multicystic dysplasia.
   (c) Hydronephrosis.
6. **Anterior wall defects**
   (a) Omphalocoele.
   (b) Gastroschisis.

14.11 Ultrasound Signs Suggesting Chromosomal Abnormality

1. Cystic hygroma.
2. Hydrops.
3. Omphalocoele.
4. Gross renal anomalies.
5. Major structural cardiac defects — particularly cushion defects.
6. Multiple structural abnormalities involving separate systems.
7. Symmetrical growth retardation.
8. Severe growth retardation.
9. Duodenal stenosis/atresia.
10. Single umbilical artery — associated with any structural anomaly.
11. Abnormal placenta — (cystic).

14.12 Cystic Structures seen in the Fetal Abdomen

1. Renal
   (a) Multicystic Dysplasia.
   (b) Hydronephrosis.
   (c) Bladder in outflow obstruction.
2. Gut obstruction
   (a) Duodenal (double bubble)   ⎤ with
   (b) Jejunal (multiple fluid filled loops) ⎰ polyhydramnios.
3. Ovarian cyst
   (a) Simple.
   (b) Complex associated with torsion.
4. Mesenteric cysts.
5. Reduplication cysts.
6. Hepatic cysts.
7. Pancreatic cysts.
8. Lymphangioma.

14.13   Major Structural Abnormalities Diagnosable Antenatally

Renal
1. Hydronephrosis
2. Multicystic dysplastic kidney
3. Other causes of macrocysts — in particular those associated with named syndromes: see section 8.
4. Autosomal recessive polycystic disease — bilaterally enlarged, highly reflective kidneys. Usually associated with oligohydramnios.
5. Autosomal dominant polycystic disease — a few cases have been reported in which US has demonstrated cysts or large kidneys with accentuation of the cortico-medullary junction.

Central Nervous System
1. Anencephaly — 50–60% of all neural tube defects. Approx. 50% have an associated spinal anomaly.
2. Spina bifida — failure of fusion of the posterior vertebral arch. It may be open or closed (membrane covers the lesion).
   Myelocoele — only CSF is present in the sac.
   Meningomyelocoele — neural tissue in the sac.
   Site: 90% lumbosacral; 6% thoracic; 3% cervical.
   Associated Arnold Chiari malformation in 90% (100% with open lesions).
   US signs of the Arnold Chiari malformation are:
   (a) Hydrocephalus.
   (b) Abnormally pointed fronto-parietal region (lemon sign).
   (c) Abnormally shaped cerebellum (banana sign) due to downward displacement of the cerebellum.

Anterior Abdominal Wall Defects
1. Gastroschisis — a defect separate to the cord insertion through which small bowel herniates. No covering membrane. Umbilical vessels not involved. Defect is usually on the right side and liver may, rarely, be involved. Low incidence of chromosome abnormalities. Incidence 1:10 000 – 1:15 000 live births.

2. **Omphalocoele** — abdominal wall defect due to failure of small bowel to reenter the abdomen. Membrane (amnion) covers the eventrated viscera (small bowel ± liver). Umbilical vessels pass through the defect. High incidence of chromosomal abnormalities. Other malformations in 30–60%. Incidence 1:2 280–1:10 000.

Congenital Diaphragmatic Hernia
Incidence 1:2 100 – 1:5 000 live births.
High association (16–56%) with other anomalies:

Cardiac	13%.
Neural tube defects	28%.
Omphalocoele	20%.
Renal	15%.

Mortality is 80%; secondary to pulmonary hypoplasia.
US signs:
Displaced heart.
Bowel within the thorax.
Polyhydramnios after 25 weeks.

Cardiac Anomalies
Major structural cardiac defects are potentially diagnosable antenatally.
The examination is best performed at 20 weeks with a repeat at 24 weeks.
A normal examination requires visualization of
1. Four chambers with an intact ventricular septum.
2. Normal A–V valves.
3. Normal semilunar valves.
4. Normal connections of the great vessels.
(The patent ductus arteriosus and foramen ovale are normal structures in the fetus.)
A fetal tachycardia, > 200 beats/min, has a high association with structural abnormalities.
A fetal bradycardia may be due to complete heart block but is more likely found in a structurally normal heart.
Complete heart block is associated with maternal SLE.

Skeletal Dysplasias

The diagnosis depends on identifying
1. Abnormal bone growth for gestational age.
2. Abnormal bone architecture.

   In the majority of cases femoral shortening is marked

LETHAL
1. Achondrogenesis.
2. Thanatophoric dwarfism.
3. Asphyxiating thoracic dysplasia — severe form.
4. Short rib polydactyly syndromes.
5. Campomelic dysplasia.
6. Homozygous achondroplasia*.

SOMETIMES LETHAL
1. Chondroectodermal dysplasia.
2. Chondrodysplasia punctata — rhizomelic type.
3. Diastrophic dwarfism.
4. Metatropic dwarfism.
5. Osteogenesis imperfecta*.
6. Hypophosphatasia* — infantile type.
7. Osteopetrosis* — AR congenita type.

NOT USUALLY LETHAL
1. Achondroplasia* — this shows a late fall in growth after 22–24 weeks.
2. Spondyloepiphyseal dysplasia congenita.
3. Mesomelic dysplasia.

14.14 Fetal Growth

Fetal measurements of growth
1. Abdominal circumference (AC).
2. Head circumference (HC).
3. Thigh circumference (not easy to reproduce therefore little used).

Growth retardation

Definition
5th centile for weight.

Incidence
approx 5% births.

Risk factors
Maternal
> Hypertension.
> Renal disease.
> Heart disease.

Placental bleeding in early pregnancy.
Multiple pregnancy.
Previous growth retarded baby.

One third of cases have no known risk factors. Perinatal mortality/morbidity 4–8× of normally grown babies. Higher incidence of abnormal physical and neurological development.

Types of growth retardation

TYPE 1

Time onset
— 2nd trimester.

Form
— symmetrical the whole of the body being affected.

Causes
1. **Genetic** (low growth potential).
2. **Chromosomal abnormalities***.
3. **Malformations.**
4. **Intrauterine infections.**
5. **Drugs** e.g. alcohol, smoking, etc.

TYPE 2

Time onset
— 3rd timester.

Form
— Asymmetric the trunk being more affected than the head.

Causes
1. **Hypertension.**
2. **Maternal renal or vascular disease.**
3. **Placental insufficiency.**
4. **Impairment of placental maturation** (failure of invasion of the spiral arteries).
5. **Idiopathic.**
* Cases of early onset of growth retardation or cases where a structural anomaly is apparent in association with growth retardation should be karyotyped (amniocentesis/placental biopsy).

Asymmetrical growth results in an elevated HC/AC ratio.

Doppler velocity waveform in the uterine and umbilical arteries show changes that can indicate fetal compromise. The fetal circulation (aorta, neck vessel etc.) similarly show changes. (Increasing vascular resistance in the abnormal shows a decreased or absent diastolic flow.)

14.15 Normal Placental Development

	Gestation age (weeks)
Entire surface of the placenta is covered with villi	implantation to 6–7
Villous placenta (chorion frondosum) develops	7–11
Atrophy of the remaining villi (chorion laeve)	7–11
Three layers of the placenta identifiable	12

1. Basal plate.
2. Placental substance.
3. Chorionic plate.

14.16 Placental Grading

The normal placenta shows ultrasound features which change as the pregnancy progresses.
Not all placentae reach grade III.
Early maturation (grade III at > 30 weeks) may indicate a failing placental unit.

PLACENTAL GRADING (Grannum *et al.*)

	Basal layer	Placental substance	Chorionic plate
Grade 0	No densities	Finely homogeneous	Straight and well defined
Grade I	No densities	Few scattered echogenic areas	Subtle undulations
Grade II	Linear arrangement of small echo-densities (basal stippling)	Echodensities (comma like)	Demarcation (early) of cotyledons directed to the basal layer
Grade III	Larger and partially confluent echogenic areas	Circular densities with central echopoor areas	Septation of cotyledons extending to the basal layer

Grannum P., Berkowitz R.I., Hobbins J.C. (1979) The ultrasonic changes in the maturing placenta and their relation to fetal pulmonic maturity. *Am. J. Obstet. Gynecol.*, **133**: 915–22.

14.17 Placenta and Membranes in Twin Pregnancies

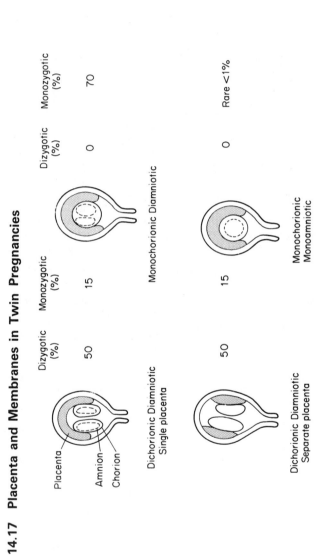

Dizygotic (%)   Monozygotic (%)   Dizygotic (%)   Monozygotic (%)

50   15   Monochorionic Diamniotic   0   70

Dichorionic Diamniotic Single placenta

Placenta
Amnion
Chorion

50   15   Monochorionic Monoamniotic   0   Rare <1%

Dichorionic Diamniotic Separate placenta

14.18 Abnormalities of the Placenta

Placenta praevia
Definition
A portion of the placenta covers the cervical os.

Incidence
(ultrasound)
20% at 20 weeks gestation (termed low lying if it does not
completely and symmetrically cover the os).
0.5% at term (due to differential growth of the uterus and
the development of the lower segment).

Incidence increases with
1. Maternal age.
2. Multiparity.
3. Previous uterine surgery.

Classification

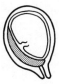
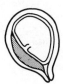
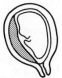

Symetrical
Complete
praevia

Asymmetrical
Complete
praevia

Marginal
Praevia

Low lying
placenta

Associations
1. Maternal haemorrhage.
2. Abnormal presentation.
3. Intrauterine growth retardation.
4. Preterm delivery.
5. Increased perinatal mortality.

N.B. 3–5 are related to premature detachment of the placenta.

14.19   Placental Haemorrhage

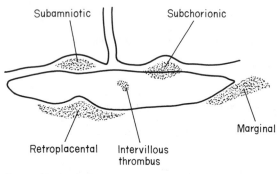

1. **Retroplacental** ⎫
2. **Marginal** ⎭ both result in abruption.
3. **Preplacental** — may be either subamniotic or subchorionic but it is often impossible to distinguish this with US.
4. **Intervillous thrombosis** — On US — intraplacental sonolucencies. Incidence increases as the placenta matures. Differential diagnosis — maternal venous lakes.

Placental Abruption
Definition
Premature separation of the normally sited placenta.
Incidence
Clinically apparent in 1% of pregnancies.
Classification
1. Marginal.
2. Retroplacental.
Maternal risk factors
1. Hypertension.
2. Vascular disease.
3. Smoking.
4. Drug abuse (cocaine etc.).
5. Fibroids.
6. Trauma.

US signs — variable, related to the size, site and time since the event. Acutely a hyperreflective focus relative to the placenta which becomes echo free by 8–14 days. Placental thickness at the site of haemorrhage increases by > 4–4.5 cm.
Outcome — < 20 weeks gestation 80% normal outcome.

14.20 Causes of a Thickened Placenta (> 4 cm)

1. Diabetes.
2. Rhesus isoimmunization.
3. Fetal hydrops.
4. Triploidy.
5. Intrauterine infections.

14.21 Causes of a Thin Placenta

Intrauterine growth retardation (IUGR).

14.22 Gestational Trophoblastic Disease

Definition
Proliferative disease of the trophoblast.
Classification
1. Hydatidiform mole.
2. Invasive mole.
3. Choriocarcinoma.
Incidence
Geographical variation.
1:1200–2000 pregnancies USA.
1:100 Hospital patients Indonesia.
Risk Factors
Increasing maternal age.
Previous hydatidiform mole.
Genetics
Two distinct genetic types.
1. Complete (classic) mole 46XX of paternal origin.
2. 46 XY of paternal origin (rare).

Ultrasound Appearances.
Large echogenic mass occupying the uterine cavity with numerous small fluid filled spaces < 15 mm.
(These features are classically seen in the second trimester.)

No fetal parts except in a partial mole.

First trimester may simulate a blighted ovum.

Raised Human Chorionic Gonadotrophin (hCG) — in 100% of cases
Association
Theca–lutein cysts (multiseptate). In 20–50% patients.
Differential Diagnosis
1. Missed abortion with hydropic degeneration of the placenta.
2. Retained products.

Incomplete Mole
Ultrasound features
1. Fetal parts seen.
2. Thickened placenta with multiple fluid spaces.
3. Multiple fetal anomalies.
4. Severe intrauterine growth retardation.

Invasive mole
Develops in approx 12–15% of cases.

Metastatic choriocarcinoma
5–8% of cases.

Choriocarcinoma
50% assoc. molar pregnancy.
25% following abortion.
22% following a normal pregnancy.
 3% following an ectopic.

14.23   The Normal Uterus

Size
(length × depth × width)
Nullip post pubertal — 7 × 4 × 5 cm
Multiparity — increases the uterine size approx 1 cm in all directions.
Postmenopausal — 3 × 2 × 2 cm
The neonatal uterus is larger than the prepubertal uterus due to maternal hormones. The endometrial cavity is visualized in 97% of babies and endometrial fluid in 23%.
In childhood the cervix is larger than the uterine body.
The endometrium thickens during the normal menstrual cycle. No endometrium is discernible in the prepubertal or postmenopausal state.

14.24 Endometrial Thickness

NORMAL
Proliferative phase — 3–5 mm; seen as a thin continuous line
early and then as an interrupted line.
Secretory phase — 5–6 mm.
Endometrium is not seen in the normal post-menopausal
woman.

Increased
1. Early intrauterine pregnancy.
2. Ectopic pregnancy.
3. Oestrogen excess — e.g. polycystic ovary syndrome.
4. Endometrial carcinoma/hyperplasia ⎫ usually irregular.
5. Endometrial polyp ⎭

14.25 Enlarged Uterus

1. Pregnancy.
2. Leiomyoma.
3. Carcinoma (endometrial).
4. Sarcoma — rare.

14.26 The Normal Ovary

Volume
Length × width × depth × 0.5223 = volume of an ellipse.
Volume increases from the antenatal period to puberty.

Child	1 ml.
Normal postpubertal state	5.3–7.6 ml.
Normal postmenopausal state	4.3 ml (range 1.5–10.3 ml).

In the normal menstrual cycle one follicle becomes dominant
with a follicular growth of 2 mm/day.

Ovulation
Occurs at a follicular size of 20–24 mm (maximum diameter)
in normal cycles. Smaller in clomiphene cycles; smaller still
in pergonal cycles.

Ultrasound Signs of Ovulation
1. Collapse of the follicle.
2. Free fluid in the Pouch of Douglas.
3. Echo-free zone around the endometrium.

Definition of Simple Cystic Structures in the Ovary

Developing follicle	0.4–1.4 cm
Mature follicle	1.5–2.9 cm
Follicular cyst	> 3 cm

14.27   Ovarian Masses

Ultrasonography is 80–90% accurate in demonstrating the size, consistency and location of pelvic masses. Gross morphology correlates well with ultrasound but poorly with histology.

Simple Cystic Structures
1. Follicular cyst.
2. Cystadenoma.
3. Polycystic ovaries
   (a) large volume, mean 14 ml,
   (b) multiple (> 5) cysts, 5–8 mm in diameter,
   (c) echogenic stroma.
   (a) & (b) are seen in 35–40% of cases. 30% have normal volume ovaries, 25% have hyperechoic ovaries and 5% have enlarged ovaries with no cysts. ↑ risk of carcinoma of the endometrium.
4. Cystic teratoma — rare.

Complex (Mainly Cystic)
1. Cystadenocarcinoma.
2. Dermoid.
3. Abscess.
4. Endometriosis.
5. Ectopic pregnancy.

Complex (Mainly Solid)
1. Cystadenocarcinoma.
2. Dermoid.
3. Granulosa cell tumour.
4. Ectopic pregnancy.

Solid
1. Adenocarcinoma.
2. Solid teratoma — malignant.
3. Fibroma.
4. Lymphoma.
5. Metastases.
6. Arrhenoblastoma.

Bibliography
Callen P.W. (1988) *Ultrasonography in Obstetrics and Gynaecology.* 2nd edn. Philadelphia: Saunders.
Hansmann M., Hackelöer B-J. & Staudach A. (1985) *Ultrasound in Obstetrics and Gynaecology.* Berlin: Springer-Verlag.
Hobbins J.C. & Benacerraf B.R. (eds) (1989) *Diagnosis and Therapy of Fetal Anomalies. Clinics in Diagnostic Ultrasound, No. 25.* Edinburgh: Churchill Livingstone.
Macklad N.F. (ed.) (1986) *Ultrasound in Perinatology. Clinics in Diagnostic Ultrasound, No. 19.* Edinburgh: Churchill Livingstone.

Notes

Notes

Chapter 15

Evaluating Statistics — Explanations of Terminology in General Use

1. **Reliability:** reproducibility of results. (These may be from the same observer or from different observers.) Assessment of this can be built in to a study of diagnostic accuracy of a technique, or evaluated beforehand.
2. **Accuracy:** 'proportion of results (positive and negative) which agree with the final diagnosis'.

$$\text{i.e.} \quad \frac{\text{true positives} + \text{true negatives}}{\text{total number of patients in the study.}}$$

N.B. This does not take false positive and false negatives into account, and is therefore less meaningful than sensitivity and specificity.

3. **Sensitivity:** 'proportion of diseased patients who are reported as positive'.

$$\text{i.e.} \quad \frac{\text{true positives}}{\text{total number of final diagnosis positive.}}$$

4. **Specificity:** 'proportion of disease-free patients who are reported as negative'.

$$\text{i.e.} \quad \frac{\text{true negatives}}{\text{total number of final diagnosis negative.}}$$

5. **Positive predictive value:** 'proportion of patients reported positive who have the disease'.

$$\text{i.e.} \quad \frac{\text{true positives}}{\text{true positives} + \text{false positives.}}$$

6. **Negative predictive value:** 'proportion of patients reported negative who do not have the disease'.

i.e. $\dfrac{\text{true negatives}}{\text{true negatives} + \text{false negatives}}.$

Differences in the prevalence of the disease in different studies can affect sensitivity and specificity. For example, if a study is conducted in a tertiary referral hospital the patients will be highly selected and this can alter the way that subtle abnormalities are interpreted as there is a high likelihood of disease being present.

Predictive values are now in common use to indicate the usefulness of an imaging test. However, these depend on sensitivity, specificity *and* prevalence and therefore only apply to settings with a similar prevalence. Formulae are available for calculation of predictive values for different prevalences — see further reading.

7. **Receiver operating characteristic (ROC) curves:** In many situations it is not possible to be definitely positive or definitely negative when reporting. With this method approximately five or six levels of certainty may be used in reporting (e.g. 1 = definitely positive, 2 = probably positive, etc.). Using each of these levels in turn as the point of cut off between a 'definitely positive' and a 'definitely negative' result, the sensitivity and specificity for each level are then plotted in the form of a graph of sensitivity against 1- specificity. The area under the curve will be 1.0 for a perfect technique (or observer) and 0.5 for an absolutely useless technique (or observer!) see figure below.

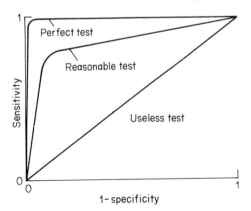

Further Reading

Freedman L.S. (1987) Evaluating and comparing imaging techniques: a review and classification of study designs. *Br. J. Radiol.*, 60: 1071–81.

Notes

Notes

PART 2

Achondroplasia

A primary defect of enchondral bone formation. Autosomal dominant (but 80% are spontaneous mutations).

Skull
1. Large skull. Small base. Small sella. Steep clivus. Small funnel-shaped foramen magnum.
2. Hydrocephalus — of variable severity.

Thorax
1. Thick, stubby sternum.
2. Short ribs with deep concavities to the anterior ends.

Axial Skeleton
1. Decreasing interpedicular distance caudally in the lumbar spine.
2. Short pedicles with a narrow sagittal diameter of the lumbar spinal canal.
3. Posterior scalloping.
4. Anterior vertebral body beak at T12/L1/L2.

Pelvis
1. Square iliac wings.
2. 'Champagne-glass' pelvic cavity.
3. Short, narrow sacrosciatic notch.
4. Horizontal sacrum articulating low on the ilia.

Appendicular Skeleton
1. Rhizomelic micromelia with bowing of long bones.
2. Widened metaphyses.
3. Ball-and-socket epiphyseal/metaphyseal junction.
4. Broad and short proximal and short proximal and middle phalanges.
5. Trident shaped hands.

Acquired Immune Deficiency Syndrome (AIDS) in Adults

A. Chest:
— > 50% present with pulmonary symptoms.
— Bronchoscopy, lavage ± transbronchial biopsy should be considered in all patients as CXR is not pathognomonic.
— The presence of mediastinal/hilar nodes or pleural effusions is serious and often indicates a serious complication such as infections (TB, fungal) or tumours (lymphoma, Kaposi's). Mediastinal/hilar nodes are not a common feature of AIDS or pneumocystis.

1. **Opportunist infections**
   (a) Pneumocystis carinii — most common life-threatening infection. Affects 60% of all AIDS patients at least once, and 25% of initial episodes are fatal (it requires intubation, 90% fatality).
   CXR— typically bilateral perihilar and/or basal reticulonodular infiltrates.
   — rapid progression to alveolar consolidation in 3–5 days.
   — rarely
   (i) asymmetrical, upper lobe
   (ii) 7% have cystic parenchymal changes which can lead to a pneumothorax
   (iii) mediastinal/hilar nodes or effusions
   (iv) miliary nodules or solitary nodule (mimics rounded consolidation)
   (b) CMV — found in 80% of autopsies but rarely the only pathogen.
   CXR — typically indistinguishable from pneumocystis or fibrosis.
   (c) Mycobacterium — affects 10%, and can occur long before other features of AIDS.
   (d) Bacterial — e.g. *H. influenzae* and *Streptococcus*.
2. **Neoplasms**
   (a) Kaposi's sarcoma — lung involvement occurs in 20% of Kaposi's, and is almost always preceded by cutaneous and/or visceral involvement. It can mimic the appearance of an opportunist infection. Transbronchial and open lung biopsy are often not diagnostic.
   (b) Pulmonary lymphoma — rare.

B. Abdomen

1. **Dysphagia** — common. Usually due to candidiasis, but occasionally due to viral oesophagitis or Kaposi's sarcoma.

2. **Diarrhoea** — common. Usually CMV colitis if mild, or cryptosporidium (protozoa) if severe. The latter produces thick mucosal folds and mild dilatation with a predilection for the duodenum and jejunum. *Giardia*, *Clostridium difficile* and *Mycobacterium* may also occur.

3. **Retroperitoneal/mesenteric lymphadenopathy**
   (a) Progressive generalized lymphadenopathy syndrome- — i.e. two or more extra-inguinal nodes persisting for more than 3 months with no obvious cause. Biopsy reveals benign hyperplasia, and CT shows clusters of small nodes less than 1 cm in diameter in the mesentery and retroperitoneum.
   (b) Kaposi's sarcoma — stomach is the commonest site but may be multi-centric and involve gut and liver.
   (c) Lymphoma — usually aggressive form of Non-Hodgkin's lymphoma. Peripheral nodes are present in 50% and extra-nodal involvement is common, particularly bowel, viscera and marrow.
   (d) Mycobacterium.

C. CNS

— 30% of AIDS have neurological signs during their illness.
— 10% of AIDS present with neurological signs, and at autopsy 80% have CNS pathology.

1. **Cerebral atrophy** — probably due to diffuse encephalitis produced by HIV (occasionally toxoplasmosis, CMV) leading to dementia.

2. **Cerebral masses** — occur in 20% of AIDS patients with neurological signs. Commonest causes are
   (a) Toxoplasmosis — affects 10% of AIDS and causes abscesses. They are commonly multiple thin walled with necrotic hypodense centres and display ring or nodular enhancement.
   (b) Lymphoma — affects 6% of AIDS. They are isodense or slightly hyperdense. 50% display uniform contrast enhancement, and 50% show ring enhancement. Solitary lesions are present in 50% of cases.

3. **Other** — white matter disease (progressive multifocal leukoencephalopathy), chronic meningitis (HIV, Cryptococcus, Mycobacterium) and myelopathy may also occur.

Further Reading

Federle M.P. (1988) A Radiologist Looks at A.I.D.S.: Imaging Evaluation Based on symptom Complexes. *Radiology*, **166**: 553–562.

Acquired Immune Deficiency Syndrome (AIDS) in Children

Majority of cases are due to transmission from an infected mother (i.v. drug user, partner of an i.v. drug user, or past history of contact with a bisexual partner) or from transfusions (in the neonatal period or because of diseases such as thalassaemia and haemophilia). 50% of those infected congenitally will present in the first year of life.

AIDS in children differs from AIDS in adults in the following ways:
1. Shorter incubation period.
2. Children are more likely to have serious bacterial infections or CMV.
3. They develop pulmonary lymphoid hyperplasia (PLH). This was previously called lymphocytic interstitial pneumonia (LIP), which is rare in adults.
4. They almost never develop Kaposi sarcoma.
5. They are less likely to be infected with *Toxoplasma*, *Mycobacterium*, *tuberculosis*, *Cryptococcus* and *Histoplasma*.

Generalized Features

Failure to thrive; weight loss; fever; generalized lymphadenopathy; hepatosplenomegaly; recurrent infections; chronic diarrhoea; parotitis.

Chest

1. *Pneumocystis carinii* pneumonia (PCP) — may be localized initially but typically there is rapid progression to generalized lung shadowing which is a mixed alveolar and interstitial infiltrate.
2. Cytomegalovirus (CMV) pneumonia.
3. Pulmonary lymphoid hyperplasia (PLH) — in 50% of patients. Insidious onset of clinical symptoms. CXR shows a diffuse, symmetrical reticulonodular or nodular pattern

(2–3 mm in diameter) which is most easily seen at the bases and periphery of the lungs, ± hilar or mediastinal lymphadenopathy. The nodules consist of collections of lymphocytes and plasma cells without any organisms. Children with PLH are more likely to have generalized lymphadenopathy, salivary gland enlargement and finger clubbing than those whose CXR changes are due to opportunistic infection and the prognosis for PLH is better.

4. Mediastinal or hilar adenopathy may be secondary to PLH, *M. tuberculosis*, *M. avium-intracellulare*, CMV, lymphoma or fungal infection.

5. Cardiomyopathy.

Abdomen

1. Hepatosplenomegaly — due to chronic active hepatitis, hepatitis A or B, CMV, Epstein–Barr virus and *M. tuberculosis*, generalized sepsis, tumour (fibrosarcoma of the liver) or congestive cardiac failure.

2. *Candida* oesophagitis.

3. Chronic diarrhoea — infectious agents are only infrequently found but included *Candida*, CMV and *Cryptosporidium*. Radiological findings are non-specific and include a malabsorption type pattern with thickening of bowel wall and mucosal folds and dilatation. Fine ulceration may be seen.

4. Peumatosis coli.

5. Mesenteric, para-aortic and retroperitoneal lymphadenopathy — due to *M. avium-intracellulare*, lymphocytic proliferation (lymph node syndrome), lymphoma or Kaposi sarcoma.

6. Renal failure and urinary tract infections.

Head

1. Encephalopathy — variable severity and progression. May be the primary manifestation of the illness and the majority of symptomatic HIV-infected children may be affected to some degree. Younger children may become microcephalic. CT show
   (a) Cerebral atrophy.
   (b) Basal ganglia and frontal lobe calcification.
   (c) Low attenuation white matter.

2. Meningitis — due to typical and atypical organisms.

3. Chronic otitis media and sinusitis.

Further Reading

Amodio J.B., Abramson S. & Berdon W.E. & Levy J. (1987) Pediatric AIDS. *Semin. Roentgenol.*, 22: 66–76.

Bradford B.F., Abdenour Jr G.E., Frank J.L., Scott G.B. & Beerman R. (1988) Usual and unusual radiologic manifestations of acquired immunodeficiency syndrome (AIDS) and human immunodeficiency virus (HIV) infection in children. *Radiol. Clin. North Am.*, 26: 341–53.

Faloon J., Eddy J., Wiener L. & Pizzo P.A. (1989) HIV in children. *J. Peds.*, 114: 1–30.

Acromegaly

The effect of excessive growth hormone on the mature skeleton.

Skull
1. Thickened skull vault.
2. Enlarged paranasal sinuses and mastoids.
3. Enlarged pituitary fossa because of the eosinophilic adenoma.
4. Prognathism (increased angle of mandible).

Thorax and Spine
1. Increased sagittal diameter of the chest with a kyphosis.
2. Vertebral bodies show an increase in the AP and transverse dimensions with posterior scalloping.

Appendicular Skeleton
1. Increased width of bones but unaltered cortical thickness.
2. Tufting of the terminal phalanges.
3. Prominent muscle attachments.
4. Widened joint spaces — especially the metacarpo-phalangeal joints — because of cartilage hypertrophy.
5. Premature osteoarthritis.
6. Increased heel pad thickness (> 21.5 mm in female; > 23 mm in male).
7. Generalized osteoporosis.

Alkaptonuria

The absence of homogentisic acid oxidase leads to the accumulation of homogentisic acid and its excretion in sweat and urine. The majority of cases are inherited as an autosomal recessive trait.

Axial Skeleton
1. Osteoporosis.
2. Intervertebral disc calcification — predominantly in the lumbar spine.
3. Disc space narrowing with vacuum phenomenon.
4. Marginal osteophytes and end-plate sclerosis.
5. Symphysis pubis — joint-space narrowing, chondrocalcinosis, eburnation and, rarely, bony ankylosis.

Appendicular Skeleton
1. Large joints show joint-space narrowing, bony sclerosis, articular collapse and fragmentation and intra-articular loose bodies.
2. Calcification of bursae and tendons.

Extraskeletal
Ochronotic deposition in other organs may have the following results
1. Cardiovascular system — atherosclerosis, infarction and murmurs.
2. Genitourinary system — prostatic enlargement with calculi.
3. Upper respiratory tract — hoarseness and dyspnoea.
4. Gastrointestinal tract — dysphagia.

Aneurysmal Bone Cyst

1. Age — 10–30 years (75% occur before epiphyseal closure)
2. Sites — ends of long bones, especially in the lower limbs. Also flat bones and vertebral appendages.
3. Appearances
   (a) Arises in unfused metaphysis or in metaphysis and epiphysis after fusion.
   (b) Well-defined lucency with thin but intact cortex.
   (c) Marked expansion (ballooning).
   (d) Thin internal strands of bone.
   (e) ± new bone in the angle between original cortex and the expanded part.
   (f) Fluid level(s) on CT.

Ankylosing Spondylitis

A mesenchymal disease mainly manifest as an inflammatory arthritis affecting synovial and cartilaginous joints and as an enthesopathy.

Axial Skeleton

1. Involved initially in 70–80%. Initial changes in the sacroiliac joints followed by the thoracolumbar and lumbosacral regions. The entire spine may be involved eventually.
2. The radiological changes in the sacroiliac joints (see section 3.12) are present at the time of the earliest spinal changes.
3. Disco-vertebral junction
   (a) Osteitis — resulting in the squaring of vertebral bodies.
   (b) Syndesmophytes — eventually leading to the 'bamboo spine' (see section 2.13).

(c) Disc calcification.
(d) Erosions and destruction — which can be central, peripheral or extensive (pseudarthrosis).
(e) Osteoporosis — with long-standing disease.
(f) Kyphosis.
4. Apophyseal joints ⎫ haziness, erosions, subchondral
5. Costotransverse joints ⎬ sclerosis and eventually
6. Costovertebral joints ⎭ ankylosis.
7. Posterior ligament calcification and ossification.

Appendicular Skeleton

1. Involved initially in 10–20% but eventually in 50% of cases. Mild and transient. Asymmetrical involvement of few joints, most frequently hips and shoulders.
2. Similar changes to rheumatoid arthritis, but synovitis is more discrete and less severe. Subchondral bone sclerosis and chondral ossification lead to bony ankylosis. (In adult rheumatoid arthritis, bony ankylosis only occurs in the carpus and tarsus.)
3. No periarticular osteoporosis.

Extraskeletal

1. Iritis in 20% — more frequent with a peripheral arthropathy.
2. Pulmonary upper lobe fibrosis and cavitation (1%).
3. Heart disease — aortic incompetence, conduction defects and pericarditis.
4. Amyloidosis.
5. Inflammatory bowel disease.

Asbestos Inhalation

Lung and/or pleural disease due to the inhalation of asbestos fibres. Disease is more common with crocidolite (blue asbestos) than chrysotile (white asbestos). Pleural disease alone 50%; pleura and lung parenchyma 40%; lung parenchyma alone 10%.

Pleura
1. Plaques or pleural thickening. Most frequent in the lower half of the thorax and tend to follow rib contours. Parietal pleura is affected. Do not occur with less than 20 years exposure.
2. Calcified plaques (in 25%) — probably related to the type of fibre. Usually diaphragmatic.
3. Effusions (in 20%) — frequently recurrent, usually bilateral and often associated with chest pain. Usually associated with pulmonary involvement.

Lung Parenchyma
1. Small nodular and/or reticular opacities which progress through three stages
   (a) Fine reticulation in the lower zones → ground glass appearance.
   (b) More prominent interstitial reticulation in the lower zones.
   (c) Reticular shadowing in the mid and upper zones with obscured heart and diaphragmatic outlines.
2. Large opacities (1 cm or greater), associated with widespread interstitial fibrosis.

Complications
1. Carcinoma of the bronchus — 6–10 × increased incidence in smokers with asbestosis and accounts for 35% of deaths.
2. Mesothelioma — 80% of all mesotheliomas are associated with asbestosis. Accounts for 10% of deaths.
3. Peritoneal mesothelioma.
4. Gastrointestinal carcinomas.
5. Laryngeal carcinoma.

Calcium Pyrophosphate Dihydrate Deposition Disease

1. Three manifestations which occur singly or in combination
   (a) Crystal-induced acute synovitis (pseudogout).
   (b) Cartilage calcification (chondrocalcinosis).
   (c) Structural joint abnormalities (pyrophosphate arthropathy).
2. Associated conditions are hyperparathyroidism and haemochromatosis (definite) and gout, Wilson's disease and alkaptonuria (less definite).
3. Chondrocalcinosis involves
   (a) Fibrocartilage — especially menisci of the knee, triangular cartilage of the wrist, symphysis pubis and annulus fibrosus of the intervertebral disc.
   (b) Hyaline cartilage — especially the wrist, knee, elbow and hip.
4. Synovial membrane, joint capsule, tendon and ligament calcification.
5. Pyrophosphate arthropathy is most common in the knee, wrist, metacarpophalangeal joint and acromioclavicular joint. It has similar appearances to osteoarthritis but with several differences
   (a) Unusual articular distribution — the wrist, elbow and shoulder are uncommon sites for osteoarthritis.
   (b) Unusual intra-articular distribution, e.g. the patellofemoral compartment of the knee and the radiocarpal compartment of the wrist.
   (c) Numerous, prominent subchondral cysts.
   (d) Marked subchondral collapse and fragmentation with multiple loose bodies simulating a neuropathic joint.
   (e) Variable osteophyte formation.

Chondroblastoma

1. Age — 5–20 years.
2. Sites — upper humerus, lower femur, upper tibia and greater tuberosity (50% occur in the lower limb).
3. Appearances
   (a) Arises in the epiphysis prior to fusion and may expand to involve the metaphysis.
   (b) Well-defined lucency with a thin sclerotic rim.
   (c) Internal calcification.

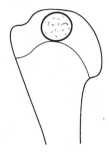

Chondromyxoid Fibroma

1. Age — 10–30 years.
2. Sites — upper end of tibia (50%); also femur and ribs.
3. Appearances
   (a) Metaphyseal ± extension into epiphysis, but never only in the epiphysis.
   (b) Round or oval, well-defined lucency with a sclerotic rim.
   (c) Eccentric expansion.
   (d) Internal calcification is uncommon.

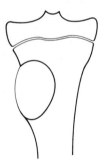

Chondrosarcoma

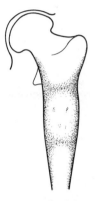

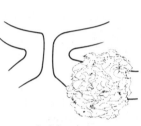

Central   Peripheral

Central
1. Age — 30–60 years.
2. Sites — femur and humerus.
3. Appearances
   (a) Metaphyseal or diaphyseal.
   (b) Lucent, expansile lesion with a sclerotic margin.
   (c) Endosteal cortical thickening or thinning.
   (d) ± cortical destruction and a soft-tissue mass.
   (e) Amorphous or punctate internal calcification.

Peripheral
1. Age — 30–60 years.
2. Sites — pelvic and shoulder girdle, upper femur and humerus.
3. Appearances
   (a) Soft-tissue mass, often arising from the cartilage tip of an osteochondroma.
   (b) Multiple calcific densities.
   (c) Ill-defined margins.
   (d) In the later stages, destruction of underlying bone.

Cleidocranial Dysplasia

Autosomal dominant. One-third are new mutations.

Skull
1. Brachycephaly. Wormian bones. Frontal and parietal bossing.
2. Wide sutures and fontanelles with delayed closure.
3. Broad mandible. Small facial bones. Delayed eruption and supernumerary teeth.
4. Basilar invagination.

Thorax
1. Aplasia or hypoplasia of the clavicles, usually the lateral portion but occasionally the middle portion.
2. Small, high scapulae.
3. Neonatal respiratory distress because of thoracic cage deformity.

Pelvis
1. Absent or delayed ossification of the pubic bones, producing apparent widening of the symphysis pubis.

Appendicular Skeleton
1. Short or absent fibulae.
2. Coxa vara or coxa valga.
3. Congenital pseudarthrosis of the femur.
4. Hand
   (a) Long 2nd and 5th metacarpals; short 2nd and 5th middle phalanges.
   (b) Cone-shaped epiphyses.
   (c) Tapered distal phalanges.
   (d) Supernumerary ossification centres.

Coal Miner's Pneumoconiosis

The effect of the inhalation of coal dust in coal workers.

Simple
1. Small round opacities, 1–5 mm in size. Widespread throughout the lungs but sparing the extreme bases and apices.
2. Less well defined than silicosis.
3. Generally less dense than silicosis, but calcification occurs in at least a few of the nodules in 10% of older coal workers.
4. 'Eggshell' calcification of lymph nodes in 1%.

Complicated, i.e. Progressive Massive Fibrosis (see Silicosis).

Complications (see Silicosis).

Cretinism (Congenital Hypothyroidism)

Appendicular Skeleton
1. Delayed appearance of ossification centres which may be (a) slightly granular, (b) finely stippled; (c) coarsely stippled or (d) fragmented. The femoral capital epiphyses may be divided into inner and outer halves.
2. Delayed epiphyseal closure.
3. Short long-bones with slender shafts, endosteal thickening and dense metaphyseal bands.
4. Coxa vara with shortened femoral neck and elevated greater trochanter.

Skull
1. Brachycephaly.
2. Multiple wormian bones.
3. Delayed development of vascular markings and diploic differentiation.
4. Delayed sutural closure.
5. Poorly developed sinuses and mastoids.

Axial Skeleton
1. Kyphosis at the thoracolumbar junction, usually associated with a hypoplastic or 'bullet-shaped' body of LV1 or LV2.

The bone changes may have completely regressed in adults.

Crohn's Disease

Colon and small bowel are affected equally. Gastric involvement is uncommon and is usually affected in continuity with disease in the duodenum. Oesophageal involvement is rare.

Small Bowel
1. Terminal ileum is the commonest site.
2. Asymmetrical involvement and skip lesions are characteristic. The disease predominates on the mesenteric border.
3. Apthoid ulcers — the earliest sign in the terminal ileum and colon.
4. Fissure ulcers — typically they are distributed in a longitudinal and transverse fashion. They may progress to abscess formation, sinuses and fistulae.
5. Blunting, thickening or distortion of the valvulae conniventes — the earliest sign in the small bowel proximal to the terminal ileum. Due to hyperplasia of lymphoid tissue producing an obstructive lymphoedema of the bowel wall.
6. 'Cobblestone' pattern — 2 possible causes.
   (a) A combination of longitudinal and transverse fissure ulcers bounding intact mucosa. Or
   (b) The bulging of oedematous mucosal folds that are not closely attached to the underlying muscularis.
7. Separation of bowel loops — due to thickened bowel wall.
8. Strictures — which may be short or long, single or multiple. Significant clinical obstruction is less commonly observed.
9. Pseudosacculation.

Colon
1. Asymmetrical involvement and skip lesions. The rectum is involved in 30–50%.
2. Aphthoid ulcers.
3. Deeper fissure ulcers which may produce a 'cobblestone' pattern.
4. Strictures.
5. Pseudosacculation.
6. Inflammatory pseudopolyps.
7. The ileocaecal valve may be thickened, narrowed and ulcerated.

Complications

1. Fistulae.
2. Perforation — which is usually localized and results in abscess formation.
3. Toxic megacolon.
4. Carcinoma
   (a) Colon — less common than in ulcerative colitis, but this may be because more patients with Crohn's disease undergo colectomy at an early stage.
   (b) Small bowel — 300 × increased incidence.
5. Lymphoma.
6. Associated conditions.
   (a) Erythema nodosum.
   (b) Arthritis
   (i) Spondyloarthritis mimicking ankylosing spondylitis. It follows a course independent of the bowel disease and precedes it in 25% of cases.
   (ii) Enteropathic synovitis, the activity of which parallels the bowel disease. The weight-bearing joints of the lower limbs, wrist and fingers are affected.
   (c) Cirrhosis.
   (d) Chronic active hepatitis.
   (e) Gallstones.
   (f) Oxalate urinary tract calculi.
   (g) Pericholangitis.
   (h) Cholangiocarcinoma.
   (i) Sclerosing cholangitis.

Cushing's Syndrome

Cushing's syndrome results from increased endogenous or exogenous cortisol.

Spontaneous Cushing's syndrome is rare and due to

Pituitary disease (Cushing's disease)	80%

90% of these are due to adenoma and 20% have radiological evidence of an intrasellar tumour.

Adrenal disease — adenoma
                        — carcinoma

Ectopic ACTH, e.g. from a carcinoma of the bronchus } 20%

Iatrogenic Cushing's syndrome is common and due to high doses of corticosteroids. The effects of excessive amounts of corticosteroids are:

1. Growth retardation in children.
2. Osteoporosis.
3. Pathological fractures which show excessive callus formation during healing; vertebral end-plate fractures, in particular, show prominent bone condensation.
4. Avascular necrosis of bone.
5. Increased incidence of infection— including osteomyelitis and septic arthritis (the knee is affected most frequently).
6. Hypertension.
7. Water retention resulting in oedema.

Cystic Fibrosis

An autosomal recessive condition in which the basic problem is one of excessively viscid mucus.

Cardiopulmonary
1. Bronchial wall thickening and mucus-filled bronchi.
2. Atelectasis — subsegmental, segmental or lobar (especially the right upper lobe).
3. Recurrent pneumonia.
4. Bronchiectasis.
5. Focal emphysema in generally overinflated lungs.
6. 'Honeycomb lung' (q.v.), ± pneumothorax (rare before puberty).
7. Low incidence of pleural effusion or empyema at all ages.
8. Cor pulmonale — more common in the older age group and often precedes death.

Gastrointestinal
1. Meconium ileus (10%), meconium peritonitis and meconium ileus equivalent (5–10%).
2. Thickened mucosal folds, nodular filling defects and small-bowel dilatation.

Liver
1. Hepatomegaly.
2. Portal hypertension.

Pancreas
1. Calcification (lithiasis).

Skeletal
1. Retarded maturation.
2. Clubbing and hypertrophic osteoarthropathy.

Sinuses
1. Chronic sinusitis — opaque maxillary antra in nearly all children over 2 years of age.
2. Nasal polyps (10–15%).
3. Mucocoele.

Down's Syndrome (Trisomy 21)

Craniofacial
1. Brachycephaly and microcephaly.
2. Hypoplasia of facial bones and sinuses.
3. Wide sutures and delayed closure. Multiple wormian bones.
4. Hypotelorism.
5. Underdeveloped teeth. No. 2] [2. Less caries than usual.

Axial Skeleton
1. Increased height and decreased AP diameter of lumbar vertebrae.
2. Atlantoaxial subluxation.
3. Incomplete fusion of vertebral arches of the lumbar spine.

Pelvis
1. Flared iliac wings with small acetabular angles resulting in an abnormal iliac index (iliac angle + acetabular angle).

Chest
1. Congenital heart disease (40%) — mainly endocardial cushion defects and aberrant right subclavian artery.
2. Eleven pairs of ribs.
3. Two ossification centres for the manubrium (90%).

Hands
1. Short tubular bones, clinodactyly (50%) and hypoplasia of the middle phalanx of the little finger (60%).

Gastrointestinal
1. Umbilical hernia.
2. Duodenal atresia or stenosis.
3. Tracheo-oesophageal fistula.
4. Anorectal anomalies.

Enchondroma

1. Age — 10–50 years.
2. Sites — hands and wrists predominate (50%). Any other bones formed in cartilage.
3. Appearances
   (a) Diaphyseal or diametaphyseal.
   (b) Well-defined lucency with a thin sclerotic rim.
   (c) Often expansile; cortex preserved.
   (d) Internal ground-class appearance ± calcification.
   (e) Especially in long bones, may be multilocular.

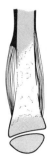

Syndromes
Ollier's disease — multiple enchondromata.
Maffucci's syndrome — enchondromata + haemangiomata.

Eosinophilic Granuloma

See 'Histiocytosis X'.

Ewing's Tumour

1. Age — 5–15 years.
2. Sites — femur, pelvis and shoulder girdle.
3. Appearances
   (a) Diaphyseal or, less commonly, metaphyseal.
   (b) Ill-defined medullary destruction.
   (c) ± small areas of new bone formation.
   (d) Periosteal reaction — lamellated (onion skin), Codman's triangle or 'sunray' spiculation.
   (e) Soft-tissue extension.
   (f) Metastases to other bones and lungs.

Extrinsic Allergic Alveolitis

An allergic reaction in the alveoli of sensitized individuals following repeated exposure to one of a number of specific antigens (see section 4.21).

Acute Exposure

1. Symptoms 4–8 hours after exposure (dyspnoea, dry cough, fever, malaise and myalgia).
2. The chest X-ray may be normal.
3. When radiological changes are present they usually parallel the severity of clinical symptoms. Changes consist of
   (a) Ground-glass, nodular or miliary shadows, 1–several mm in diameter, diffusely throughout both lungs but with some sparing of the apices and bases. Usually poorly defined.
   (b) Alveolar shadows, particularly in the lower zones, following heavy exposure to antigen.
   (c) Septal lines.
   (d) Hilar lymphadenopathy is rare but may be more frequent in mushroom-worker's lung.
   4. Removal from antigen exposure results in resolution of the radiological changes over 1–several weeks.

Chronic Exposure

1. Persistent exposure to low doses of antigen.
2. The diffuse nodular pattern is replaced by the changes characteristic of diffuse interstitial fibrosis.
   (a) Reticular pattern   ⎫ but with
   (b) Loss of lung volume   ⎬ marked upper-zone
   (c) 'Honeycomb' pattern ⎭ predominance.

Fibrous Dysplasia

Unknown pathogenesis. Medullary bone is replaced by fibrous tissue.

1. Diagnosis usually made between 3 and 15 years.
2. May be monostotic or polyostotic. In polyostotic cases the lesions tend to be unilateral; if bilateral then asymmetrical.
3. Most frequent sites are femur, pelvis, skull, mandible, ribs (most common cause of a focal expansile rib lesion) and humerus. Other bones are less frequently affected.
4. Radiological changes include
   (a) A cyst-like lesion in the diaphysis or metaphysis with endosteal scalloping ± bone expansion. No periosteal new bone. The epiphysis is only involved after fusion. Thick sclerotic border — 'rind' sign. Internally the lesion shows a ground-glass appearance ± irregular calcifications together with irregular sclerotic areas.
   (b) Bone deformity, e.g. shepherd's crook deformity of the proximal femur.
   (c) Growth disparity.
   (d) Accelerated bone maturation.
   (e) Skull shows mixed lucencies and sclerosis mainly on the convexity of the calvarium and the floor of the anterior fossa.
   (f) Leontiasis ossea is a sclerosing form affecting the face ± the skull base and producing leonine facies. In such cases extracranial lesions are rare. Involvement may be asymmetrical.
5. Associated endocrine abnormalities include
   (a) Sexual precocity (+ skin pigmentation) — in 30% of females with the polyostotic form. This constitutes the McCune–Albright syndrome.
   (b) Acromegaly, Cushing's syndrome, gynaecomastia and parathyroid hyperplasia (all rare).

Giant Cell Tumour

1. Age — 20–40 years (only 3% occur before epiphyseal closure).
2. Sites — long bones, distal femur especially; occasionally the sacrum or pelvis. Spine rarely.
3. Appearances
   (a) Epiphyseal and metaphyseal, i.e. subarticular.
   (b) A lucency with an ill-defined endosteal margin.
   (c) Eccentric expansion ± cortical destruction and soft-tissue extension.
   (d) Cortical ridges or internal septa produce a multilocular appearance.

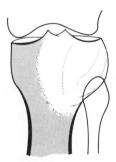

Gout

Caused by monosodium urate monohydrate or uric acid crystal deposition. Idiopathic (in the majority of patients) or associated with many other disorders, e.g. myeloproliferative diseases, drugs and chronic renal disease. Idiopathic gout may be divided into three stages

Asymptomatic Hyperuricaemia
1. No radiological signs but renal calculi or arthritis will develop in 20%.

Acute Gouty Arthritis
1. Mono- or oligoarticular; occasionally polyarticular.
2. Predilection for joints of the lower extremities, especially the 1st metatarsophalangeal joint (70%), intertarsal joints, ankles and knees. Other joints are affected in long-standing disease.
3. Soft-tissue swelling and joint effusion during the acute attack, with disappearance of the abnormalities as the attack subsides.

Chronic Tophaceous Gout

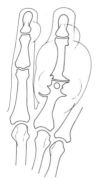

1. In 50% of patients with recurrent acute gout.
2. Eccentric, asymmetrical nodular deposits of calcium urate (tophi) in the synovium, subchondral bone, helix of the ear and in the soft tissues of the elbow, hand, foot, knee and forearm. Calcification of tophi is uncommon; ossification is rare.
3. Joint space is preserved until late in the disease.
4. Little or no osteoporosis until late, when there may be disuse osteoporosis.
5. Bony erosions are produced by tophaceous deposits and may be intra-articular, periarticular or well away from the joint. The latter two may be associated with an obvious soft-tissue mass. Erosions are round or oval, with the long axis in line with the bone. They may have a sclerotic margin. Some erosions have an overhanging lip of bone, which is strongly suggestive of the condition.
6. Severe erosive changes result in an arthritis mutilans.

Complications

1. Urolithiasis — in 10% of gout patients (higher in hot climates).
2. Renal disease
   (a) Acute urate nephropathy — precipitation of uric acid in the collecting ducts. Usually follows treatment with cytotoxic drugs.
   (b) Chronic urate nephropathy — rare.

Haemangioma

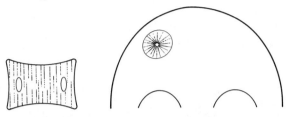

1. Age — 10–50 years.
2. Sites — vertebra (dorsal lumbar) or skull vault.
3. Appearances
   (a) Vertebra — coarse vertical striations, usually affecting only the body but the appendages are, uncommonly, also involved.
   (b) Skull — radial spiculation ('sunburst') within a well-defined vault lucency. 'Hair-on-end' appearance in tangential views.

Haemochromatosis

A genetically determined primary abnormality of iron metabolism. Also occurs secondary to alcoholic cirrhosis or multiple blood transfusions, e.g. in thalassaemia or chronic excessive oral iron ingestion.

Clinically — cirrhosis, skin pigmentation, diabetes (bronze diabetics), arthropathy and, later, ascites and cardiac failure.

Bones and joints
1. Osteoporosis.
2. Chondrocalcinosis — due to calcium pyrophosphate dihydrate deposition (q.v.).
3. Arthropathy — resembles the arthropathy of calcium pyrophosphate deposition disease (q.v.), but shows a predilection for the metacarpophalangeal joints (especially the 2nd and 3rd), the midcarpal joints and the carpometacarpal joints. It also exhibits distinctive beak-like osteophytes and is less rapidly progressive.

Liver and Spleen
1. Mottled increased density of liver and spleen due to the deposition of iron.

Haemophilia

Classical (Factor VIII deficiency) or Christmas disease (Factor IX deficiency). Both are X-linked recessive traits, i.e. manifest in males and carried by females.

Joints
1. Knee, elbow, ankle, hip and shoulder are most frequently affected.
2. Soft-tissue swelling due to haemarthrosis which may appear to be unusually dense owing to the presence of haemosiderin in the chronically thickened synovium.
3. Periarticular osteoporosis.
4. Erosion of articular surfaces, with subchondral cysts.
5. Preservation of joint space until late.
6. Accelerated maturation and growth of epiphyses resulting in disparity of size between epiphysis and diaphysis.
7. Contractures.

Bones
1. Osteonecrosis — especially in the femoral head and talus.
2. Haemophilic pseudotumour — in the ilium, femur and tibia most frequently
   (a) Intraosseous — a well-defined medullary lucency with a sclerotic margin. It may breach the cortex. ± periosteal reaction and soft-tissue component.
   (b) Subperiosteal — periosteal reaction with pressure resorption of the cortex and a soft-tissue mass.
   3. Fractures — secondary to osteoporosis.

Soft Tissues
1. Pseudotumour — slow growing.
2. Ectopic ossification.

Further Reading
Stoker D.J. & Murray R.O. (1974) Skeletal changes in haemophilia and other bleeding disorders. *Semin. Roentgenol.*, 9: 185–93.

Histiocytosis X

A disease characterized by intense proliferation of reticulohisti-ocytic elements. Younger patients have more disseminated disease. There are three clinical subgroups.

Eosinophilic Granuloma
1. Accounts for 50% of histiocytosis.
2. Commonest in 4–7 year olds, who present with bone pain, local swelling and irritability.
3. 50–75% have solitary lesions. When multiple, usually only two or three. Long bones, pelvis, skull and flat bones are the most common sites involved.
4. Radiological changes in the skeleton include
   (a) Well-defined lucency in the medulla ± thin sclerotic rim. ± endosteal scalloping. True expansion is uncommon except in ribs and vertebral bodies. ± overlying periosteal reaction.
   (b) Multilocular lucency, without expansion, in the pelvis.
   (c) Punched-out lucencies in the skull vault with little or no surrounding sclerosis. May coalesce to give a 'geographical skull'.
   (d) Destructive lesions in the skull base, mastoids, sella or mandible ('floating teeth').
   (e) Vertebra plana, with intact intervertebral discs.
5. Lung involvement in < 10% and associated with a worse prognosis.
   (a) Hilar lymphadenopathy.
   (b) Miliary shadowing.
   (c) 'Honeycomb lung'.

Hand–Schüller–Christian Disease
1. Commonest in 1–3 year olds.
2. Osseous lesions together with mild to moderate visceral involvement which includes lymphadenopathy, hepato-splenomegaly, skin lesions, diabetes insipidus, exoph-thalmos and pulmonary disease.
3. Bone lesions are similar to eosinophilic granuloma, but more numerous and widely distributed.

Letterer–Siwe Disease
1. Major visceral involvement with less prominent bone involvement during the first year of life.
2. Bone lesions are poorly defined.

Homocystinuria

An autosomal recessive inborn error of metabolism. A lack of cystathionine synthetase results in the accumulation of homocystine and methionine, with a deficiency of cystathionine and cystine.
1. Mental defect (60%).
2. Tall, stature, slim build and arachnodactyly, with a morphological resemblance to Marfan's syndrome.
3. Pectus excavatum or carinatum, kyphoscoliosis, genu valgum and pes cavus.
4. Osteoporosis.
5. Medial degeneration of the aorta and elastic arteries.
6. Arterial and venous thromboses.
7. Lens subluxation — usually downward.

Hurler's Syndrome

A mucopolysaccharidosis transmitted as an autosomal recessive trait. Clinical features become evident at the end of the first year — dwarfism, mental retardation, coarse facial features, corneal opacification, deformed teeth and hepatosplenomegaly. Respiratory infections and cardiac failure usually lead to death in the first decade.

Craniofacial
1. Scaphocephalic macrocephaly.
2. ± hydrocephalus.
3. J-shaped sella (prominent sulcus chiasmatus).

Axial Skeleton
1. Oval vertebral bodies with an antero-inferior beak.
2. Kyphosis and a thoracolumbar gibbus.
3. Posterior scalloping with widened interpedicular distance.
4. Short neck.

Appendicular Skeleton
1. Thickened diaphyses.
2. Angulated, oblique growth plates, e.g. those of the distal radius and ulna are angled toward each other.
3. Coxa valga (common). Genu valgum (always).
4. Trident hands with a coarse trabecular pattern. Proximal tapering of metacarpals.

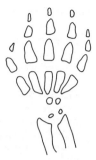

Cardiovascular System
1. Cardiac failure due to intimal thickening of coronary arteries or valves.

N.B. Hunter's syndrome is very similar clinically and radiologically, but the differences are:
   (a) X-linked recessive transmission (i.e. no affected females).
   (b) Later onset (2–6 yrs) and slower progression (death in the 2nd or 3rd decade).
   (c) No corneal clouding.

Hyperparathyroidism, Primary

Causes
1. Adenoma of one gland (90%). (2% of adenomas are multiple.)
2. Hyperplasia of all four glands (5%). (More likely if there is a family history.)
3. Carcinoma of one gland.
4. Ectopic parathormone — e.g. from a carcinoma of the bronchus.
5. Multiple endocrine adenopathy syndrome (type 1) — hyperplasia or adenoma associated with pituitary adenoma and pancreatic tumour.

Bones
1. Osteopenia — uncommon. When advanced there is loss of the fine trabeculae and sometimes a ground-glass appearance.
2. Subperiosteal bone resorption — particularly affecting the radial side of the middle phalanx of the middle finger, medial proximal tibia, lateral and occasionally medial end of clavicle, symphysis pubis, ischial tuberosity, medial femoral neck, dorsum sellae, superior surface of ribs and proximal humerus. Severe disease produces terminal phalangeal resorption and, in children, the 'rotting fence-post' appearance of the proximal femur.
3. Diffuse cortical change — cortical tunnelling eventually leading to a 'basketwork' appearance. 'Pepper-pot skull'.
4. Brown tumours — the solitary sign in 3% of cases. Most frequent in the mandible, ribs, pelvis and femora.
5. Bone softening — basilar invagination, wedged or codfish vertebrae, kyphoscoliosis, triradiate pelvis. Pathological fractures.

Soft tissues
1. Calcification in soft tissues, pancreas, lung and arteries.

Joints
1. Marginal erosions — predominantly the distal interphalangeal joints, the ulnar side of the base of the little-finger metacarpal and the hamate. No joint-space narrowing.
2. Weakened subarticular bone, leading to collapse.
3. Chondrocalcinosis (calcium pyrophosphate dihydrate deposition disease) and true gout.
4. Periarticular calcification, including capsular and tendon calcification.

Kidney
1. Nephrocalcinosis.
2. Calculi (in 50%).

Hypercalcaemia
1. Asymptomatic (in 15%) or overt (in 8%).

Gastrointestinal Tract
1. Peptic ulcer.
2. Pancreatitis.

Hypoparathyroidism

1. Short stature, dry skin, alopecia, tetany ± mental retardation.
2. Skeletal changes affecting the entire skeleton.
3. Minimal, generalized increased density of the skeleton, but especially affecting the metaphyses.
4. Calcification of paraspinal ligaments (secondary to elevation of plasma phosphate, which combines with calcium, resulting in heterotopic calcium phosphate deposits).
5. Basal ganglia calcification — uncommon.

Hypophosphatasia

Autosomal recessive. Deficiency of serum and tissue alkaline phosphatase, with excessive urinary excretion of phosphoethanolamine. 50% die in early infancy.

Neonatal Form
1. Most severely affected. Stillborn or die within 6 months.
2. Clinically — hypotonia, irritability, vomiting respiratory insufficiency, failure to thrive, convulsions and small stature with bowed legs.
3. Radiologically
   (a) Profoundly deficient mineralization with increased liability to fractures.
   (b) Irregular lack of metaphyseal mineralization affecting especially the wrists, knees and costochondral junctions.

Infantile Form
1. Initially asymptomatic, but between 2 weeks and 6 months shows the same symptoms as the neonatal form. Most survive.
2. Radiologically
   (a) Cupped and frayed metaphyses with widened growthplates.
   (b) Demineralized epiphyses.
   (c) Defective mineralization of skull, including sutures which appear widened.
   (d) Premature sutural fusion → craniostenosis with brachycephaly.

Childhood Form
1. Presents 6 months–2 years with bowed legs, genu valgum, delayed walking, bone pain, dental caries and premature loss of teeth.
2. Radiologically
   (a) Mild rickets.
   (b) No craniostenosis.

Adult Form
1. Osteomalacia — both clinically and radiologically.

Hypothyroidism

See 'Cretinism'.

Juvenile Chronic Arthritis

Three main clinical subgroups account for 70% of cases.

Systemic Onset
1. Most common at 1–5 years. M = F.
2. Severe extra-articular clinical manifestations include pyrexia, rash, lymphadenopathy and hepatosplenomegaly.
3. Joint involvement is late, but eventually a polyarthritis affects especially the knees, wrists, carpi, ankles and tarsi.

Polyarticular Onset
1. Onset at any age. More common in females.
2. Arthritis predominates with a similar distribution to the systemic onset, but also including the small joints of the fingers and toes. The cervical spine is involved frequently and early.
3. Prolonged disease leads to growth retardation and abnormal epiphyseal development.

Pauciarticular or Monoarticular Onset (most common presentation)
1. Most commonly presents at 1–5 years.
2. Four or less joints involved at the onset — knees, ankles and hips most commonly.
3. ± iridocyclitis.

Less Common Chronic Arthritides in Children
1. Seropositive juvenile onset rheumatoid arthritis — closely resembles the adult disease. Most common over 10 years of age and more common in girls.
2. Juvenile ankylosing spondylitis.
3. Juvenile psoriatic arthritis.
4. Enteropathic arthritis.

Radiological changes
1. Periarticular soft-tissue swelling.
2. Osteopenia — juxta-articular, diffuse or band-like in the metaphyses; the latter particularly in the distal femur, proximal tibia, distal radius and distal tibia.
3. Accelerated bone growth with large epiphyses and early fusion of growth-plates.
4. Over- or undergrowth of diaphyses.
5. Periostitis — common. Mainly periarticular in the phalanges, metacarpals and metatarsals, but when diaphyseal will eventually result in enlarged rectangular tubular bones.
6. Erosions and joint-space narrowing are late manifestations.
7. Epiphyseal compression fractures.
8. Subluxation and dislocation — most commonly in the hip leading to protrusio acetabuli. Atlanto-axial subluxation is most frequent in seropositive juvenile onset rheumatoid arthritis.
9. Bony ankylosis — especially in the carpus and tarsus.

Lymphoma

Intrathoracic Lymphadenopathy

1. 66% of patients with Hodgkin's disease have intrathoracic disease and 99% of these have intrathoracic lymphadenopathy.
2. 40% of patients with non-Hodgkin's lymphoma have intrathoracic disease and 90% of these have intrathoracic lymphadenopathy.
3. Nodes involved are (in order of frequency) anterior mediastinal, paratracheal, tracheobronchial, bronchopulmonary and subcarinal. Involvement tends to be bilateral and asymmetrical, although unilateral disease is not uncommon.
4. Nodes show a rapid response to radiotherapy and 'eggshell' calcification of lymphnodes may be observed following radiotherapy.

Pulmonary Disease

1. More common in Hodgkin's disease than non-Hodgkin's lymphoma.
2. Very unusual without lymphadenopathy, but may be the first evidence of recurrence after radiotherapy.
3. Most frequently one or more large opacities with an irregular outline. ± air bronchogram.
4. Collapse due to endobronchial lymphoma or, less frequently, extrinsic compression. (Collapse is less common than in bronchial carcinoma.)
5. Lymphatic obstruction → oedema or lymphangitis carcinomatosa.
6. Miliary or larger opacities widely disseminated throughout the lungs.
7. Cavitation — eccentrically within a mass and with a thick wall. (More common than in bronchial carcinoma.)
8. Calcification following radiotherapy.
9. Soft-tissue mass adjacent to a rib deposit.
10. Pleural and pericardial effusions.

Gastrointestinal Tract

Involvement may be the primary presentation (5% of all lymphomas) or be a part of generalized disease (50% at autopsy). In descending order of frequency, the stomach, small intestine, rectum and colon may be involved.

Stomach

1. Primary lymphoma accounts for 2.5% of all gastric neoplasms and 2.5% of lymphomas present with a stomach lesion. Non-Hodgkin's lymphoma accounts for 80%.
2. The radiological manifestations comprise
   (a) Diffuse mucosal thickening and irregularity ± decreased distensibility and peristaltic activity. ± multiple ulcers.
   (b) Smooth nodular mass ± central ulceration. Surrounding mucosa may be normal or show thickened folds.
   (c) Single or multiple ulcers with irregular margins.
   (d) Thickening of the wall with narrowing of the lumen. If the distal stomach is involved there may be extension into the duodenum.
   (e) Duodenal ulcer associated with a gastric mass.

Small Intestine

1. Usually secondary to contiguous spread from mesenteric lymph nodes. Primary disease only in non-Hodgkin's lymphoma.
2. Usually more than one of the following signs is evident
   (a) Irregular mucosal infiltration → thick folds ± nodularity.
   (b) Irregular polypoid mass ± barium tracts within it or central ulceration.
   (c) Annular constriction — usually a long segment.
   (d) Aneurysmal dilatation, with no internal mucosal pattern.
   (e) Polyps — multiple and small or solitary and large. The latter may induce an intussusception.
   (f) Multiple ulcers.
   (g) Non-specific malabsorption pattern.
   (h) Fistula.
   (i) Perforation.

Colon and Rectum

1. Rarely involved. Caecum and rectum more frequently involved than the rest of the colon.
2. Radiologically the disease may show
   - (a) Polypoidal mass — which may induce an intussusception.
   - (b) Diffuse infiltration of the wall.
   - (c) Constricting annular lesion.

Retroperitoneal Lymphadenopathy

1. The typical lymphographic appearances are
   - (a) Enlarged nodes.
   - (b) Foamy or 'ghost-like' internal architectural pattern.
   - (c) Discrete filling defects.
   - (d) Non-filling of lymph nodes.

Skeleton

1. Radiological involvement in 10–20% of patients with Hodgkin's disease (50% at autopsy).
2. Involvement arises either from direct spread from contiguous lymph nodes or infiltration of bone marrow (spine, pelvis, major long bones, thoracic cage and skull are sites of predilection).
3. Patterns of bone involvement are
   - (a) Predominantly osteolytic.
   - (b) Mixed lytic and sclerotic.
   - (c) Predominantly sclerotic — de novo or following radiotherapy to a lytic lesion.
   - (d) 'Moth-eaten' — characteristic of round cell malignancies.
4. In addition the spine may show
   - (a) Anterior erosion of a vertebral body due to involvement of an adjacent paravertebral lymph node.
   - (b) Solitary dense vertebral body (ivory vertebra).
5. Hypertrophic osteoarthropathy.

Central Nervous System
1. Primary lymphoma of brain (microgliomatosis) accounts for 1% of brain tumours.
2. The cerebrum, brainstem and cerebellum are affected (in order of frequency).
3. Two patterns may be recognized at CT
   (a) Large round or oval space-occupying lesion showing increased attenuation and surrounding oedema. Marked homogeneous enhancement (although avascular at angiography). Multifocal in 50%.
   (b) Cuff of tissue around the lateral ventricles with marked enhancement.

Further Reading
Craig O. & Gregson R. (1981). Primary lymphoma of the gastrointestinal tract. *Clin. Radiol.*, 32: 63–71.
Felson B. (ed.) (1980) The lymphomas and leukaemias. Part I. *Semin. Roentgenol.*, 15 (3).
Felson B. (ed.) (1980) The lymphomas and leukaemias. Part 2, *Semin. Roentgenol.*, 15 (4).
Privett J.T.J., Rhys Davies E. & Roylance J. (1977) The radiological features of gastric lymphoma. *Clin. Radiol.*, 28: 457–63.
Strickland B. (1967) Intrathoracic Hodgkin's disease. Part II. Peripheral manifestations of Hodgkin's disease in the chest. *Br. J. Radiol.*, 40: 930–8.
Thomson J.C.G. & Brownell B. (1981) Computed tomographic appearances in microgliomatosis. *Clin. Radiol.*, 32: 367–74.

Marfan's Syndrome

A connective tissue disorder transmitted as an autosomal dominant trait, but with extremely variable expression.
1. Tall stature, long slim limbs and arachnodactyly.
2. Joint laxity.
3. Scoliosis (60%) and kyphosis.
4. Pectus excavatum or carinatum.
5. Narrow facies with a narrow, high arched palate.
6. Lens subluxation — usually upwards.
7. Ascending aortic dilatation ± dissection. Less commonly aneurysms of the descending thoracic or abdominal aorta or pulmonary artery.

Morquio's Syndrome

A mucopolysaccharidosis transmitted as an autosomal recessive trait. Clinical presentation during the second year, with decreased growth, progressive skeletal deformity, corneal opacities, lymphadenopathy, cardiac lesions and deafness.

Axial Skeleton
1. Universal vertebra plana. Wide discs.
2. Hypoplastic dens.
3. Hypoplastic dorsolumbar vertebra which may be displaced posteriorly.
4. Central anterior vertebral body beaks.
5. Short neck.
6. Dorsal scoliosis and dorsolumbar kyphosis.

Appendicular Skeleton
1. Defective irregular ossification of the femoral capital epiphyses leading to flattening.
2. Genu valgum.
3. Short, wide tubular bones with irregular metaphyses. Proximal tapering of the metacarpals.
4. Irregular carpal and tarsal bones.

Cardiovascular System
1. Late onset aortic regurgitation.

Multiple Endocrine Neoplasia (MEN) Syndromes

Autosomal dominant. Classification.

MEN I (Wermer's Syndrome)
1. Hyperparathyroidism (90%).
2. Pancreatic islet cell tumours (60%)
   Gastrinomas (60%) — usually slow growing: →
   Zollinger–Ellison syndrome.
   Insulinomas — symptoms of hypoglycaemia.
   VIPomas — secreting vasoactive intestinal peptide →
   explosive, watery diarrhoea with hypokalaemia and achlor-
   hydria.
   Glucagonomas — produce a syndrome of diabetes mellitus,
   necrolytic migratory erythema, anaemia, weight loss and
   thrombo-embolic complications.
3. Pituitary tumours (5%) — hormone secreting and non-
   secreting.
4. Thyroid adenoma.
5. Adrenal adenoma.
6. Carcinoid tumour.

MEN IIa (Sipple's Syndrome)
1. Medullary carcinoma of the thyroid (100%).
2. Phaeochromocytoma (50%).
3. Hyperparathyroidism (10%).

MEN IIb
1. Marfanoid appearance (100%).
2. Multiple mucosal neuromas (100%).
3. Medullary carcinoma of the thyroid (100%).
4. Phaeochromocytoma (50%).

Multiple Myeloma/Plasmacytoma

Plasma cell neoplasms of bone are solitary (plasmacytoma;
3% of all plasma cell tumours) or multiple (multiple myeloma;
94% of all plasma cell tumours). 3% of all plasma cell
tumours are solely extraskeletal.

Plasmacytoma
1. A well-defined, grossly expansile bone lesion arising, most
   commonly, in the spine, pelvis or ribs.
2. It may also exhibit soft-tissue extension, internal septa or
   pathological fracture.

Multiple Myeloma
Radiological manifestations are skeletal and extraskeletal.

SKELETAL
1. 80–90% have an abnormal skeleton at the time of diagnosis.
2. The skeleton may
   (a) be normal — uncommon;
   (b) show generalized osteopenia only — rare;
   (c) show osteopenia with discrete lucencies
       (i) The lucencies are usually
           — widely disseminated at the time of diagnosis (spine, pelvis, skull, ribs and shafts of long bones);
           — uniform in size (c.f. metastases, which are usually of varying size);
           — well-defined, with a narrow zone of transition.
       (ii) Vertebral body collapse, occasionally with disc destruciton. ± paravertebral shadow. Involvement of pedicles is late.
       (iii) Rib lesions tend to be expansile and associated with extrapleural soft-tissue masses.
       (iv) Pathological fractures occur and healing is accompanied by much callus.
   (d) show a permeating, mottled pattern of bone destruction similar to other round cell malignancies, e.g. Ewing's sarcoma, anaplastic metastatic carcinoma, leukaemia and reticulum cell sarcoma.
   (e) show multiple sclerotic lesions which mimic osteoblastic metastases (2%).

EXTRASKELETAL
1. Hypercalcaemia (30%).
2. Soft-tissue tumours in sinuses, the submucosa of the pharynx and trachea, cervical lymph nodes, skin and gastrointestinal tract.
3. Hepatosplenomegaly.

Further Reading
Meszaros W.T. (1974) The many facets of multiple myeloma. *Semin. Roentgenol.*, 9: 219–28.

Neurofibromatosis

Autosomal dominant but 50% are spontaneous mutations.
There are at least two distinct forms:
1. Classical Von Recklinghausen (peripheral) neurofibromatosis accounts for over 90% of all cases and its major
   features are (six or more) *café au lait* spots, peripheral
   neurofibromas and Lisch nodules (pigmented iris hamartomas).
2. Bilateral acoustic (central) neurofibromatosis is associated
   with few, if any, *café au lait* spots and no Lisch nodules.
   These patients have other central nervous system tumours,
   particularly meningiomas.

Skull and Brain
1. Hemihypertrophy or hemiatrophy of the cranium. Macrocranium.
2. Dyplastic sphenoid — absent greater wing ± lesser wing
   (empty orbit), absent posterolateral wall of the orbit. May
   produce proptosis.
3. Lytic defects in the calvarium, especially in or near the
   lambdoid suture.
4. Optic nerve gliomas (common). Optic nerve sheath meningiomas (rare).
5. Neuromas, especially acoustic neuromas. If bilateral they
   are virtually pathognomonic of the condition.
6. Meningiomas.
7. Heavy calcification of the choroid plexuses is rare but
   classical.

Thorax
1. Rib notching, 'twisted ribbon' ribs and splaying of ribs.
2. Interstitial pulmonary fibrosis progressing to a 'honeycomb
   lung'.

Axial Skeleton

1. Sharp angular kyphoscoliosis (in 10%) with dysplastic vertebral bodies.
2. Posterior scalloping due to dural ectasia.
3. Enlarged intervertebral foramina and eccentric unilateral scalloping due to localized neurofibromas.

Appendicular Skeleton

1. Overgrowth or, less commonly, undergrowth of long bones.
2. Overtubulation or undertubulation (due to cortical thickening).
3. Anterior and lateral bowing of the tibia is common and is usually evident in the first year. It frequently progresses to —
4. Pseudarthrosis.
5. Intraosseous neurofibromas present as subperiosteal or cortical lucencies with a smooth expanded outer margin.
6. Cortical pressure resorption from an adjacent soft-tissue neurofibroma.
7. Cortical defects may also be due to dysplastic periosteum.

Other

1. Soft-tissue tumours.
2. Renal artery stenosis or aneurysm.
3. Phaeochromocytoma (in 1%).

Further Reading

Huson S.M. (1987) The different forms of neurofibromatosis. *Br. Med. J.*, 294: 1113–4.

Klatte E.C., Franken E.A. & Smith J.A. (1976) The radiographic spectrum in neurofibromatosis. *Sem. Roentgenol.*, 11: 17–33.

Neuropathic Arthropathy

Disease	Sites of involvement
Diabetes mellitus	Metatarsophalangeal, tarsometatarsal and intertarsal joints
Steroid treatment	Hips and knee
Syringomyelia	Shoulder, elbow, wrist and cervical spine
Tabes dorsalis	Knee, hip, ankle and lumbar spine
Congenital insensitivity to pain	Ankle and intertarsal joints
Myelomeningocoele	Ankle and intertarsal joints
Leprosy	Hands (interphalangeal), feet (metatarsophalangeal) and lower limbs
Chronic alcoholism	Metatarsophalangeal and interphalangeal joints

Radiological changes include
1. Variable progression, but often rapid. In the early stages can resemble osteoarthritis.
2. Joint effusion.
3. Osteochondral fractures and fragmentation of articular surfaces.
4. Intra-articular bony debris.
5. Excessive callus formation.
6. Subluxations and dislocations.
7. Bone density is normal but in diabetes and syringomyelia superadded infection is not uncommon, resulting in juxta-articular osteoporosis.
8. Bone resorption can produce a 'cup and pencil' appearance.

Non-Accidental Injury

Skeletal

1. Fractures in 11–55% and significantly more common in the younger child. Typically multiple, in varying stages of healing and explained by an implausible history.

2. Shaft fractures are more common than metaphyseal fractures although the latter are characteristic.

3. Metaphyseal fractures are due to tractional and torsional stresses on limbs and histologically there is a transmetaphyseal disruption of the most immature metaphyseal primary spongiosa. The most subtle indication of injury is a transverse lucency within the subepiphyseal region of the metaphysis. It may be visible in only one projection and its appearance is influenced by the severity of the bony injury, the degree of displacement of the fragments and the chronicity of the process. Peripherally the fracture line may undermine and isolate a thicker fragment of bone and it is this thick peripheral margin of bone that produces the corner fractures and bucket handle configurations.

4. Rib fractures comprise 5–27% of all fractures in abused children. Posterior rib fractures have a higher specificity for abuse than antero-lateral fractures. In the absence of prematurity, birth injury, metabolic disorders, bone dysplasias and major trauma e.g. road traffic accidents, rib fractures may be considered specific for abuse. 80% are occult.

5. Skull fractures which are linear and in the parietal bone are most common but others are more suggestive of non-accidental injry:
   (a) Multiple fractures.
   (b) Non-parietal fractures.
   (c) Complex fractures.
   (d) Depressed fractures.
   (e) Diastatic fractures greater than 5 mm in width.
   (f) Growing fractures (leptomeningeal cysts).
   A depressed occipital fracture is virtually pathognomonic of abuse.

6. In infants and young children certain fractures have a high specificity for abuse owing to their unusual locations. These include scapular injuries, injuries involving the small bones of the hands and feet and spinal injuries.

7. Dislocations are rarely encountered in abused children. Malalignment of bones sharing an articulation usually indicates a growth plate injury rather than dislocation. When dislocations do occur they are likely secondary to massive injury and are accompanied by adjacent fracture.

Intracranial Injuries

Shaking is the most important mechanism in the production of intracranial injury in child abuse. The spectrum of injuries include:

    (a) Subdural haematoma, especially posterior interhemispheric collections due to tearing of the small bridging veins which cross the subdural space.

    (b) Intraventricular haemorrhage — when gross is usually associated with massive intracranial injury.

    (c) Subarachnoid haemorrhage.

    (d) Cerebral oedema — generalized or focal and is the most common CT alteration in all types of paediatric head injury.

    (e) Cerebral contusion — seen usually along the cerebral convexities, particularly in the frontal and parasagittal regions, conforming to the sites of greatest stress during acceleration–deceleration movements.

        Commonly associated with subdural haematomata.

    (f) Cerebral atrophy — depending on the site of the original injury may be focal or diffuse and evident as early as 1 month following the acute injury.

    (g) Post-traumatic hydrocephalus.

Visceral Trauma

Commonly occurs after the child is able to move about. Mortality of 50% for visceral injuries associated with child abuse. The most likely mechanism of injury is a direct blow or the effect of rapid deceleration after being hurled. The most common injuries involve the hollow viscera, mesenteries liver and pancreas.

Further Reading

Hobbs C.J. (1984) Skull fracture and the diagnosis of abuse. *Arch. Dis. Childh.* 59: 246–52.

Kleinman P. (1987) *Diagnostic Imaging of Child Abuse.* Baltimore: Williams & Wilkins.

Merten, D.F., Radkowski M.A. & Leonidas J.C. (1983) The abused child: a radiological rappraisal. *Radiology*, 148: 377–81.

Worlock P., Stower M. & Barbor P. (1986) Patterns of fractures in accidental and non-accidental injury in children: a comparative study. *Br. Med. J.*, 293: 100–3.

Zimmerman R.A., Bilaniuk L.T., Bruce D., Schut L., Uzzell B. & Goldberg H.I. (1979) Computed tomography of craniocerebral injury in the abused child. *Radiology*, 130: 687–90.

Non-ossifying Fibroma (Fibrous Cortical Defect)

1. Age — 10–20 years.
2. Sites — femur and tibia.
3. Appearances

    (a) Diametaphyseal, becoming diaphyseal as the bone grows.

    (b) Well-defined lucency with a sclerotic margin.

    (c) Eccentric ± slight expansion; in thin bones, e.g. fibula, it occupies the entire width of the bone.

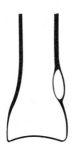

Ochronosis

See 'Alkaptonuria'.

Osteoblastoma

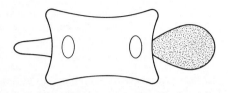

1. Age — 10–20 years.
2. Sites — vertebra (neural arch predominantly) and, less commonly, in the long bones.
3. Appearances
   (a) Well-defined lucency with a sclerotic rim.
   (b) May be expansile, but the cortex is preserved.
   (c) ± internal calcification.
   (d) May be purely sclerotic in the spine.
   (e) In long bones it is metaphyseal or diaphyseal.

Osteochondroma (Exostosis)

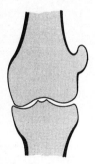

1. Age — 10–20 years.
2. Sites — distal femur, proximal tibia, proximal humerus, pelvis and scapula. When there are multiple osteochondromata the condition is termed diaphyseal aclasis.
3. Appearances
   (a) Metaphyseal.
   (b) Well-defined eccentric protrusion with the parent cortex and trabeculae continuous with that of the tumour.
   (c) Tumour is usually directed away from the end of the bone and migrates away from the end as growth proceeds.
   (d) The cartilage cap is not visible in childhood, but becomes calcified in the adult.
   (e) If large → failure of correct modelling.
   (f) Rapid growth of a stable lesion suggests transformation to a chondrosarcoma (less than 1% of cases).

Osteogenesis Imperfecta

A clinically heterogeneous condition due to disorders of collagen. There are several distinct genetic entities and the current classification is as shown below:

Type 1
Osseous fragility (variable from minimal to severe); blue sclerae; presenile deafness due to otosclerosis (in 20%). Multiple fractures and intracranial bleeding may result in stillbirth or perinatal death. Gracile, osteoporotic bones often with deformity secondary to fractures and mechanical stresses. Rapid fracture healing ± exuberant callus. Flattened or biconcave vertebral bodies. Wormian bones, although these may be obliterated in adulthood. Autosomal dominant.
   Subgroup A: with normal teeth.
   Subgroup B: with dentinogenesis imperfecta.

Type II
Lethal perinatal. Extremely severe osseous fragility.
   Subgroup A: extremely osteopenic skull; broad beaded ribs; short, broad 'concertina' shaped long bones; platyspondyly. New mutation, autosomal dominant.
   Subgroup B: better ossification of skull; thin, wavy ribs with only a few fractures; short, broad 'concertina' shaped long bones; vertebral body height similar to or greater than disc space. Autosomal recessive.
   Subgroup C: poor ossification of skull; thin, irregularly shaped ribs, short, poorly modelled long bones with multiple angulations; normal vertebral body height. Autosomal recessive or new dominant mutation.

Type III
Rare. Moderate to severe osseous fragility; normal sclerae; severe deformity of long bones and spine result in severe dwarfing; cystic expansion of ends of long bones with increasing age. Wormian bones. Markedly elongated lumbar pedicles. White sclerae. Autosomal recessive, or new dominant mutation.

Type IV
Rare. Osseous fragility with normal sclerae and severe deformity of long bones and spine. Autosomal dominant.

Further Reading

Sillence D.O. (1981) Osteogenesis imperfecta. An expanding panorama of variants. *Clin. Orthop.*, 159: 11–25.

Sillence D.O., Senn A. & Danks D.M. (1979) Genetic heterogeneity in osteogenesis imperfecta. *J. Med. Genet.*, 16: 101–16.

Smith R., Francis M.J.O. & Houghton G.R. (1983) *The Brittle Bone Syndrome: Osteogenesis Imperfecta*. Butterworth: London.

Thompson E.M., Young I.D., Hall C.M. & Pembrey M.E. (1987) Recurrence risk and prognosis in severe sporadic osteogenesis imperfecta. *J. Med. Genet.*, 24: 390–405.

Osteogenic Sarcoma

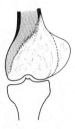

1. Age — 10–25 years with a second peak in the 7th decade (flat bones).
2. Sites — distal femur, proximal tibia, proximal humerus and pelvis.
3. Predisposing factors — Paget's disease, radiotherapy, osteochondroma, fibrous dysplasia, osteogenesis imperfecta, osteopetrosis and bone infarct.
4. Association — bilateral retinoblastoma.
5. Appearances
   (a) Metaphyseal; epiphyseal and diaphyseal are unusual.
   (b) May be predominantly lytic, sclerotic or mixed.
   (c) Wide zone of transition with normal bone.
   (d) Cortical destruction with soft tissue extension.
   (e) ± internal calcification of bone.
   (f) Periosteal reaction — 'sunray' spiculation, lamellated and/or Codman's triangle.
6. Unusual variants:
   (a) Parosteal — broad based, sessile, juxtacortical tumour with irregular margins. Less malignant. Femur is most common site. Older age group, 20–40 years.
   (b) Telangiectatic — lytic, permeating tumour extending into the soft tissues.
   (c) Multicentric.

Further Reading

Kumar R., David R., Madewell J.E. & Lindell Jr M.M. (1987) Radiographic spectrum of osteogenic sarcoma. *Am. J. Roentgenol.*, 148: 767–72.

Osteoid Osteoma

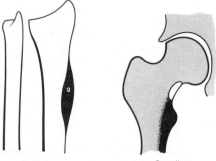

Cortical   Cancellous

1. Age – 10–30 years.
2. Sites — most commonly femur and tibia.
3. Appearances

   Cortical
   (a) Central lucent nidus (less than 1 cm) ± dense calcified centre.
   (b) Dense surrounding bone.
   (c) Eccentric bone expansion ± periosteal reaction.

   Cancellous
   (a) Usually femoral neck.
   (b) Lucent lesion with bone sclerosis a distance away. The head and neck may be osteoporotic.

Osteomalacia

Increased uncalcified osteoid in the mature skeleton.
1. Decreased bone density.
2. Looser's zones — bilaterally symmetrical transverse lucent bands of uncalcified osteoid which, later in the disease, have sclerotic margins. Common sites are the scapulae, femoral necks and shafts, pubic rami and ribs.
3. Coarsening of the trabecular pattern with ill-defined trabeculae.
4. Bone softening — protrusio acetabulae, bowing of long bones, biconcave vertebral bodies and basilar invagination.

Osteopetrosis

A defect of bone resorption due to decreased osteoclastic activity. A number of forms have been recognized.

Benign or Tarda, AD
1. Often asymptomatic individuals in whom a chance diagnosis is made on radiographs taken for some other purpose. Some have a mild anaemia and there may be cranial nerve compressions. Predisposition to fractures. Tooth extraction may be complicated by osteomyelitis.
2. Increasing bone sclerosis during childhood, with some sparing of the peripheral skeleton.
3. 'Bone-within-bone' appearance — usually disappearing by the end of the second decade.
4. 'Rugger jersey' spine.

Malignant or Congenita, AR
1. Manifestations during infancy — failure to thrive and evidence of marrow failure due to bone overgrowth i.e. anaemia, thrombocytopenia and hepatosplenomegaly. Pathological fractures. Cranial nerve palsies due to bony compression. Death in the first decade.
2. Generalized bone sclerosis with transverse metaphyseal bands.
3. 'Bone-within-bone' appearance.
4. 'Rugger jersey' spine.
5. Later, flask-shaped ends of the long bones.

Intermediate, AR

With Renal Tubular Acidosis, AR
1. Presents in early childhood with failure to thrive and hypotonia due to renal tubular acidosis. Anaemia, cranial nerve lesions and fractures are variable features.
2. Radiology is similar to the benign form but tends to normality in later childhood. Basal ganglia and periventricular calcification are consistent findings which differentiate this form from the others.

Further Reading

Beighton P. (1988) *Inherited Disorders of the Skeleton*, pp. 163–9. Edinburgh: Churchill Livingstone.

Beighton P. & Cremin B.J. *Sclerosing Bone Dysplasias*, pp. 19–31. Berlin: Springer-Verlag.

Paget's Disease

A condition characterized by excessive abnormal remodelling of bone. Increasing prevalence with age — rare in patients less than 40 years old, 3% of the population in middle age and 10% of the population in old age. The disease predominates in the axial skeleton — spine (75%), skull (65%), pelvis (40%) — and proximal femur (75%). (The percentages represent patients with Paget's disease in whom these sites are affected.) Monostotic disease does occur. There are 3 stages.

Active (Osteolytic)

1. Skull — osteoporosis circumscripta, especially in the frontal and occipital bones.
2. Long bones — a well-defined, advancing radiolucency with a V-shaped margin which begins subarticularly.

Osteolytic and Osteosclerotic

1. Skull — osteoporosis circumscripta with focal areas of bone sclerosis.
2. Pelvis — mixed osteolytic and osteosclerotic areas.
3. Long bones — epiphyseal and metaphyseal sclerosis with diaphyseal lucency.

Inactive (Osteosclerotic)

1. Skull — thickened vault. 'Cotton wool' areas of sclerotic bone. The facial bones are not commonly affected (c.f. fibrous dysplasia).
2. Spine — especially the lumbar spine. Enlargement of vertebrae and coarsened trabeculae. Cortical thickening produces the 'picture frame' vertebral body. Ivory vertebra.
3. Pelvis — widening and coarsened trabeculation of the pelvic ring, with splitting of the iliopectineal line may progress to widespread changes in the pelvis which are commonly asymmetrical.

4. Long bones — sclerosis due to coarsened, thickened trabeculae. Cortical thickening with encroachment on the medullary canal. The epiphyseal region is nearly always involved.

Complications
1. Bone softening — bowed bones, basilar invagination and protrusio acetabuli.
2. Fractures — transverse with a predilection for the convex aspect of the bone and which usually only partially traverse the bone.
3. Sarcomatous change — in 1% of patients (5–10% if there is widespread involvement). Femur, pelvis and humerus most commonly affected. Osteogenic sarcoma (50%), fibrosarcoma (25%) and chondrosarcoma (10%) are the most common histological diagnoses. They are predominantly lytic.
4. Degenerative joint disease — most frequent in the hip and knee.
5. Neurological complications — nerve entrapment and spinal-cord compression.
6. High output cardiac failure.
7. Extramedullary haemopoiesis.
8. Osteomyelitis.

Plasmacytoma

See 'Multiple myeloma/plasmacytoma'.

Polycystic Disease, Infantile

Autosomal recessive. Polycystic kidneys, with periportal hepatic fibrosis and bile duct obstruction.

Polycystic Disease of the Newborn
1. Presents in the first few days with renal failure and/ or respiratory distress because of elevated diaphragms. Majority die in a few days.
2. Bilateral large smooth kidneys with dense striated nephrograms (because of dilated tubules).
3. Calyces are not usually demonstrated but are normal.
4. Markedly hyperechoic kidneys on US with loss of corticomedullary differentiation.

Polycystic Disease of Childhood
1. Presents at 3–5 years.
2. Renal cysts are less prominent and hepatic fibrosis is greater. Presentation is, therefore, with portal hypertension.
3. Kidneys may be similar to the newborn type (although not so massive) or to the adult type. Multiple hepatic cysts.

Polycystic Disease, Adult

Autosomal dominant. Presents in 3rd–4th decade and terminal renal failure occurs within 10 years. May be diagnosed by screening family members and has been identified antenatally.

Kidneys
1. Bilateral, but asymmetrical, enlarged lobulated kidneys. Unilateral in 8%.
2. Multiple smooth defects in the nephrogram with elongation and deformity of calyces giving a 'spider leg' appearance. Cysts may produce filling defects in the renal pelvis. ± calcification in cyst walls.
3. Multiple cysts on US.
4. Increased incidence of renal cell carcinoma (may be bilateral).

Other Organs
1. Cystic changes in the liver (in 30%) and, less commonly, in the pancreas and spleen.
2. Displacement of bowel.
3. Intracranial aneurysms in 10%.

Pseudohypoparathyroidism

End organ unresponsiveness to parathormone. X-linked dominant transmission.
1. Short stature, round face, thickset features, mental retardation and hypocalcaemia.
2. Short 4th and 5th metacarpals and metatarsals.
3. Basal ganglia calcification (50%).
4. Soft-tissue calcification.

Pseudopseudohypoparathyroidism

Similar clinical and radiological features to pseudohypoparathyroidism but with a normal plasma calcium.

Psoriatic Arthropathy

Occurs in 5% of psoriatics and may antedate the skin changes.
There are five clinical and radiological types.
1. Polyarthritis with predominant involvement of the distal
   interphalangeal joints.
2. Seronegative polyarthritis simulating rheumatoid arthritis.
3. Monoarthritis or asymmetrical oligoarthritis.
4. Spondyloarthritis which can mimic ankylosing spondylitis.
5. Arthritis mutilans (commonly associated with severe skin
   changes).

The radiological changes comprise

1. Involvement of synovial and cartilaginous joints and
   entheses.
2. Joints most frequently affected are the interphalangeal
   joints of the hands and feet, the metacarpophalangeal
   and metatarsophalangeal joints, the sacro-iliac joints and
   those in the spine. The large joints are relatively spared.
   Involvement is asymmetrical.
3. Preserved bone density.
4. Soft-tissue swelling— periarticular or fusiform of a digit.
5. The joint space is narrowed in the large joints and
   widened in the small joints because of severe destruction
   of subchondral bone.
6. Erosions which are initially periarticular and progress to
   involve the entire articular surface. 'Cup and pencil'
   deformity. Severe destructive changes result in an arthritis
   mutilans. Erosions also occur at entheses.
7. Bony proliferation (a) adjacent to the erosions and (b) at
   tendon and ligament insertions.
8. Periosteal new bone — particularly in the hands and feet.
9. Ankylosis — especially at the interphalangeal joints of
   the hands and feet.
10. Distal phalangeal tuft resorption — almost always with
    severe nail changes.
11. Sacro-iliitis and spondylitis with paravertebral ossifi-
    cation.

Pulmonary Embolic Disease

Clinical conditions which predispose to venous thrombo-embolism are
1. Surgical procedures, especially major abdominal and gynaecological surgery and hip operations.
2. Trauma.
3. Prolonged bed-rest.
4. Neoplastic disease.
5. Pregnancy and the puerperium.
6. Oestrogens.

Pulmonary embolism is massive if more than 50% of the major pulmonary arteries are involved and minor if less than 50% are involved. Duration of embolism in the pulmonary arteries may be acute (< 48 hours), subacute (several days or weeks) or chronic (months or years).

Acute or Subacute Massive Embolism
1. The chest X-ray is most commonly normal.
2. Asymmetrical oligaemia — often best diagnosed by comparison with a previous chest X-ray. The main pulmonary artery may be enlarged.

Acute Minor
1. Although segmental oligaemia ± dilatation of the segmental artery proximal to the obstruction may be observed, this is uncommon and the chest X-ray is often normal.
2. Pulmonary infarction follows in about 33%. The signs are non-specific but include
   (a) Subpleural consolidation — segmental or subsegmental. Single or multiple.
   (b) Segmental collapse and later linear (plate) atelectasis.
   (c) Pleural reaction with a small effusion.
   (d) Elevation of the hemidiaphragm on the affected side.
   (e) Cavitation of the infarct.

3. Infarction is more common the right side and in the lower zones.

N.B. The ventilation-perfusion radionuclide lung-scan is an extremely useful investigation for the diagnosis of pulmonary embolism, especially as the chest X-ray is so commonly normal. The characteristic abnormality is a segmental perfusion defect at the periphery of the lung with no corresponding ventilation defect, i.e. a mismatched defect. This is pathognomonic of pulmonary embolism. When the chest X-ray shows collapse or infarction the lung scan shows a corresponding ventilation and perfusion defect, i.e. a matched effect. This is a non-specific finding seen with any pulmonary mass lesion.

Pulmonary arteriography is reserved for those patients in whom embolectomy is being considered.

Chronic
1. 'Plump' hila with peripheral arterial pruning, i.e. the signs of pulmonary arterial hypertension.
2. ± multiple areas of linear atelectasis.

Further Reading
Bedont R.A. & Armstrong II J.D. (1989) Imaging of venous thromboembolic disease. *Current Imaging*, 1: 154–60.
Kerr I.H., Simon G. & Sutton G.C. (1971) The value of the plain radiograph in acute massive pulmonary embolism. *Br. J. Radiol.*, 44: 751–7.
Robinson P.J. (1989) Lung scintigraphy — doubt and certainty in the diagnosis of pulmonary embolism. *Clin. Radiol.*, 40: 557–60.

Reiter's Syndrome

Sexually transmitted or following dysentery. Males predominate.
1. Urethritis ± cystitis ± prostatitis.
2. Circinate balanitis (30%).
3. Conjunctivitis (30%).
4. Keratoderma blennorrhagica.
5. Arthritis (radiological changes in 80% of cases)
   (a) Involvement of synovial and cartilaginous joints and entheses.

(b) Asymmetrical involvement of the lower limbs — most commonly the knees, ankles, small joints of the feet and calcaneum. The spine and sacro-iliac joints are involved less frequently.

(c) Soft-tissue swelling.

(d) Osteoporosis is a feature of the acute disease but not of recurrent or chronic disease.

(e) Erosions which are initially periarticular and progress to involve the central portion of the articular surface.

(f) Periosteal new bone.

(g) New bone formation at ligament and tendon insertions.

(h) Sacro-iliitis and spondylitis with paravertebral ossification.

Renal Osteodystrophy

Due to renal glomerular disease — mostly bilateral reflux nephropathy pyelonephritis and chronic glomerulonephritis. It consists of osteomalacia or rickets + secondary hyperparathyroidism + osteosclerosis.

Children

1. Changes most marked in the skull, pelvis, scapulae, vertebrae and metaphyses of tubular bones.

2. Vertebral sclerosis may be confined to the upper and lower thirds of the bodies — 'rugger jersey' spine.

3. Soft-tissue calcification — less common than in adults.

4. Rickets — but the epiphyseal plate is less wide and the metaphysis is less cupped than in vitamin-D dependent rickets.

5. Secondary hyperparathyroidism — subperiosteal erosions and a 'rotting fence-post' appearance of the femoral necks. ± slipped upper femoral epiphysis.

6. Delayed skeletal maturation.

Adults

1. Hyperparathyroidism (q.v.).

2. Soft-tissue calcification is common, especially in arteries.

3. Osteosclerosis, including 'rugger jersey' spine.

4. Osteomalacia is mainly evident as Looser's zones.

Rheumatoid Arthritis

A multisystem collagen disorder in which joint disease is variably associated with other systemic manifestations.

1. A symmetrical arthritis of synovial joints, especially the metacarpophalangeal and proximal interphalangeal joints of the hands and feet, wrists, knees, ankles, elbows, glenohumeral and acromioclavicular joints and hips. The synovial articulations of the axial skeleton may also be affected, especially the apophyseal and atlantoaxial joints of the cervical spine. Less commonly the sacroiliac and temperomandibular joints are involved.

2. Cartilaginous joints, e.g. discovertebral junctions outside the cervical spine, symphysis pubis and manubriosternal joints, and entheses are less frequently and less severely involved (c.f. seronegative spondyloarthropathies).

3. The sequence of pathological/radiological changes at synovial joints is
   (a) Synovial inflammation and effusion → soft-tissue swelling and widened joint space.
   (b) Hyperaemia and disuse → juxta-articular osteoporosis; later generalized.
   (c) Destruction of cartilage by pannus → joint-space narrowing.
   (d) Pannus destruction of unprotected bone at the insertion of the joint capsule → periarticular erosions.
   (e) Pannus destruction of subchondral bone → widespread erosions and subchondral cysts.
   (f) Capsular and ligamentous laxity → subluxation, dislocation and deformity.
   (g) Fibrous and bony ankylosis.

4. Periosteal reaction — uncommon.

5. Secondary degenerative arthritis in the major weight-bearing joints.

Complications

1. Joint complications
   (a) Deformity and subluxation.
   (b) Pyogenic arthritis.
   (c) Tendon rupture.
   (d) Baker's cyst — which may rupture.
   (e) Cord or root compression due to cervical subluxation.
   (f) Hoarseness — due to involvement of the crico-arytenoid joints.
2. Subcutaneous nodules.
3. Anaemia.
4. Pulmonary complications
   (a) Pleural effusion.
   (b) Rheumatoid nodules.
   (c) Fibrosing alveolitis.
   (d) Caplan's syndrome.
5. Cardiac complications
   (a) Pericarditis ± effusion.
6. Ocular complications
   (a) Episcleritis.
   (b) Uveitis.
   (c) Sjögren's syndrome.
7. Arteritis
   (a) Raynaud's phenomenon.
   (b) Leg ulcers.
   (c) Visceral ischaemia.
8. Felty's syndrome (splenomegaly, leucopenia and rheumatoid arthritis).
9. Peripheral and autonomic neuropathy.
10. Amyloidosis.
11. Complications of therapy.

Rickets

Increased uncalcified osteoid in the immature skeleton.

Changes at the Growth Plate and Cortex
1. Widened growth plate (a).
2. Fraying, splaying and cupping of the metaphysis, which is of reduced density (b).
3. Thin bony spur extending from the metaphysis to surround the uncalcified growth plate (c).
4. Indistinct cortex because of uncalcified subperiosteal osteoid (d).
5. Rickety rosary — cupping of the anterior ends of the ribs and, on palpation, abnormally large costochondral junctions.
6. Looser's zones uncommon in children.

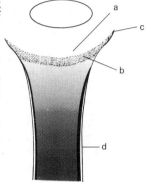

Changes Due to Bone Softening (Deformities)
1. Bowing of long bones.
2. Triradiate pelvis.
3. Harrison's sulcus — indrawing of the lower part of the chest wall because of soft ribs.
4. Scoliosis.
5. Biconcave vertebral bodies.
6. Basilar invagination.
7. Craniotabes — flattening of the occiput and accumulating osteoid in the frontal and parietal regions.

General Changes
1. Retarded bone maturation and growth.
2. Decreased bone density — uncommon.

Sarcoidosis

A multisystem granulomatous disorder of unknown aetiology.
Commonest presentations are:

erythema nodosum	30%
routine chest X-ray	25%
respiratory symptoms	20%
ocular symptoms	8%
other skin lesions	5%.

Intrathoracic Sarcoidosis (in 90%)
The chest X-ray at presentation may be:

normal	8%
bilateral hilar lymphadenopathy (BHL)	50%
bilateral hilar lymphadenopathy + pulmonary infiltrate	30%
pulmonary infiltrate ± fibrosis	12%.

1. Lymphadenopathy — bilateral hilar ± uni- or bilateral paratracheal lymphadenopathy. Anterior mediastinal lymph nodes are also involved in 16%. Unilateral hilar lymphadenopathy in 1–5%. 'Eggshell' calcification occurs in 1–5% and takes about 6 years to develop.
2. Parenchymal shadowing includes
   (a) Micronodular shadows < 2 mm ⎫ predominantly
   (b) Larger shadows < 5 mm, ill defined, ⎬ mid
       mimicking consolidation or odema ⎭ zones.
   (c) Large nodules, 1–4 cm, ill defined, multiple, bilateral and in any zone.
   (d) Coarse fibrosis — typically in the mid and upper zones.
3. Pleural involvement in 5–7%. Effusion in 2%.
4. Pneumothorax — secondary to chronic lung fibrosis.
5. Bronchostenosis in 1–2% — extrinsic compression or endobronchial granuloma.

Skin Sarcoidosis
1. Erythema nodosum — almost always in association with bilateral hilar lymphadenopathy.
2. Lupus pernio, plaques, subcutaneous nodules and scar infiltration.

Ocular Sarcoidosis

1. Most commonly manifests as acute uveitis + bilateral hilar lymphadenopathy + erythema nodosum.

Hepatic and Gastrointestinal Sarcoidosis

1. Hepatic granulomas in 66%, but symptomatic hepatobiliary disease is rare.
2. Gastric and peritoneal granulomas occur but are asymptomatic.

Neurologic Sarcoidosis

1. Neuropathies — especially bilateral lower motor neurone VII nerve palsies.
2. Cerebral sarcoidosis is evident in 14% of autopsies of patients dying of sarcoidosis, but in only 1–5% clinically. Most commonly it produces nodular granulomatous masses in the basal meninges or adhesive meningitis, which result in cranial nerve palsies and/or hydrocephalus. Granulomas in the brain parenchyma present as space-occupying lesions. (On CT scanning they have a high attenuation, are homogeneously enhancing and peripherally situated.)

Joint Sarcoidosis

1. A transient, symmetrical arthropathy involving knees, ankles and, less commonly, the wrists and interphalangeal joints.

Bone Sarcoidosis

1. In 3% of patients and most frequently associated with skin lesions.
2. Hands and feet are most commonly affected.
   (a) Enlarged nutrient foramina in phalanges and, occasionally, metacarpals and metatarsals.
   (b) Coarse trabeculation, eventually assuming a lacework, reticulated pattern. Initially metaphyseal and eventually affecting the entire bone.
   (c) Larger, well-defined lucencies.
   (d) Resorption of distal phalanges.
   (e) Terminal phalangeal sclerosis.
   (f) Periarticular calcification.

   (g) Subperiosteal bone resorption — simulating hyperparathyroidism.
   (h) Periosteal reaction.
   (i) Soft-tissue swelling — dactylitis.
3. In the remainder of the skeleton
   (a) Well-defined lucencies with a sclerotic margin.
   (b) Paraspinal masses with an extradural block at myelography.
   (c) Destructive lesions of the nasal and jaw bones.

Sarcoidosis Elsewhere
1. Peripheral lymphadenopathy in 15%.
2. Hypercalcaemia (10%) and hypercalciuria (60%).
3. Splenomegaly in 6%.
4. Uveoparotid fever (uveitis, cranial nerve palsy, fever and parotitis).

Further Reading
Freundlich I.M., Libshitz, H.I., Glassman L.M. & Israel H.L. (1970) Sarcoidosis: typical and atypical thoracic manifestations and complications. *Clin. Radiol.*, 21: 376–83.
Kendall, B.E. (1978) Radiological findings in neurosarcoidosis. *Br. J. Radiol.*, 51: 81–92.
Rockoff S.D. & Rohatgi P.K. (1985) Unusual manifestations of thoracic sarcoidosis. *Am. J. Roentgenol.*, 144: 513–28.

Scleroderma (Progressive Systemic Sclerosis)

A multisystem connective tissue disorder, the course of which varies from acute and fulminating to mild and chronic.

Soft Tissues
1. Raynaud's phenomenon (60%).
2. Skin thickening — initially of the fingers (and less often the toes) and of the mouth; progresses to shiny taut skin.
3. Subcutaneous calcification — especially in the fingertips and over bony prominences.
4. Myopathy or myositis.

Joints
1. Eventually 50% of patients have articular involvement. Fingers, wrists and ankles are commonly affected.
2. Terminal phalangeal resorption is associated with soft-tissue atrophy.
3. Erosions at the distal interphalangeal, 1st carpometacarpal, metacarpophalangeal and metatarsophalangeal joints.

Mandible
1. Thickening of the periodontal membrane ± loss of the lamina dura.

Ribs
1. Symmetrical erosions on the superior surfaces which predominate along the posterior aspects of the 3rd–6th ribs.

Respiratory System
1. Lung involvement in 10–25%.
2. Aspiration pneumonitis secondary to gastro–oesophageal reflux.
3. Interstitial lung disease and fibrosis, more marked in the lower zones.

Gastrointestinal System

1. Oesophageal abnormalities (50%) — dilatation, atonicity, poor or absent peristalsis and free gastro-oesophageal reflux through a widely open gastro-oesophageal junction.
2. Small bowel (75%) — dilated, atonic, thickened mucosal folds and pseudosacculation.
3. Colon (75%) — atonic with pseudosacculations on the antimesenteric border.

Heart

1. Cardiomegaly (30%) — due to myocardial ± pericardial involvement. ± pericardial effusion.
2. Cor pulmonale may develop secondary to the interstitial lung disease.

Scurvy

The result of vitamin-C deficiency.

1. Onset at 6 months–2 years. Rare in adults.
2. Earliest signs are seen at the knees.
3. Osteoporosis (usually the only sign seen in adults).
4. Loss of epiphyseal density with a pencil-thin cortex (Wimberger's sign) (a).
5. Dense zone of provisional calcification — due to excessive calcification of osteoid (b).
6. Metaphyseal lucency (Trümmerfeld zone) (c).
7. Metaphyseal corner fractures through the weakened lucent metaphysis (Pelkan spurs) resulting in cupping of the metaphysis (d).
8. Periosteal reaction due to subperiosteal haematoma (e).

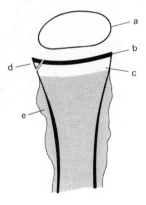

Sickle-cell Anaemia

Skeletal
1. Marrow hyperplasia produces widening of medullary cavities, decreased bone density, coarsening of the trabecular pattern, and cortical thinning and expansion. The changes are most marked in the axial skeleton.
   - (a) Skull — coarse granular osteoporosis with widening of the diploe which spares the occiput below the internal occipital protuberance. 'Hair-on-end' appearance (5%). Focal lucencies (but probably due to infarcts).
   - (b) Spine — osteoporosis, exaggerated vertical trabeculae and biconcave vertebral bodies (but see also 2(c) below).
2. Vascular occlusion due to sickling results in osteonecrosis.
   - (a) Sickle-cell dactylitis (hand–foot syndrome) — in children aged 6 months–2 years. Symmetrical soft-tissue swelling, patchy lucency and sclerosis of the shafts of metacarpals, metatarsals and phalanges, and periosteal reaction.
   - (b) Long bones — diaphyseal or epiphyseal infarcts. The femoral head is affected in 12% of patients (60% in sickle/haemoglobin C (SC) disease).
   - (c) Spine — square-shaped compression infarcts of the vertebral end-plates are virtually diagnostic.
3. Growth disturbances — retarded growth, delayed closure of epiphyses and tibiotalar slant.
4. Fractures.
5. Osteomyelitis and pyogenic arthritis — due to salmonellae in over 50% of cases.

Extraskeletal
1. Extramedullary haemopoiesis — but more common in thalassaemia.
2. Cholelithiasis.
3. Splenic infarction.
4. Cardiomegaly and congestive cardiac failure — because of anaemia.
5. Renal papillary necrosis.

Silicosis

Occurs in miners, quarry workers, masons, pottery workers, sand blasters, foundry workers and boiler scalers. The duration and degree of exposure determine the time of onset of disease

(a) Chronic silicosis — disease after 20–40 years of exposure.

(b) Accelerated silicosis — disease after 5–15 years of exposure.

(c) Acute silicoproteinosis — heavy exposure over a short period of time (several months–5 years), e.g. in sand blasters.

Simple

1. Nodular shadows, pin-point to pea-sized, which are first seen around the right hilum but later are disseminated throughout both lungs within relative sparing of the extreme bases and apices. Exceptionally, they may be restricted to the upper zones.
2. Inhalation of pure silica produces very sharp, dense nodules. Mixed dusts are less well defined and of lower density. Density increases with the size of the nodule. Goldminers have very dense nodular shadows.
3. Nodules may calcify, especially in goldminers.
4. Minor hilar lymph-node enlargement, but only obvious when calcification occurs (in 5%). Anterior and posterior mediastinal lymph nodes may also enlarge.
5. Kerley A and B lines — more pronounced with mixed dusts.
6. Silicoproteinosis presents as diffuse alveolar disease.

Complicated, i.e. Progressive Massive Fibrosis (PMF)

1. Superimposed on the changes of simple silicosis.
2. The rapid development of massive, ill-defined, dense, oval or round shadows. Usually bilateral and fairly symmetrical in the upper two-thirds of the lungs.
3. They begin peripherally and increase in size and density as they move towards the hilum, leaving emphysematous lung at the periphery.
4. May cavitate or calcify.

Complications
1. Infections — chronic bronchitis and tuberculosis.
2. Pneumothorax — but usually limited by thickened pleura.
3. Cor pulmonale — a common cause of death.
4. Caplan's syndrome — in patients with rheumatoid disease. Well-defined, peripheral nodules 0.5–5 cm in diameter. Calcification and cavitation may occur.

Simple Bone Cyst

1. Age — 5–15 years.
2. Sites — proximal humerus and femur (75% of cases) and apophysis of the greater trochanter.
3. Appearances
   (a) Metaphyseal, extending to the epiphyseal plate. It migrates away from the metaphysis with time.
   (b) Well-defined lucency with a thin sclerotic rim.
   (c) Usually central.
   (d) Thinned cortex with slight expansion (never more than the width of the epiphyseal plate).
   (e) Thin internal septa.

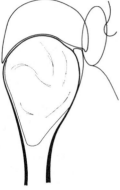

Steroids

See 'Cushing's syndrome'.

Systemic Lupus Erythematosus

Musculoskeletal
1. Polyarthritis — bilateral and symmetrical, involving the small joints of the hand, knee, wrist and shoulder. Soft-tissue swelling and periarticular osteoporosis of the proximal interphalangeal and metacarpophalangeal joints simulate rheumatoid arthritis, but periarticular erosions are not a usual feature.
2. Easily correctable deformities of the hand which cause little functional disability.
3. Osteonecrosis — most frequently of the femoral head.
4. Terminal phalangeal sclerosis and resorption.

Cardiorespiratory
1. Pleural effusion (60%), which is often recurrent. Often accompanied by a pleurisy resulting in elevation of a hemidiaphragm and plate atelectasis at the base.
2. Uraemic pulmonary oedema.
3. Acute lupus pneumonitis.
4. Diffuse interstitial disease — uncommon.
5. Cardiomegaly — due to pericarditis with effusion, myocardial disease or fluid overload in renal failure.

Abdomen
1. Hepatosplenomegaly.
2. Renal disease eventually results in small, smooth, non-functioning kidneys.

Thalassaemia

Skeletal

1. Marrow hyperplasia is more pronounced than in sickle-cell anaemia (q.v.). The changes in thalassaemia major are more severe than in thalassaemia minor. Initially both axial and appendicular skeleton are affected but as marrow regresses from the appendicular skeleton at puberty the changes in the latter diminish.
    (a) Skull — granular osteoporosis, widening of the diploe, thinning of the outer table and 'hair-on-end' appearance. Involvement of the facial bones produces obliteration of the paranasal sinuses, hypertelorism and malocclusion of the teeth. These changes are rarely a feature of other haemoglobinopathies and are important differentiating signs.
    (b) Spine — osteoporosis, exaggerated vertical trabeculae and fish-shaped vertebrae.
    (c) Ribs, clavicles and tubular bones of the hands and feet show the typical changes of marrow hyperplasia (see Sickle-cell anaemia).
2. Growth disturbances.
3. Fractures.

Extraskeletal

1. Extramedullary haemopoiesis — including hepatosplenomegaly.
2. Cardiomegaly.

Tuberous Sclerosis

Autosomal dominant. 25–50% are fresh mutations.
Mental retardation in 60%. 30% die in the first 5 years; 75% are dead by 20 years.

Central Nervous System

1. Cortical and/or subependymal periventricular nodules. Calcification in 50–80%, but not visible until after infancy.
2. Ventricular dilatation, with or without obstruction.
3. Gliomas in 6%.
4. Retinal tumours (phakomas) in 50%; 60% are bilateral.

Skin
1. Adenoma sebaceum, subungual fibromas, shagreen patches and *cafe-au-lait* spots.

Kidneys
1. Hamartomas (angiomyolipomas) in 50–80%. Single or multiple, uni- or bilateral. (N.B. approx. 50% of patients with an angiomyolipoma have no other evidence of tuberous sclerosis.)

Skeleton
1. Calvarium, spine and pelvis — sclerotic islands in 40–50%.
2. Hands and feet — cystic defects and periosteal new bone, especially in the phalanges. The changes are more marked in the hands.

Lungs
1. Interstitial lung disease progressing to 'honeycomb lung' in 5%. Never before 20 years. A frequent cause of death.

Heart
1. Cardiac rhabdomyomas. The chest X-ray is normal or shows non-specific cardiac enlargement.

Further Reading
Medley B.E., McLeod R.A. & Wayne Houser O. (1976) Tuberous sclerosis. *Semin. Roentgenol.*, 11: 35–54.

Turner's Syndrome

Females with XO chromosome pattern.
1. Small stature with retarded bone maturation.
2. Mental retardation in 10%.
3. Osteoporosis.

Chest
1. Cardiovascular abnormalities — present in 20%, and 70% are coarctation.
2. Broad chest; mild pectus excavatum; widely spaced nipples.

Abdomen
1. Ovarian dysgenesis.
2. Renal anomalies — 'horseshoe kidney' and bifid renal pelvis are the most common.

Axial Skeleton
1. Scoliosis and kyphosis.
2. Hypoplasia of the cervical spine.

Appendicular Skeleton
1. Cubitus valgus in 70%.
2. Short 4th metacarpal and/or metatarsal in 50%, ± short 3rd and 5th metacarpals.
3. Madelung's deformity.
4. Enlargement of the medial tibial plateau ± small exostosis inferiorly.
5. Pes cavus.
6. Transient congenital oedema of the dorsum of the feet.

Ulcerative Colitis

1. Diseased colon is affected in continuity with symmetrical involvement of the wall.
2. Rectum involved in 95%. The rectum may appear normal if steroid enemas have been administered.
3. Granular mucosa and mucosal ulcers.
4. 'Thumbprinting' due mucosal oedema.
5. Blunting of haustral folds progresses to a narrowed, shortened and tubular colon if the disease becomes chronic.
6. Widening of the retrorectal space.
7. Inflammatory pseudopolyps due to regenerating mucosa. Found in 10–20% of ulcerative colitics and usually following a previous severe attack. Filiform polyps occur in quiescent phase.
8. Patulous ileocaecal valve with reflux ileitis (dilated terminal ileum).

Complications

1. Toxic megacolon — in 7–10%.
2. Strictures — much less common than in Crohn's disease and must be differentiated from carcinoma.
3. Carcinoma of the colon — 20–30 × increased incidence if extensive colitis has been present for more than 10 years.
4. Associated conditions
   (a) Erythema nodosum, aphthous ulceration and pyoderma gangrenosum.
   (b) Arthritis — similar to Crohn's disease (q.v.).
   (c) Cirrhosis.
   (d) Chronic active hepatitis.
   (e) Pericholangitis.
   (f) Sclerosing cholangitis.
   (g) Bile duct carcinoma.
   (h) Oxalate urinary calculi.

Index

Part 1 is indexed by sections
Part 2 is indexed by page numbers
References in **bold** type are to principal sections

Abdomen **6.1–6.45**
 in AIDS 413
  in children 415
 fetal: cystic structures **14.12**
 gasless **6.3**
Abdominal abscess 6.1
Abdominal calcification, neonatal 7.7
Abdominal mass
 in child **6.6**
 gasless abdomen 6.3
 in neonate **6.5**
Abdominal surgery: pleural effusion 4.35
Abdominal tumours: pneumoperitoneum
  6.2
Abdominal viscus, hollow: perforation
  4.38
Abdominal wall, anterior, defects 14.13
 raised AFP 14.10
Abdomino-perioneal resection 8.26
Abetalipoproteinaemia 6.30
Abortion
 incomplete **14.4**
 missed 14.4, 14.22
  raised serum alphafeto protein (AFP)
   14.10
 threatened **14.4**
Abscess, *see individual abscesses*
Accuracy **15**(404)
Acetabular fractures 3.13
Achalasia
 dysphagia 6.10
 oesophageal strictures 6.14, 6.15
 pneumonia, slowly resolving/recurrent
  4.10
 posterior mediastinal masses 4.51
 tertiary oesophageal contractions 6.16
Achondrogenesis 1.6
 antenatal diagnosis 14.13
 large head 12.19
Achondroplasia **411**
 antenatal diagnosis 14.13
 basilar invagination 12.13
 cupping of metaphyses 1.46
 dwarfing skeletal dysplasia 1.5
 homozygous 1.6, 14.13

 J-shaped sella 12.24
 large head 12.19
 narrow spinal canal 2.19
 vertebral body,
  beaks 2.15
  scalloping 2.16
Acidosis, metabolic: neonatal respiratory
      distress 4.46
Acinar disease **4.15**
Acinar nodules 4.15
Acoustic neuroma
 CT 12.33, 12.34
 petrous bone destruction 12.10
Acquired Immune Deficiency Syndrome (AIDS)
 in adults **412–414**
 in children **414–416**
Acrocephalopolysyndactyly (Carpenter
      syndrome) 12.15
Acrocephalosyndactyly (Apert's syndrome)
      1.56, 12.15
Acrocephaly 12.15
Acrodysostosis
 accelerated skeletal maturation 1.2
 narrow spinal canal 2.19
Acromegaly **416**
 arthritis + preserved/widened joint
      space 3.6
 chondrocalcinosis 3.11
 expanded pituitary fossa 12.23
 heel pad thickness increase 416, 9.7
 kidneys, bilateral large smooth 8.10
 osteoporosis 1.29
 skull vault density increase 12.7
 thymic hyperplasia 4.54
 vertebral body,
  enlargement 2.7
  scalloping 2.16
Acro-osteolysis 1.54, 12.16
 of Hajdu and Cheney 1.54, 12.16
Actinomycosis
 gastrocolic fistula 6.20
 ileal lesions 6.35
 lung cavities 4.27
 retroperitoneal fibrosis 8.26
 rib lesion + soft-tissue mass 4.44

Acute tubular necrosis (ATN)
   bilateral large smooth kidneys 8.10
   nephrographic pattern 8.18
Adamantinoma
   cystic 11.14
   site of origin 1.17
Addison's disease
   adrenal calcification 7.22
   osteoporosis 1.29
   small heart 5.2
   thymic hyperplasia 4.54
Adenocarcinoma, mucinous: calcified
      pulmonary metastasis 4.29
Adenoid enlargement 11.17
   chronic upper airway obstruction 4.2
Adenoma
   gastrointestinal bleeding localization
      13.21
   thyroid imaging 13.9
   see also individual adenomata
Adenomyomatosis: gallbladder filling
      defect 7.2
Adhesions, small bowel 6.29
Adnexal mass 14.6
Adrenalectomy 13.19
Adrenal gland
   adenoma 7.23, 13.19
   calcification **7.22**
   carcinoma,
      calcification 7.22
      CT 7.23
      skeletal metastases 1.16
      unilateral visualization 13.19
   cyst 7.23
   cystic disease 7.22
   haemorrhage 7.22, 7.23
      abdominal mass in neonate 6.5
   infarct 13.19
   masses, CT **7.23**
   metastases 7.23
      imaging 13.19
   nodular hyperplasia 7.23
   post-traumatic haemorrhage 7.23
   tumours 7.23
      accelerated skeletal maturation 1.2
      bone metastases 1.16
      gynaecomastia 9.1
   visualization, unilateral **13.19**
Adult respiratory distress syndrome (shock
      lung)
   post-chest trauma 4.45
   pulmonary oedema 4.17
Air embolism
   gas in portal veins 7.4
   subclavian vein catheterization 5.20
Air-space, opacification 4.13
Air-space disease
   localized **4.16**
   widespread **4.15**
Alcohol
   abuse: gas in stomach wall 6.23
   avascular necrosis 1.40

Alcoholic pancreatitis 7.20
Alcoholism 455
   tertiary oesophageal contractions
      6.16
Aldosteronism 13.19
Alkaptonuria **417**
   fusion/bridging symphysis pubis 3.15
   intervertebral disc calcification 2.12
   soft-tissue calcification 9.2
   syndesmophytes 2.13
Allergic alveolitis, drug-induced 4.48
Alphafeto protein (AFP) **14.10**
Alveolar cell carcinoma
   localized air-space disease 4.16
   opacity with air bronchogram 4.28
   pulmonary nodule, solitary 4.25
   widespread air-space disease 4.15
Alveolar microlithiasis 4.22
   multiple pulmonary calcifications
      4.29
Alveolar shadowing 4.15
Alveolitis
   allergic, drug-induced 4.48
   fibrosing 4.23
   see also Extrinsic allergic alveolitis
Amiodarone 7.16
Amnion, in twin pregnancies **14.17**
Amoebiasis
   colonic polyps 6.36
   lung cavities 4.27
   toxic megacolon 6.39
Amoebic abscess
   focal hypodense CT liver lesion 7.13
   hepatic calcification 7.6
   hepatomegaly 7.5
Amoebic colitis
   aphthous ulcers 6.42
   'thumbprinting' in colon 6.41
Amoeboma: colonic strictures 6.37
Amyloidosis
   duodenal folds,
      decreased/absent 6.25
      thickened 6.26
   generalized low density liver CT 7.15
   hepatomegaly 7.5
   kidneys, bilateral large smooth 8.10
   malabsorption 6.33
   nephrogram 8.18
   non-dilated small bowel, thickened folds
      6.30, 6.31
   small bowel dilatation 6.28
   splenomegaly 7.18
   stomach abnormality + thickened small
      bowel folds 6.31
Anaemia
   left ventricle enlarged 5.6
   pulmonary arteries enlarged 5.15
   see also individual anaemias
Anencephaly
   antenatal diagnosis 14.13
   raised serum alphafeto protein (AFP)
      14.10

Aneurysm
  aortic, *see* Aortic aneurysm
  basilar artery 12.28
  carotid 12.12
  circle of Willis: calcification 12.25,
      12.28, 12.30
  coronary artery 5.7
  expanded pituitary fossa 12.23
  gated blood pool imaging 13.14
  giant 12.26, 12.33
    CT 12.34
  infraclinoid 11.1, 11.8
  intracranial calcification 12.26
  ophthalmic artery 11.7
  pulmonary artery: hilar enlargement
      4.30
  renal artery 8.2, 8.20
  sella erosion and osteoporosis 12.25
  soft-tissue calcification 9.2
  ventricular 5.7
  vertebrobasilar 12.12
Aneurysmal bone cyst **418**, 1.18
  distal phalangeal destruction 1.54
  extradural spinal mass 2.22
  lucent bone lesions,
    grossly expansile 1.23
    medullary + eccentric expansion 1.22
    subarticular 1.24
  mandible 11.14
  peak age incidence 1.18
  vertebra,
    collapse 2.2
    enlarged body 2.7
    pedicle erosion 2.5
Angina pectoris
  myocardial perfusion imaging 13.13
  unstable: gated blood pool imaging
      13.14
Angiodysplasia 13.21
Angiofibroma, adolescent 11.17
Angiogram, brain isotope **13.11**
Angioma
  calcification 12.30
  spinal block 2.21
  spinal mass 2.23
Angiomyolipoma 485, 7.23, 7.13
Angioneurotic oedema: thickened
      duodenal folds 6.26
Angio-oedema: upper airway obstruction
      4.1
Aniridia 6.6
Ankylosing spondylitis **418–419**
  aortic valve calcification 5.9
  arthritis + bone density preservation
      3.4
  atlanto-axial subluxation 2.11
  intervertebral disc calcification 2.12
  protrusio acetabuli 3.13
  pseudoarthrosis 1.38
  pulmonary upper zone fibrosis 4.33
  sacroiliitis, bilateral symmetrical 3.12
  soft-tissue calcification 9.2

  symphysis pubis fusion/bridging 3.15
  syndesmophytes 2.13
  vertebrae, block 2.9
  vertebral body squaring 2.8
Annular pancreas, *see* Pancreas, annular
Anomalous pulmonary venous drainage 5.3
  see also Total anomalous pulmonary
      venous drainage (TAPVD)
Anorectal anomalies: symphysis pubis
      widening 3.14
Anterior cardiophrenic angle masses 4.49
Anticoagulants: widespread air-space
      disease 4.15
Anticonvulsants: osteomalacia/rickets 1.30
Anti-inflammatory drugs: avascular
      necrosis 1.40
Antrochoanal polyp 11.17
  chronic upper airway obstruction 4.2
Antrum, *see* Maxillary antrum
Anus, imperforate, *see* Imperforate anus
Aorta
  ascending, aneurysm 4.49
  coarctation, *see* Coarctation of aorta
  posterior mediastinal masses 4.51
  unfolded (atherosclerotic) 5.10
  unfolded/dilated/ruptured 4.51
Aortic aneurysm 5.10
  anterior mediastinal mass 4.49
  bronchial stenosis/occlusion 4.7
  dysphagia 6.10
  large aortic arch 5.10
  middle mediastinal mass 4.50
  retroperitoneal fibrosis 8.26
  right sided diaphragmatic humps 4.39
  traumatic 4.45
  vertebral body scalloping 2.17
Aortic arch
  double 4.2
  interrupted,
    neonatal cyanosis 5.18
    neonatal pulmonary venous
        congestion 5.17
  large **5.10**
  right-sided **5.12**, 6.11
    dysphagia 6.10
  small **5.11**
Aortic calcification 4.32
Aortic dissection 4.45
Aortic incompetence
  large aortic arch 5.10
  left ventricle enlarged 5.6
Aortic stenosis
  aortic arch enlargement 5.10
  critical: neonatal pulmonary venous
      congestion 5.17
  left ventricle, enlarged 5.6
  myocardial perfusion imaging 13.13
Aortic thrombosis: rib notching 1.51
Aortic valve
  bicuspid, calcification 5.9
  calcification 5.9
  disease: gross cardiac enlargement 5.1

Apert's syndrome (acrocephalosyndactyly) 12.15
  carpal fusion 1.56
Aphthous ulcers 427, **6.42**
Aplastic anaemia, drug-induced 4.48
Appendicitis
  acute 13.22
  pneumoperitoneum 6.2
Appendix
  abscess,
    abdominal mass in child 6.6
    bladder fistula 8.29
  carcinoids 6.29, 6.31, 6.35
Aqueduct stenosis 12.18, 12.19
Arachnodactyly **1.53**
Arachnoid cyst
  CT 12.33, 12.34
  extradural spinal mass 2.22
Arachnoiditis: spinal block 2.21
Argyrosiderosis 4.21
Armillifer: soft-tissue calcification 9.2
Arnold–Chiari malformation
  congenital hydrocephalus: large head 12.19
  raised intracranial pressure 12.18
  spina bifida with 14.13
  ultrasound signs 14.13
Arrhenoblastoma 14.27
Arterial insufficiency: periosteal reactions 1.33
Arterial obstruction: protein-losing enteropathy 6.34
Arteriovenous fistula
  renal induced hypertension 8.20
  subclavian vein catheterization 5.20
Arteriovenous malformation
  cerebral,
    brain isotope angiogram 13.11
    brain surface enhancement 12.31
    calcification 12.26
    CT 12.34
  enlarged optic foramen 11.7
  intraorbital calcification 11.9
  premature closure of growth plate 1.3
  pulmonary nodule,
    multiple 4.26
    solitary 4.25
  rib notching 1.51
  superior orbital fissure enlargement 11.8
Arteritis
  avascular necrosis 1.40
  renal induced hypertension 8.20
Arthritides
  atlanto-axial subluxation 2.11
  bone scans 13.4
  carpal fusion 1.56
  in children **444–445**
  chondropathic 3.2
  depositional 3.2
  inflammatory 3.2
  periosteal reaction 1.36
  subarticular lucent lesions 1.24
  see also individual diseases

Arthritis
  + bone density preservation **3.4**
  crystal induced 3.1
  gouty, *see* Gouty arthritis
  inflammatory 3.2
    arthritis + preserved/widened joint space 3.6
  juvenile chronic, *see* Juvenile chronic arthritis
  major types **3.2**
  mono- **3.1**
  + osteoporosis **3.3**
  + periosteal reaction **3.5**
  + preserved/widened joint space **3.6**
  pyogenic,
    arthritis + osteoporosis 3.3
    arthritis + periosteal reaction 3.1, 3.5
    avascular necrosis 1.40
    carpal fusion 1.56
    monoarthritis 3.1
    periosteal reaction 3.1
  rheumatoid, *see* Rheumatoid arthritis
  tuberculous, *see* Tuberculous arthritis
Arthritis mutilans **3.7**
Arthrogryposis multiplex congenita: carpal fusion 1.56
Arthropathy
  calcium pyrophosphate 1.24
  in haemochromatosis 437
  see also individual diseases
Articular (hyaline) cartilage calcification 421, **3.11**
Aryepiglottic fold cyst 4.2
Asbestos inhalation 420, 4.21
  cardiac calcification 5.8
  gallium uptake 13.7
  gastric carcinoma 6.17
  honeycomb lung 4.20
  oesophageal strictures 6.15
  pleural calcification 420, 4.42
  pleural effusion 420, 4.36
Ascites **6.4**
  bilateral elevated hemidiaphragms 4.41
  chylous 6.4
  in fetus 14.9
  gasless abdomen 6.3
  rectosigmoid junction, anterior indentation 6.43
Aseptic necrosis: bone scans 13.4
Aspartylglucosaminuria 1.7
Aspergillosis
  bronchial stenosis/occlusion 4.7
  lung cavities 4.27
Asphyxia: neonatal pulmonary venous congestion 5.17
Asphyxiating thoracic dysplasia of Jeune 4.46, 14.13
  dwarfing skeletal dysplasia 1.5
  lethal neonatal dysplasia 1.6
Aspiration
  chronic: bronchiectasis 4.14
  lung cavities 4.27
  pulmonary oedema 4.17, 4.18

repeated: slowly resolving/recurrent pneumonia 4.10
Aspiration pneumonia
  increased density of hemithorax 4.8
  pulmonary opacities 4.23
Aspiration pneumonitis: post-chest trauma 4.45
Asthma
  bilateral hypertransradiant hemithoraces 4.6
  bronchial occlusion 4.7
  pneumomediastinum 4.38
Astrocytoma (cystic glioma)
  accelerated skeletal maturation 1.2
  brain isotope angiogram 13.11
  calcification 12.30
  cerebellar 12.32
    CT 12.32
  intracranial calcification 12.26, 12.30
Atelectasis 4.4
  adhesive 4.15
  bronchial occlusion 4.7
  cicatrisation 4.15
  neonatal respiratory distress 4.46
  relaxation 4.15
Atheroma: soft-tissue calcification 9.2
Atherosclerosis 5.10
  carotid siphon 12.26, 12.28, 12.30
  intracranial calcification 12.26
Atlanto-axial subluxation 445, 2.11
Atlanto-occipital fusion 12.13
  basilar invagination 12.13
Atlas, anomalies 12.13
Atrial myxoma, *see* Myxoma
Atrial septal defect (ASD)
  gross cardiac enlargement 5.1
  neonatal cyanosis 5.18
  right atrium enlargement 5.3
  right ventricle enlargement 5.4
  + shunt reversal: enlarged left atrium 5.5
  valve calcification 5.9
Atrioventricular (AV) fistula: enlarged left ventricle 5.6
Atrioventricular canal: enlarged right atrium 5.3
Atrio-ventricular shunts: fetal hydrops 14.9
Atrium, *see* Left atrium; Right atrium
Autosomal dominant polycystic disease 14.13
Autosomal recessive polycystic disease 14.13
Avascular necrosis 1.39, 1.40
  idiopathic 1.40
  skull vault lucent lesions 12.4
Axis, anomalies 12.13
Azygos vein, enlarged 5.14

'Backwash' ileitis 6.35
Bagassosis 4.21
'Bag of worms' 4.25

Ball-valve thrombus: enlarged pulmonary veins 5.16
'Bamboo spine' 418
Barotrauma, opaque maxillary antrum 11.12
Barrett's oesophagus 6.14
  strictures 6.15
  ulceration 6.13
Barytosis 4.21
  pulmonary opacities 4.22, 4.23
Basal angle 12.13
Basal Cell Naevus Syndrome 12.32
Basal ganglia calcification **12.29**
  in AIDS 415
Basilar artery, aneurysm 12.28
Basilar invagination **12.13**
'Beak sign' 6.21
Beckwith–Wiedemann syndrome
  dysphagia 6.11
  large head 12.19
  Wilms' tumour 6.6
Behçet's disease
  aphthous ulcers 6.42
  oesophageal ulceration 6.13
Beri-beri: enlarged pulmonary arteries 5.15
Bertin, septum of, enlarged 8.11
Berylliosis: bilateral hilar enlargement 4.31
β-blockers 4.48
Beta cell insulinoma 7.21
Bezoar 6.17, 6.21
Bile ducts
  gas in 7.3
  malignancy 7.3
Biliary atresia: osteomalacia/rickets 1.30)
Biliary cirrhosis, primary : hypertrophic osteoarthropathy 1.34
Biliary fistula, spontaneous 7.3
Biliary obstruction: malabsorption 6.33
Biliary tree
  dilatation: focal hypodense CT liver lesion 7.13
  gas in 6.1, **7.3**, 7.12
Birth trauma 4.49
  non-accidental injury vs. 1.37
Bismuth infection: soft-tissue calcification 9.2
Bladder
  calcification **8.28**
  calculus 8.28, 8.30
  carcinoma,
    bladder fistula 8.29
    dilated ureter 8.25
    squamous cell 8.28
    transitional cell 8.27, 8.28
  diverticulum: bone scans 13.2
  extrophy: widening of symphysis pubis 3.14
  filling defect **8.27**
  fistula **8.29**
  foreign body 8.28, 8.30
  gas in 8.4

Bladder *(cont.)*
  outflow obstruction,
    in child **8.30**
    fetal 14.12
    hydronephrosis in child 8.17
  tumour, bone metastases 1.16
  wall, gas in 8.4
Bladder neck obstruction 8.30
  fetal hydrops 14.9
Blalock operation: rib notching 1.51
Blalock–Taussig shunt 4.18
Blastomycosis
  pulmonary calcification 4.29
  pulmonary opacities 4.23
  rib lesion + soft-tissue mass 4.44
Bleeding diatheses
  periosteal reaction 1.36
  pleural effusion 4.34
  small bowel thickened folds 6.30
Blood dyscrasia, haematemesis 6.9
Blood group incompatibility 14.9
Blood pool imaging, gated **13.14**
'Boat-shaped' skull 12.15
Bochdalek hernia
  CT mediastinal mass containing fat 4.52
  posterior mediastinal masses 4.51
  right sided diaphragmatic humps 4.39
Bone 1.1–1.57
  accelerated skeletal maturation **1.2**
  asymmetrical maturation **1.4**
  brittle **1.29**
  coarse trabecular pattern **1.14**
  decreased density, regional 1.27
  density increase,
    generalized **1.8**
    generalized, in adults **1.9**
    skull base 12.9
    skull vault **12.7, 12.8**
  density preservation + arthritis 3.4
  disease,
    diffuse infiltrative 1.28
    of occiput, atlas, axis 12.13
    spinal block 2.21
  healing benign/malignant,
    lucent + marginal sclerosis 1.19
    multiple sclerotic lesions 1.11
    solitary sclerotic lesion 1.10
  lesions, post-traumatic 1.24
  lucent lesions,
    + calcium/bone **1.25**
    grossly expansile **1.23**
    subarticular **1.24**
    see also Skull vault
  lucent medullary lesions, (ill-defined)
    1.21
  lucent medullary lesions, well-defined,
    eccentric expansion **1.22**
    marginal sclerosis **1.19**
    no marginal sclerosis **1.20**
  multiple sclerotic lesions **1.11**
  petrous, destruction **12.10, 12.11**

premature closure of growth plate **1.3**
resorption, subperiosteal 442
retarded skeletal maturation **1.1**
sclerosis with periosteal reaction **1.12**
softening, changes due to 474
solitary lesions with lucent centre **1.13**
solitary sclerotic lesions **1.10**
'Bone in bone' appearance 463, 12.7
Bone cyst
  aneurysmal, *see* Aneurysmal bone cyst
  bone scan 13.5
  mandibular 11.14
  simple **482**
    lucent lesion in medulla 1.19
    peak age incidence 1.18
    site of origin 1.17
Bone dysplasia
  abnormal modelling of long bones 12.6
  cupping of metaphyses 1.46
  + increased skull density **12.6**
  retarded skeletal maturation **1**.1
  sclerosing 11.10
    skull vault thickening 12.5
  skull, defective mineralization 12.20
  skull vault, defective ossification 12.17
  see also Skeletal dysplasia
Bone infarct 1.10, 1.11
Bone island
  multiple sclerotic lesions 1.11
  positive radiograph + bone scan 13.5
  solitary sclerotic lesion 1.10
Bone metastases **1.16**
  bone sclerosis + periosteal reaction
    1.12
  clavicle (outer end) erosion/absence 1.49
  distal phalangeal destruction 1.54
  lucent lesions,
    with calcium/bone 1.25
    grossly expansile 1.23
    subarticular 1.24
  most common radiological appearances
    1.16
  'moth-eaten' bone 1.25
  pedicle destruction 2.5
  periosteal reactions 1.31, 1.32
  rib lesions 1.50
  sacral scalloping 2.18
  spinal mass,
    extradural 2.22
    intradural 2.23
  vertebral body, ivory 2.10
  vertebral collapse 2.2, 2.3
Bone neoplasms
  benign 1.19
    lucent bone lesions with calcium/bone
      1.25
    lucent lesions, grossly expansile 1.23
    lucent medullary bone lesion 1.19, 1.20
    pedicle erosion/destruction/absence
      2.5
    vertebral body enlargement 2.7

extradural spinal mass 2.22
lucent lesions,
  with calcium/bone 1.25
  grossly expansile 1.23
osteomalacia/rickets 1.30
primary,
  peak age incidence **1.18**
  sites of origin **1.17**
sympathetic monoarthritis 3.1
Bone sarcoma 1.10
  ill-defined lucent medullary lesions 1.21
  lucent bone lesions with calcium/bone
    1.25
Bone scans
  abnormal + normal/minimal
    radiographic changes **13.4**
  increased uptake **13.1**
    not due to skeletal abnormality **13.2**
  normal + positive radiograph **13.5**
  photopenic areas (defects) **13.3**
Bowel
  abnormalities of rotation **6.8**
  fluid-filled 6.3
  malrotation 6.8, 6.27
  non-rotation 6.8
  reverse rotation 6.8
  wall, gas 6.1
  wash-out 6.3
Bowel, small
  adhesions 6.29
  aphthous ulcers 427, **6.42**
  carcinoma: strictures 6.29
  'cobblestone' pattern 427
  dilated **6.28**
  fissure ulcers 427
  inflammation: thickened folds 6.30
  intramural haematoma: thickened folds
    6.30
  ischaemia 6.28, 6.29
    thickened folds 6.30
  lymphoma 447, 6.28, 6.29, 6.31, 6.32,
    6.34
  mechanical obstruction 6.28
  metastases,
    multiple nodules 6.32
    strictures 6.29
    thickened folds 6.31
  multiple nodules **6.32**
  nodular lymphoid hyperplasia 6.32
  non-dilated, thickened folds in **6.30,
    6.31**
  polyposis 6.32
  proximal obstruction 6.21
  resection 6.28, 6.33
  sarcoma 6.29
  stagnant loop/stricture 6.33
  strictures **6.29**
  thick folds 6.28, **6.30, 6.31**
  tumours,
    strictures 6.29
    thickened folds 6.31
  vasculitis 6.30

venous obstruction 6.30
  *see also individual anatomical regions,
    entries beginning* Intestinal
Brachial plexus, trauma 4.45
Bradycardia, fetal 14.13
Brain **12.21–12.33**
  surface enhancement 12.31
Brain death 13.11
Brain isotope angiogram **13.11**
Brainstem glioma 12.32
  CT 12.32
Breast
  abscess 10.10
  benign vs. malignant lesions, *see*
    Mammography
  calcification 10.2, 10.3
  cyst 10.5, 10.6
  disease: ultrasound **10.11**
  giant cyst 10.7
  haematoma 10.3, 10.8
  intraductal papilloma 10.5
  intramammary lymph nodes 10.4, 10.5,
    10.6, 10.8
  lipoma 10.4, 10.7
  lymphatic obstruction 10.10
  metastases: opacities on mammogram
    10.6
  oedematous **10.10**
  papillomatosis 10.6
  sebaceous cyst 10.5, 10.7
  venous obstruction 10.10
Breast carcinoma
  bone metastases 1.16, 1.50
  extradural spinal mass 2.22
  focal rib lesions (metastases) 1.50
  gastric metastases 6.17
  inflammatory, increased uptake on bone
    scans 13.2
  mammography, *see* Mammography
  oedema 10.10
  pleural effusion 4.36
  pulmonary metastases 4.25, 4.36
  screening **10.12**
  single well-defined opacity on
    mammogram 10.5
  skull base metastases 12.12
  spinal metastases 2.2
  ultrasound 10.11
Brodie's abscess 1.12
  lucent bone lesion in medulla 1.19
  solitary bone lesions with lucent centre
    1.13
Bronchial adenoma: bronchial stenosis/
    occlusion 4.7
Bronchial atresia: bronchial stenosis/
    occlusion 4.7
Bronchial carcinoma
  asbestosis 420
  bronchial stenosis/occlusion 4.7
  chronic upper airway obstruction 4.3
  consolidation + bulging of fissures 4.13
  extradural spinal mass 2.22

Bronchial carcinoma (*cont.*)
  gallium uptake 13.7
  gynaecomastia 9.1
  hilar enlargement, unilateral 4.30
  hypertrophic osteoarthropathy 1.34
  lung cavities 4.27
  metastases: distal phalangeal destruction 1.54
  middle mediastinal mass 4.50
  oesophageal strictures 6.14
  pleural effusion 4.34, 4.36
  pulmonary nodule, solitary 4.25
  rib lesion + soft-tissue mass 4.44
  rib lesions, focal (metastases) 1.50
  secondary penumonia 4.11
  skull base metastases 12.12
  spinal metastases 2.2
  superior vena cava enlargement 5.13
  ventilation perfusion mismatch 13.12
Bronchial cartilage deficiency 4.14
Bronchial fibrosis: bronchial stenosis/occlusion 4.7
Bronchial laceration/fracture 4.7, 4.45
Bronchial obstruction 4.11
  bronchiectasis 4.14
  pneumonia, slowly resolving/recurrent 4.10
  unilateral pulmonary oedema 4.18
Bronchial occlusion 4.1, **4.7**
Bronchial perforation 4.38
Bronchial stenoses **4.7**
  bilateral hypertransradiant hemithoraces 4.6
Bronchiectasis **4.14**
  cystic 4.20
    honeycomb lung 4.20
    lung cavities 4.27
    ring shadows 4.47
  hypertrophic osteoarthropathy 1.34
  pneumonia, slowly resolving/recurrent 4.10
Bronchiolitis, acute: bilateral hypertransradiant hemithoraces 4.6
Bronchogenic cyst
  CT mediastinal cyst 4.53
  lung cavities 4.27
  middle mediastinal mass 4.50
  pulmonary nodule 4.25
Bronchogram, air 4.15, 4.25
  opacities **4.28**
Broncho-pleural fistula: pneumothorax 4.37
Bronchospasm, drug-induced 4.48
Bronchus
  foreign body 4.7, 4.14
  fractured 4.7, 4.45
Brown tumour of hyperparathyroidism 442, 11.14
  focal rib lesion 1.50
  lucent bone lesions 1.20
    grossly expansile 1.23

skull vault lucency 12.1
treated, localized density in skull vault 12.8
Brucellosis
  hepatic calcification 7.6
  hepatomegaly 7.5
  splenic calcification 7.19
  splenomegaly 7.18
Brunner's glands, hypertrophied 6.24
Budd–Chiari malformation
  colloid liver scan 13.15
  duodenal folds thickened 6.26
  generalized low density liver CT 7.15
  hepatomegaly 7.5
  low density CT liver 7.17
  small bowel thickened folds 6.30
Budgerigar fancier's lung 4.21
Bulbar palsy: dysphagia 6.10
Bullae, unilateral lung 4.5
Buphthalmos 11.5
Burkitt's lymphoma: loss of lamina dura of teeth 11.16
Burns
  avascular necrosis 1.40
  distal phalangeal destruction 1.54
  premature closure of growth plate 1.3
  soft-tissue calcification 9.3
  soft-tissue ossification 9.6
Bursitis: soft-tissue calcification 9.5
Busulphan therapy 4.29
Byssinosis 4.21

Cachexia: slowly resolving/recurrent pneumonia 4.10
Caecum
  carcinoids 6.35
  tuberculosis 6.35
Caffey's disease, *see* Infantile cortical hyperostosis
Calcium, inhalation (pneumoconiosis) 4.21, 4.22
Calcium hydroxyapatite deposition disease 9.5
  monoarthritis 3.1
Calcium pyrophosphate dihydrate deposition disease **421**, 9.5
  arthritis + bone density preservation 3.4
  chondrocalcinosis 3.11
  intervertebral disc calcification 2.12
  monoarthritis 3.1
  subarticular lucent bone lesions 1.24
Calculi, *see* Bladder, calculi; Renal calculi
Calculus disease, renal cysts 8.14
Callus
  excessive formation **1.15**
  sclerotic bone lesions,
    multiple **1.11**
    solitary **1.10**
Campomelic dwarfism 1.6
Campomelic dysplasia 14.13

Camurati–Engelmann disease (diaphyseal dysplasia) 1.8
  skull density increase 12.6
Canada-Cronkhite syndrome
  colonic polyps 6.36
  multiple nodules in small bowel 6.32
Candida infections, in AIDS 415
Capillary haemangioma: focal hyperechoic ultrasound liver 7.10
Capitate–hamate fusion 1.56
Caplan's syndrome: multiple pulmonary nodules 482, 4.26
Carbon monoxide poisoning
  basal ganglia calcification 12.29
  intracranial calcification 12.27
Carcinogenic dusts 4.21
Carcinoid syndrome 4.25
Carcinoid tumours
  'bull's eye' lesions in stomach 6.22
  focal hyperdense CT liver lesion 7.14
  ileal lesions 6.35
  MIBG imaging 13.18
  small bowel,
    strictures 6.29
    thickened folds 6.31
Carcinomatosis: pulmonary opacities 4.23
Carcinosarcoma: oesophageal strictures 6.15
Cardia, obstruction 6.16
Cardiac anomalies: antenatal diagnosis 14.13
Cardiac arrhythmia
  drug-induced 4.48
  fetal hydrops 14.9
  subclavian vein catheterization 5.20
Cardiac calcification 5.8
Cardiac defects, fetal 14.11
Cardiac enlargement, gross 5.1
Cardiac failure
  azygos vein enlarged 5.14
  congestive,
    ascites 6.4
    hepatomegaly 7.5
    neonatal cyanosis 5.18
  left, enlarged right ventricle 5.4
  oedematous breast 10.10
  pleural effusion 4.34
  pulmonary oedema 4.17
Cardiac output, decreased 5.11
Cardiac tamponade 5.20
Cardiomegaly 5.17
  neonatal asphyxia 5.17
  neonatal cyanosis 5.18
Cardiomyopathy
  congestive: myocardial perfusion imaging 13.13
  fetal hydrops 14.9
  gross cardiac enlargement 5.1
  hypertrophic 13.13
  ischaemic 13.14
  left ventricle enlargement 5.6
Cardiovascular disease: fetal hydrops 14.9

Cardiovascular system 5.1–5.20
  involvement in syndromes 5.19
Carinal cyst: middle mediastinal mass 4.50
Carotid aneurysm 12.12
Carotid siphon: atherosclerosis 12.26, 12.28, 12.30
Carotid stenosis/occlusion 13.11
Carpal fusion 1.56
Carpenter syndrome (acrocephalopolysyndactyly) 12.15
Cartilage, calcification: bone scans 13.2
Cartilage neoplasms: lucent bone lesions 1.25
Cataract 11.9
Cathartic colon 6.37
Catheter embolism: subclavian vein catheterization 5.20
Catheterization, subclavian vein, complications 5.20
Caustic ingestion: oesophageal ulceration 6.13
Cavernous haemangioma: focal hypoechoic ultrasound liver 7.11
Cavernous sinus thrombosis: exophthalmos, unilateral 11.1
Central nervous system
  in AIDS 413
  anomalies, antenatal diagnosis 14.13
  tumour, intradural spinal mass 2.23
Cephalhaematoma: skull vault density increase 12.8
Cerebellum, tumours 12.32
Cerebral abscess
  brain isotope angiogram 13.11
  calcification 12.26
  CT 12.33, 12.34
Cerebral arteriovenous malformation, *see* Arteriovenousmalformation
Cerebral atrophy 13.11
  in AIDS 413, 415
  non-accidental injury 457
Cerebral contusion: non-accidental injury 457
Cerebral cyst
  brain isotope angiogram 13.11
  CT 12.33, 12.34
Cerebral disease: pulmonary oedema 4.17
Cerebral gigantism: accelerated skeletal maturation 1.2
Cerebral haemorrhage: neonatal respiratory distress 4.46
Cerebral infarction
  increased uptake on bone scans 13.2
  infection localization 13.6
  surface enhancement of brain 12.31
Cerebral masses
  accelerated skeletal maturation 1.2
  in AIDS 413
  brain isotope angiogram 13.11
  CT appearances 12.34
  CT attenuation 12.33

Cerebral metastases
  calcification 12.26
  CT 12.33, 12.34
Cerebral oedema
  neonatal respiratory distress 4.46
  non-accidental injury 457
  raised intracranial pressure 12.18
Cerebral palsy: scoliosis 2.1
Cerebral sarcoidosis 476
Cerebrovascular accident: pulmonary
    oedema 4.17
Cerebrovascular occlusion 13.11
Cervical ribs 2.9
Cervix, carcinoma 6.45
  bone metastases 1.16
  dilated ureter 8.25
Chagas' disease
  dysphagia 6.10
  tertiary oesophageal contractions 6.16
Chédiak–Higashi syndrome: bronchiectasis
    4.14
Chemotherapy
  mammographic changes 10.9
  slowly resolving/recurrent pneumonia
    4.10
Chest
  in AIDS 412
    in children 414–415
  radiograph, following chest trauma 4.45
  trauma,
    chest radiograph 4.45
    closed: pleural effusion 4.36
    pneumomediastinum 4.38
Chest wall arteriovenous malformation:
    rib notching 1.51
Chicken pox
  pneumonia 4.29
  widespread air-space disease 4.15
Child abuse, *see* Non-accidental injury
Childbirth: pneumomediastinum 4.38
Children
  abdominal masses 6.6
  AIDS in 414–416
  arthritides, *see* Juvenile chronic arthritis
  bone density increase, generalized 1.8
  chronic upper airway obstruction 4.2
  megacolon in 6.40
  orbital masses 11.2
  posterior fossa neoplasms 12.32
  ring shadows 4.47
  skull vault thickening 12.5
China clay, pneumoconiosis 4.21
Choanal atresia 4.46
  acute upper airway obstruction 4.1
  chronic upper airway obstruction 4.2
  dysphagia 6.11
Cholangiocarcinoma: focal hypodense CT
    lesions 7.13
Cholangitis, recurrent pyogenic 7.12
Cholecystectomy: non-visualization of
    gallbladder 7.1, 13.16
Cholecystitis
  emphysematous 7.3

non-visualization of gallbladder 7.1,
    13.16
  periportal hyperechoic ultrasound 7.12
Cholecystoenterostomy 7.3
Choledochal cyst
  abdominal mass 6.5, 6.6
  gasless abdomen 6.3
  intestinal obstruction in neonate 6.7
Choledochoenterostomy 7.3
Cholesteatoma
  acquired 12.11
  congenital 12.10
  CT 12.34
  parasellar calcification 12.28
Cholesterosis 7.2
Chondroblastoma **422**
  lucent bone lesions,
    + calcium/bone 1.25
    in medulla 1.19, 1.20
    subarticular 1.24
  peak age incidence 1.18
  site of origin 1.17
Chondrocalcinosis (articular cartilage
    calcification) 421,437, **3.11**
Chondrodysplasia, metaphyseal 1.5
Chondrodysplasia punctata 1.5, 1.6, 14.13
  coronal cleft vertebral bodies 2.14
  irregular/stippled epiphyses 1.39
Chondrodystrophy: large head 12.19
Chondroectodermal dysplasia, *see*
    Ellis–van Creveld syndrome
Chondroma: peak age incidence 1.18
Chondromyxoid fibroma **422**
  lucent bone lesions with calcium/bone
    1.25
  lucent medullary lesion + eccentric
    expansion 1.22
  peak age incidence 422, 1.18
  site of origin 1.17
Chondrosarcoma **423**
  bone sclerosis + periosteal reaction
    1.12
  focal rib lesion 1.50
  ill-defined lucent medullary lesions 1.21
  juxta-cortical 9.3
  lucent bone lesions with calcium/bone
    1.25
  'moth-eaten' bone 1.25
  peak age incidence 423, 1.18
  pulmonary metastases 4.25
  site of origin 1.17
Chordoma
  CT 12.33, 12.34
  extradural spinal mass 2.22
  intracranial calcification 12.26
  parasellar,
    calcification 12.28
    superior orbital fissure 11.8
  peak age incidence 1.18
  petrous bone destruction 12.10
  prevertebral soft-tissue mass 11.18
  sacral scalloping 2.18
  sella erosion and osteoporosis 12.25

Chorioangioma: fetal hydrops 14.9
Choriocarcinoma 14.22
  anterior mediastinal mass 4.49
  metastatic 14.22
  widespread air-space disease 4.15
Chorion, in twin pregnancies 14.17
Choroid plexus papilloma 12.26, 12.32
  CT 12.33
Christmas disease (Factor IX deficiency)
  438
Chromophobe 12.23, 12.26, 12.28
Chromosomal abnormalities
  fetal,
    growth retardation 14.14
    raised serum AFP 14.10
  fetal hydrops 14.9, 14.11
  retarded skeletal maturation 1.1
  ultrasound sign suggesting **14.11**
  see also individual disorders
Chylolymphatic cyst: CT mediastinal mass
  containing fat 4.52
Chylothorax: neonatal respiratory distress
  4.46
Circle of Willis, aneurysm 12.25, 12.28,
  12.30
Cirrhosis
  ascites 6.4
  colloid liver scan 13.15
  duodenal folds thickened 6.26
  generalized hyperechoic ultrasound 7.9
  gynaecomastia 9.1
  hepatomegaly 7.5
  hypertrophic osteoarthropathy 1.34
  low density liver CT 7.15, 7.17
  non-dilated small bowel, thickened folds
    6.30
  pleural effusion 4.35
  primary biliary 1.34
  protein-losing enteropathy 6.34
Clavicle
  erosion/absence of outer end **1.49**
  fracture 4.45
Claw osteophytes 2.13
Cleft palate: dysphagia 6.11
Cleidocranial dysplasia **424**, 12.17
  basilar invagination 12.13
  clavicle, erosion/absence of outer end
    1.49
  large head 12.19
  pseudoarthrosis 1.38
  widening of symphysis pubis 3.14
Cloaca, extroversion 6.8
'Cloverleaf' skull 12.15
Coal miner's pneumoconiosis **425**, 4.21
  'eggshell' calcification of lymph nodes
    4.32
  pulmonary opacities 4.23
Coarctation of aorta
  left ventricle enlargement 5.6
  neonatal pulmonary venous congestion
    5.17
  renal induced hypertension 8.20
  rib notching 1.51

  small aortic arch 5.11
Coccidioidomycosis
  bilateral hilar enlargement 4.31
  hepatic calcification 7.6
  intracranial calcification 12.27
  lung cavities 4.27
  pneumonia + enlarged hilum 4.11
  pulmonary calcification 4.29
  pulmonary nodules, multiple 4.26
  pulmonary opacities 4.23
  unilateral hilar enlargement 4.30
Cockayne's syndrome: basal ganglia
  calcification 12.29
Codman triangle 1.31
Coeliac disease 6.33
  dilated small bowel 6.28
  hypertrophic osteoarthropathy 1.34
  malabsorption 6.33
  oesophageal strictures 6.15
  protein-losing enteropathy 6.34
  small bowel thickened folds 6.30
  splenic imaging 13.17
Colitis, total active: gasless abdomen 6.3
Collagen diseases
  duodenal folds thickened 6.26
  gas in wall of colon 6.38
  honeycomb lung 4.20
  pleural effusion 4.34
  soft-tissue calcification 9.3
Colloid cyst
  CT 12.33, 12.34
  thyroid imaging 13.9
Colloid formation 13.2
Colloid liver scans, photopenic (cold)
  areas **13.15**
Colon
  aphthous ulcers 427, **6.42**
  atresia, in neonate 6.7
  carcinoma 428, 487, 6.36
    bladder fistula 8.29
    colonic polyps 6.36
    gastrocolic fistula 6.20
    megacolon 6.40
    protein-losing enteropathy 6.34
    skeletal metastases 1.16
    strictures 6.37
    vesico-intestinal fistula 8.4
  cathartic 6.37
  fistula, malabsorption 6.33
  fluid-filled 6.3
  gas in wall **6.38**
  immaturity: intestinal obstruction 6.7
  infarction 6.38
  ischaemia 6.37
  lymphoma,
    strictures 6.37
    'thumbprinting' 6.41
  metastases: 'thumbprinting' 6.41
  obstruction,
    megacolon 6.39, 6.40
    in neonate 6.7
  polyps **6.36**
  pseudo-obstruction 6.39

Colon (*cont.*)
  small left colon syndrome 6.7
  strictures **6.37**
    megacolon 6.40
    'thumbprinting' **6.41**
    villous adenoma **6.34**, 6.36
Common bile duct
  duodenal ulcer perforation 7.3
  obstruction 13.16
Computerized tomography (CT)
  adrenal masses **7.23**
  central nervous system in lymphoma
    449
  cerebral masses 449, **12.34**
    attenuation **12.33**
  liver,
    focal hyperdense lesion **7.14**
    focal hypodense lesion **7.13**
    generalized increased density, pre-
      contrast **7.16**
    generalized low density **7.15**
    low density patches, post-contrast
      7.17
  mediastinal cysts **4.53**
  mediastinal masses containing fat **4.52**
  mesenteric cystic lesion **6.46**
  optic nerve glioma vs. orbital
    meningioma **11.4**
  orbital masses in children **11.2**
  pancreatic mass, focal **7.21**
  posterior fossa neoplasms in children
    12.32
  renal cysts **8.15**
  renal lesions, focal hypodense **8.13**
  retroperitoneal cystic mass **6.45**
  thymic mass **4.54**
Congenital cholesteatoma 12.10
Congenital disorders
  accelerated skeletal maturation 1.2
  retarded skeletal maturation 1.1
Congenital fibrous band (of Ladd) 6.7
Congenital glaucoma 11.5
Congenital heart disease
  bilateral hypertransradiant hemithoraces
    4.6
  cyanotic: hypertrophic osteoarthropathy
    1.34
  retarded skeletal maturation 1.1
Congenital insensitivity to pain 455, 1.37,
    1.54
Congenital lobar emphysema 4.46
Congenital myositis ossificans progressiva
    9.4, 9.6
Connective tissue diseases
  haematemesis 6.9
  renal induced hypertension 8.20
  rib notching 1.52
Conn's adenoma 7.23
Conn's syndrome 7.23
Constrictive pericarditis, *see* Pericarditis,
    constrictive
Contrast media

pulmonary oedema 4.17
pulmonary opacities 4.22
Copper deficiency
  fraying of metaphyses 1.45
  non-accidental injury vs. 1.37
Corona radiata 4.25
Coronary artery
  aneurysm: bulge on left heart border
    5.7
  calcification 5.8
  left, anomalous 5.17
Corpus callosum, lipoma 12.30
Corrosives
  dypshagia 6.10
  gas in stomach wall 6.23
  linitis plastica 6.19
  oesophageal strictures 6.14
Cortical atrophy, cerebral 13.11
Cor triatriatum: enlarged pulmonary veins
    5.16
'Cottage loaf' cardiac configuration 5.13
Cranial fossa, posterior: neoplasms **12.32**
Cranial ossification, delayed/defective
    12.13
Cranial sutures
  diastasis 12.18, 12.20
  infiltration 12.20
  wide **12.20**
Craniodiaphyseal dysplasia 1.8, 12.6
Craniofacial dysostosis (Crouzon
    syndrome) 12.15
Craniolacunia 12.18
Craniometaphyseal dysplasia 1.8, 12.6
  Erlenmeyer flask deformity 1.47
Craniopharyngioma 12.23
  CT **12.33**, **12.34**
  cystic 12.30
  intracranial calcification 12.26
  parasellar calcification 12.28
  sella erosion and osteoporosis 12.25
Craniostenosis **12.15**
  raised intracranial pressure 12.18
  unilateral exophthalmos 11.1
Craniotubular dysplasia: bone density
    increase 1.8
Craniotubular hyperostoses 1.8
Cretinism **426**
  defective ossification of skull vault
    12.17
  irregular/stippled epiphyses 1.39
  megacolon 6.40
  small/absent sinuses 11.11
  solitary dense metaphyseal band 1.43
  vertebral bodies, beaks 2.15
  see also Hypothyroidism
Cri-du-chat syndrome: cardiovascular
    involvement 5.19
Crohn's disease **427–428**
  aphthous ulcers 6.42
  bladder fistula 8.29
  cobblestone duodenal cap 427, 6.24
  colonic polyps 6.36

colonic strictures 6.37
complications 428
duodenal folds,
  decreased/absent 6.25
  thickened 6.26
gastric folds, thickened 6.18
gastrocolic fistula 6.20
hypertrophic osteoarthropathy 1.34
ileal lesions 6.35
infection localization 13.6
linitis plastica 6.19
malabsorption 6.33
oesophageal strictures 6.15
oesophageal ulceration 6.13
protein-losing enteropathy 6.34
retroperitoneal fibrosis 8.26
retrorectal space widening 6.44
sacroiliitis, bilateral symmetrical 3.12
small bowel,
  dilatation 6.28
  multiple nodules 6.32
  strictures 6.29
  thickened folds 6.31
'thumbprinting' in colon 6.41
toxic megacolon 6.39
vesico-intestinal fistula 8.4
Crouzon syndrome (craniofacial
    dysostosis) 12.15
Crown–rump length 14.1, 14.2
Cryptococcosis
  intracranial calcification 12.27
  pulmonary opacities 4.23
Cryptogenic fibrosing alveolitis:
    honeycomb lung 4.20
CT, *see* Computerized tomography (CT)
Cushing's adenoma 7.23
Cushing's syndrome **429**
  adrenal mass 7.23
  avascular necrosis 1.40
  excessive callus formation 1.15
  expanded pituitary fossa 12.23
  generalized low density liver CT 7.15
  mediastinal lipomatosis 4.52
  osteoporosis 1.29
  retarded skeletal maturation 1.1
  rib lesion + soft-tissue mass 4.44
  teeth, loss of lamina dura 11.16
Cushion defects, endocardial 14.11
Cyanosis, neonatal **5.18**
Cyanotic heart disease
  'hair-on-end' skull vault 12.14
  hypertrophic osteoarthropathy 1.34
  renal vein thrombosis 8.21
Cyst, *see individual cysts*
Cystadenocarcinoma
  calcified pulmonary metastasis 4.29
  mucinous, CT 7.21
  ovarian 14.27
  pancreatic calcification 7.20
Cystadenoma
  mucinous, CT 7.21
  ovarian 14.27

pancreatic calcification 7.20
Cystic adamantinoma 11.14
Cystic adenoma of lung: fetal hydrops
    14.9
Cystic adenomatoid malformation 4.46,
    4.47
Cystic bronchiectasis, *see* Bronchiectasis,
    cystic
Cystic disease, renal, *see* Kidney; Renal
    cysts
Cystic duct obstruction: non-visualization
    of gallbladder 7.1
Cysticercosis
  intracranial calcification 12.27
  soft-tissue calcification 9.2
Cystic fibrosis **430**
  bronchial occlusion 4.7
  duodenal folds, decreased/absent 6.25
  generalized low density liver CT 7.15
  honeycomb lung 4.20
  hypertrophic osteoarthropathy 1.34
  malabsorption 6.33
  pancreatic calcification 7.20
  pneumonia, slowly resolving/recurrent
      4.10
  pneumothorax 4.37
  right ventricle enlargement 5.4
  ring shadows 4.47
Cystic glioma 12.30
  see also Astrocytoma
Cystic hygroma 14.11
  prevertebral soft-tissue mass 11.18
Cystic pneumatosis 6.23
Cystic tumours 4.53
Cystinuria: renal calculi 8.3
Cystitis
  cyclophosphamide-induced 8.28
  emphysematous 8.4
  gas in bladder 8.4
Cystosarcoma phylloides 10.5, 10.7
Cytomegalovirus (CMV) infection
  in AIDS 412
    in children 414
  basal ganglia calcification 12.29
  fetal hydrops 14.9
  intracranial calcification 12.27
  oesophageal ulceration 6.13

Dacroadenitis 11.2
Dandy–Walker cyst 12.19
Degenerative spondylosis: intervertebral
    disc calcification 2.12
Dehydration
  renal vein thrombosis 8.21
  small heart 5.2
Dentigerous cyst
  dental 11.14
  maxillary antrum 11.13
De Quervain's thyroiditis 13.9
Dermatitis herpetiformis 6.33
  dilated small bowel 6.28

Dermatomyositis
  gas in wall of colon 6.38
  soft-tissue calcification 9.3, 9.4, 9.5
Dermoid
  anterior mediastinal mass 4.49
  calcified cerebral 12.26
  CT 12.33, 12.34
  exophthalmos, unilateral 11.1
  implantation: distal phalangeal
      destruction 1.54
  intraorbital 11.9
  orbital masses, CT 11.2
  ovarian 14.27
  spinal mass 2.23
Diabetes mellitus 455
  arthritis mutilans 3.7
  avascular necrosis 1.40
  distal phalangeal destruction 1.54
  gas in stomach wall 6.23
  gas in urinary tract 8.4
  glomerulosclerosis 8.20
  maternal: polyhydramnios 14.8
  osteoporosis 1.29
  pneumonia, slowly resolving/recurrent
      4.10
  renal papillary necrosis 8.19
  seminal vesicle/vas deferens calcification
      8.31
  soft-tissue calcification 9.2
  tertiary oesophageal contractions 6.16
  thickened placenta 14.20
Diabetic ketoacidosis:
      pneumomediastinum 4.38
Diaphragma sellae 12.23
Diaphragmatic eventration 4.40, 4.49
Diaphragmatic hernia
  bowel malrotation 6.8
  congenital 14.13
    gasless abdomen 6.3
  CT mediastinal mass containing fat
      4.52
  fetal hydrops 14.9
  hemithorax, increased density 4.8
  neonatal respiratory distress 4.46
  ring shadows 4.47
Diaphragmatic hump
  anterior mediastinal mass 4.49
  right sided **4.39**
Diaphragmatic rupture 4.40, 4.45
Diaphragmatic splinting 4.40
Diaphyseal aclasis: Madelung deformity
      1.57
Diaphyseal dysplasia
      (Camurati–Engelmann disease)
      1.8, 12.6
Diarrhoea in AIDS 413
  in children 415
Diastasis, suture 12.18, 12.20
Diastematomyelia: widened interpedicular
      distance 2.20
Diastrophic dwarfism, *see* Dwarfism
Diffuse idiopathic skeletal hyperostosis
      (DISH)

anterior longitudinal ligament
      ossification 2.13
  intervertebral disc calcification 2.12
Disaccharidase deficiency: malabsorption
      6.33
Dislocations 457
Disseminated intravascular coagulopathy:
      widespread air-spacedisease 4.15
Diverticula
  anterior urethral 8.30
  bladder 13.2
  gastric 7.23
  oesophageal/pharnygeal **6.12**
  vesical 8.30
Diverticular disease 13.21
  bladder fistula 8.29
  retroperitoneal fibrosis 8.26
  vesico-intestinal fistula 8.4
Diverticulitis
  pneumoperitoneum 6.2
  retrorectal space widening 6.44
Diverticulosis
  intramural: oesophageal ulceration 6.13
  jejunal: malabsorption 6.33
Dorsum sellae, erosion 12.18
'Double bubble' sign 6.7, 6.27, 14.12
'Double track sign' 6.21
Down's syndrome **431**
  atlanto-axial subluxation 2.11
  cardiovascular involvement 5.19
  dilated duodenum 6.27
  intestinal obstruction in neonate 6.7
  irregular/stippled epiphyses 1.39
  retarded skeletal maturation 1.1
  small/absent sinuses 11.11
  vertebral bodies,
    anterior scalloping 2.17
    beaks 2.15
  wormian bones 12.16
Drowning, near: pulmonary oedema 4.17
Drugs, conditions due to
  gynaecomastia 9.1
  honeycomb lung 4.20
  lung disease **4.48**
  oesophageal ulceration 6.13
  paralytic ileus 6.21
  pituitary fossa expanded 12.23
  pulmonary oedema 4.17
Dumb-bell tumour 2.16
Duodenal cap, cobblestone **6.24**
Duodenitis 13.21
  cobblestone duodenal cap 6.24
  duodenal folds thickened 6.26
Duodenum
  atresia 6.27
    gasless abdomen 6.3
  bands 6.27
  carcinoma,
    cobblestone duodenal cap 6.24
    strictures 6.29
  dilated **6.27**
  folds,
    decreased/absent **6.25**

thickened **6.26**
intramural haematoma 6.26
ischaemia 6.26
lymphoma 6.24, 6.26
metastases: thickened duodenal folds
6.26
nodular lymphoid hyperplasia 6.24
obstruction,
fetal 14.12
in neonate 6.7
stenosis/atresia,
in neonate 6.7
suggesting chromosomal abnormality
14.11
ulcer,
cobblestone duodenal cap 6.24
haematemesis 6.9
perforated, gas in urinary tract 8.4
perforating into common bile duct
7.3
see also Peptic ulcer
webs/stenosis 6.27
Dwarfism
campomelic 1.6
deprivational: wide sutures 12.20
diastrophic 1.5, 1.46
antenatal diagnosis 14.13
narrow spinal canal 2.19
Laron: retarded skeletal maturation 1.1
metatropic,
antenatal diagnosis 14.13
coronal cleft vertebral bodies 2.14
cupping of metaphyses 1.46
dwarfing skeletal dysplasia 1.5
large head 12.19
platyspondyly 2.4
Russell–Silver 1.4
skeletal dysplasia **1.5**
thanatophoric 1.6
antenatal diagnosis 14.13
large head 12.19
platyspondyly 2.4
Dysbaric osteonecrosis: avascular necrosis
1.40
Dyschondrosteosis (Leri–Weil disease):
Madelung deformity 1.57
Dysentery
hypertrophic osteoarthropathy 1.34
toxic megacolon 6.39
Dysostosis multiplex, conditions exhibiting
1.7
Dysphagia
adult **6.10**
in AIDS 413
neonate **6.11**
Dysplasia, lethal neonatal **1.6**
Dystrophia myotonica: small pituitary
fossa 12.22

Ear
carcinoma 12.1
middle,

carcinoma 12.11
petrous bone destruction **12.11**
rhabdomyosarcoma 12.11
Ebstein's anomaly
enlarged right atrium 5.3
gross cardiac enlargement 5.1
neonatal cyanosis 5.18
Ectopia vesicae 8.29
Ectopic pregnancy 14.4, **14.6**, 14.7
endometrial thickening 14.24
ovarian mass 14.27
'Eggshell' calcification of lymph nodes
4.32
Ehlers–Danlos syndrome
cardiovascular involvement 5.19
haematemesis 6.9
soft-tissue calcification 9.3
vertebral body scalloping 2.16
Eisenmenger's complex: enlarged left
atrium 5.5
Elliptocytosis: 'hair-on-end' skull vault
12.14
Ellis–van Creveld syndrome
(chondroectodermal dysplasia)
1.5
antenatal diagnosis 14.13
cardiovascular involvement 5.19
carpal fusion 1.56
dwarfing skeletal dysplasia 1.5
Embryonal carcinoma: anterior
mediastinal mass 4.49
Emphysema
compensatory: unilateral
hypertransradiant hemithorax 4.5
congenital lobar,
neonatal respiratory distress 4.46
unilateral hypertransradiant
hemithorax 4.5
infected bullae 4.27
interstitial,
pneumatocoeles 4.9
ring shadows 4.47
interstitial gastric 6.23
mediastinal 4.45
pneumothorax 4.37
obstructive,
bilateral hypertransradiant
hemithoraces 4.6
unilateral hypertransradiant
hemithorax 4.5
pneumothorax 4.37
pulmonary upper zone fibrosis 4.33
small heart 5.2
surgical,
bronchial/tracheal injury 4.45
chest radiograph 4.45
unilateral: unilateral pulmonary oedema
4.18
Emphysematous cystitis 8.4
Empyema
neonatal respiratory distress 4.46
pleural calcification 4.42
subdural 12.31

Empyema *(cont.)*
  unilateral elevated hemidiaphragm 4.40
Encephalitis
  accelerated skeletal maturation 1.2
  in AIDS 413
  expanded pituitary fossa 12.23
  surface enhancement of brain 12.31
Encephalocoele 11.17, 12.18
  raised serum alphafeto protein (AFP)
    14.10
Encephalopathy, in AIDS, in children 415
Enchondroma **432**
  distal phalangeal destruction 1.54
  focal rib lesion 1.50
  lucent bone lesions with calcium/bone
    1.25
  lucent medullary lesion 1.19, 1.20
    + eccentric expansion 1.22
  site of origin 1.17
Endocardial fibroelastosis
  neonatal pulmonary venous congestion
    5.17
  right atrium enlarged 5.3
Endocarditis, infective 13.17
Endochondroma: lucent lesions, grossly
    expansile 1.23
Endocrine disorders
  accelerated skeletal maturation 1.2
  retarded skeletal maturation 1.1
Endodermal sinus tumours: anterior
    mediastinal mass 4.49
Endometrial carcinoma 14.24
  uterus enlargement 14.25
Endometrial polyp 14.24
Endometrial thickening 14.2, 14.6, 14.24
Endometrial thickness, increased **14.24**
Endometriosis 6.37, 14.27
  bladder filling defect 8.27
  indentation of rectosigmoid junction
    6.43
Endomyocardial fibrosis: enlarged right
    atrium 5.3
Endosteal hyperostosis 1.8, 12.6
Endotracheal tube, misplaced 4.7
Enteric cyst: posterior mediastinal masses
    4.51
Enteric duplication cysts 6.44, 6.46
Enteric hyperoxaluria 8.3
Enterogenous cyst: dysphagia 6.10
Eosinophilia, pulmonary 4.48
Eosinophilic enteritis
  duodenal folds thickened 6.26
  linitis plastica 6.19
  malabsorption 6.33
  protein-losing enteropathy 6.34
  small bowel thickened folds 6.30, 6.31
  stomach abnormality + thickened small
    bowel folds 6.31
  stomach folds thickened 6.18
Eosinophilic granuloma **432**, **439**
  lucent bone lesions with calcium/bone
    1.25

lucent medullary bone lesion 1.20
skull vault 12.2
vertebral collapse 2.3
  solitary 2.2
  see also Histiocytosis X
Epanutin therapy 9.7
Ependymoma 12.32
  CT 12.32, 12.33, 12.34
  spinal mass 2.23
  spinal metastases 2.23
  vertebral body scalloping 2.16
Epidermoid
  calcification 12.26
  cerebral 12.33
  CT 12.34
  distal phalangeal destruction 1.54
  skull vault lucency + sclerosis 12.3
Epidermolysis bullosa
  distal phalangeal destruction 1.54
  dysphagia 6.10
  oesophageal strictures 6.14
Epiglottic cyst 4.2
Epiglottitis, acute: acute upper airway
    obstruction 4.1
Epiphrenic diverticulum 6.12
Epiphyses
  granular/fragmented 1.1
  irregular/stippled **1.39**
Epispadias: widening of symphysis pubis
    3.14
Epistaxis: opaque maxillary antrum 11.12
Erlenmeyer flask deformity **1.47**
Erosive osteoarthritis: distal phalangeal
    destruction 1.54
Erythroblastosis fetalis 7.4
Escherichia coli
  cystitis 8.4
  pneumatocoeles 4.9
Ethmoid carcinoma 11.7, 11.17
  pneumocephalus 12.21
Ethmoid sinus, fracture 12.21
Eunuchoidism 1.29
Ewing's tumour **432**
  bone sclerosis + periosteal reaction
    1.12
  focal rib lesion 1.50
  ill-defined lucent medullary lesions 1.21
  lucent bone lesions with calcium/bone
    1.25
  'moth-eaten' bone 1.25
  peak age incidence 1.18
  periosteal reactions 1.31
  pulmonary nodules 4.26
  site of origin 1.17
Excretion urography: non-visualization of
    kidney **8.5**
Exercise induced ischaemia 13.13
Exomphalos 6.8
Exophthalmos, unilateral **11.1**
Exostoses **459**
  bone scan 13.5
  multiple 1.3

Extrapleural haematoma 4.45
Extrapleural masses 4.43
Extrinsic allergic alveolitis **433**, 4.21
  acute, pulmonary opacities 4.23
  bilateral hilar enlargement 4.31
  honeycomb lung 4.20
  pulmonary opacities 4.23
  pulmonary upper zone fibrosis 4.33

Face **11.1–11.18**
Fahr's disease 12.29
Fallot's tetralogy 1.51
  neonatal cyanosis 5.18
  pulmonary valve calcification 5.9
  right-sided aortic arch 5.12
Familial polyposis coli 6.17, 6.36
Fanconi syndrome: osteomalacia/rickets
    1.30
Farmers' lung 4.21
Fat embolism
  avascular necrosis 1.40
  post-chest trauma 4.45
  pulmonary opacities 4.23
  ventilation perfusion mismatch 13.12
  widespread air-space disease 4.15
Fat necrosis, breast 10.3
Felty's syndrome 473
  splenomegaly 7.18
Femoral neck, 'rotting fence-post' 471
Femoral shortening 14.13
Femur
  avascular necrosis 1.40
  intercondylar notch erosion/enlargement
    3.9
Fetal hydrops 14.9, 14.11
  thickened placenta 14.20
Fetomaternal transfusion: fetal hydrops
    14.9
Fetus
  abdomen: cystic structures **14.12**
  anomaly 14.8
  chromosomal abnormality: ultrasound
    signs **14.11**
  dating, measurement for **14.1**
  growth **14.14**
  structural abnormalities diagnosable
    antenatally **14.13**
Fibrin balls 4.43
Fibroadenoma 10.3
  calcification 10.2
  giant 10.7
  mammogram,
    multiple well-defined opacities 10.6
    single well-defined opacity 10.5
  typical appearance 10.4
Fibroadenoma lipoma 10.8
Fibrocartilage 421
Fibrosarcoma
  ill-defined lucent medullary lesions 1.21
  lucent bone lesions with calcium/bone
    1.25

peak age incidence 1.18
rib lesion + soft-tissue mass 4.44
site of origin 1.17
Fibrosing alveolitis
  bilateral elevated hemidiaphragms 4.41
  interstitial ossification 4.29
  pulmonary opacities 4.23
Fibrous cortical defect, *see* Non-ossifying
    fibroma
Fibrous dysplasia **434**
  basilar invagination 12.13
  brain isotope angiogram 13.11
  distal phalangeal destruction 1.54
  exophthalmos, unilateral 11.1
  lucent bone lesions with calcium/bone
    1.25
  lucent lesions, grossly expansile 1.23
  lucent medullary lesions 1.19
  mandibular lesion, cystic 11.14
  opaque maxillary antrum 11.12
  orbital hyperostosis 11.10
  osteomalacia/rickets 1.30
  polyostotic 1.2
  pseudoarthrosis 1.38
  rib lesion, focal 1.50
  sclerotic bone lesions,
    multiple 1.11
    solitary 1.10
  site of origin 1.17
  skull base density increase 12.9
  skull vault,
    increased density 12.7, 12.8
    lucency + sclerosis 12.3
    thickening 12.5
  small/absent sinuses 11.11
Fifth nerve neuroma 12.10
Filariasis: ascites 6.4
Fingers, hypoplasia 1.5
Flail chest 4.45
Fluid overload
  pleural effusion 4.35
  pulmonary oedema 4.17
Fluorosis
  generalized increased bone density 1.8,
    1.9
  periosteal reaction 1.33
  skull vault, density increase 12.7
  soft-tissue calcification 9.2
  symphysis pubis fusion/bridging 3.15
Follicular cyst 14.27
Follicular growth 14.26
Foreign body
  acute upper airway obstruction 4.1
  bladder 8.28, 8.30
  bronchial occlusion 4.7
  bronchiectasis 4.14
  chest radiograph 4.45
  dysphagia 6.10
  intracranial 12.26
  pulmonary, post-chest trauma 4.45
Forrest report, breast cancer screening
    10.12

Fourth ventricle tumours 12.32
Fracture
  avascular necrosis 1.40
  bone scans 13.4, 13.5
  healing 1.12
  increased uptake on bone scans 13.1
  non-accidental injury 456
  non-union 1.38
Fraley syndrome 8.11, 8.24
Friedländer's pneumonia 4.13
Friedreich's ataxia
  cardiovascular involvement 5.19
  scoliosis 2.1
Frontal sinus
  congenital absence 11.11
  fracture 12.21
  mucocoele 12.3
  oestoma 12.8
Frontometaphyseal dysplasia 1.8, 12.6
Frostbite
  distal phalangeal destruction 1.54
  premature closure of growth plate 1.3
Fucosidosis 1.7
Fundoplication 6.15
Fungal diseases
  pneumonia 4.10
  pulmonary opacities 4.23

Galactocoele 10.8
Gallbladder
  calculi 7.2
  carcinoma 7.2
  ectopic 7.1
  filling defect **7.2**
  gas in 7.3
  non-visualization **7.1, 13.16**
  porcelain (calcified) 7.6
  'strawberry' (cholesterosis) 7.2
  stricture 7.2
Gallium uptake **13.7**
Gallstone 7.2
  passage into bowel 7.3
Ganglioneuroma 6.6
  adrenal calcification 7.22
  posterior mediastinal mass 4.51
Gangliosidosis 1.7
Gardner's syndrome 6.17, 6.36
  multiple nodules in small bowel 6.32
  sclerotic bone lesions 1.11
Garré's sclerosing osteomyelitis 1.12
Gas
  biliary tree 6.1, **7.3**, 7.12
  bladder and bladder wall 8.4
  bowel wall 6.1
  colon wall **6.38**
  extraluminal intr-abdominal **6.1**
  portal veins 6.1, **7.4**
  retroperitoneal 6.1
  stomach wall **6.23**
  urinary tract 6.1, **8.4**
Gastrectomy: malabsorption 6.33

Gastric adenoma 13.21
Gastric diverticulum 7.23
Gastric emphysema, interstitial 6.23
Gastric ulcer
  haematemesis 6.9
  see also Peptic ulcer
Gastrinoma 451, 6.18, 7.21
Gastritis 13.21
  emphysematous 6.23
  thick gastric folds 6.18
Gastrocolic fistula **6.20**
Gastroenteritis, eosinophilic 6.18
Gastrointestinal atresia: fetal hydrops 14.9
Gastrointestinal bleeding 13.6
  localization **13.21**
  Meckel's diverticulum 13.21, 13.22
Gastrointestinal fistula 6.5
Gastrointestinal metastases 13.21
Gastrointestinal obstruction, fetal 14.12
Gastrointestinal perforation, fetal hydrops 14.9
Gastrointestinal tract **6.1–6.45**
  duplication 6.5
Gastrointestinal tumours
  ascites 6.4
  bone metastases 1.16
  gallium uptake 13.7
Gastro-oesophageal reflux 6.14, 6.15
Gastroschisis 6.8
  antenatal diagnosis 14.13
  raised AFP 14.10
Gastroscopy, gas in stomach wall after 6.23
Gated blood pool imaging **13.14**
Gaucher's disease
  avascular necrosis 1.40
  coarse trabecular bone pattern 1.14
  Erlenmeyer flask deformity 1.47
  erosion of medial metaphysis 1.48
  hepatomegaly 7.5
  splenomegaly 7.18
Genito-urinary tumours: bone metastases 1.16
Geode 1.19
'Geographical' skull 439, 12.2
Germ cell tumour: thymic mass 4.54
Germinal cellneoplasms, anterior mediastinal mass 4.49
Gestational age 14.1
  assessment **14.1**
Gestational sac
  normal growth rate 14.2
  in normal pregnancy 14.2
Gestational trophoblastic disease **14.22**
Giant aneurysm, *see* Aneurysm
Giant cell tumour 435
  distal phalangeal destruction 1.54
  lucent bone lesions,
    grossly expansile 1.23
    subarticular 1.24
  lucent medullary lesion + eccentric expansion 1.22

mandible 11.14
osteomalacia/rickets 1.30
peak age incidence 1.18
site of origin 1.17
vertebral body enlargement 2.7
vertebral collapse 2.2
Giardiasis
duodenal folds thickened 6.26
malabsorption 6.33
small bowel thickened folds 6.31
Gigantism
bilateral large smooth kidneys 8.10
cerebral 1.2
vertebral body enlargement 2.7
Glaucoma, congenital 11.5
Glioblastoma: spinal metastases 2.23
Glioblastoma multiforme, brain isotope
angiogram 13.11
Glioma
brain isotope angiogram 13.11
CT 12.33, 12.34
exophthalmos, unilateral 11.1
intracranial calcification 12.26
surface enhancement of brain 12.31
Globus hystericus: dysphagia 6.10
Glomerular disease: osteomalacia/rickets
1.30
Glomerulonephritis
acute, nephrogram 8.18
bilateral large smooth kidneys 8.10
bilateral small smooth kidneys 8.8
hypertension 8.20
renal calcification 8.2
renal vein thrombosis 8.21
Glomus jugulare 12.11
CT 12.34
Glomus tumour: distal phalangeal
destruction 1.54
Glossoptosis: dysphagia 6.11
Glottis, carcinoma 4.3
Glucagonoma 451, 7.21
Glycogen storage disease
density increase in CT liver 7.16
erosion of medial metaphysis 1.48
generalized hyperechoic ultrasound liver
7.9
generalized low density liver CT 7.15
osteoporosis 1.29
Goitre
dysphagia 6.10
multinodular: thyroid imaging 13.9
retropharyngeal 11.18
retrosternal 4.49
Gonadal tumours: accelerated skeletal
maturation 1.2
Goodpasture's syndrome
bilateral large smooth kidneys 8.10
widespread air-space disease 4.15
Gorlin's syndrome 11.14
Gout 435
arthritis + bone density preservation
3.4

arthritis + preserved/widened joint
space 3.6
avascular necrosis 1.40
chondrocalcinosis 3.11
chronic tophaceous 436
complications 436
intervertebral disc calcification 2.12
monoarthritis 3.1
soft-tissue calcification 9.3, 9.5
subarticular lucent bone lesions 1.24
Gouty arthritis 435, 3.12
bilateral asymmetrical sacroiliitis 3.12
Granulomatous disease, chronic:
bronchiectasis 4.14
Granulosa cell tumour 14.27
Graves thyrotoxicosis: thymic hyperplasia
4.54
Growth hormone deficiency: retarded
skeletal maturation 1.1
Growth plate, premature closure 1.3
Growth retardation, fetal 14.8, 14.14,
14.21
risk factors 14.14
suggesting chromosomal abnormality
14.11
symmetrical 14.11
Guinea worm: soft-tissue calcification 9.2
Gynaecological ultrasound 14.1–14.27
Gynaecomastia 9.1

Haemangioblastoma, CT 12.33
Haemangioendothelioma: focal hyperdense
CT lesion 7.14
Haemangioma 437
abdominal mass in child 6.6
bowel 13.22
coarse trabecular bone pattern 1.14
exophthalmos, unilateral 11.1
hepatic,
calcified 7.6
colloid liver scan 13.15
CT 7.13
intraorbital calcification 11.9
mandibular lesion, cystic 11.14
orbital masses, CT 11.2
peak age incidence 1.18
periosteal reactions 1.31
skull vault 12.1
'hair-on-end' 437, 12.14
lucency + sclerosis 12.3
soft-tissue calcification 9.3
spinal mass, extradural 2.22
of spine, photopenic area on bone scan
13.3
splenic calcification 7.19
vertebral body enlargement 2.7
vertebral collapse 2.2
Haemangiopericytoma
osteomalacia/rickets 1.30
retroperitoneal cystic mass 6.45
Haemangiosarcoma, intrahepatic 7.13

Haematemesis **6.9**
Haematoma
    bowel 6.26, 6.30
    breast 10.3, 10.8
    cerebral, CT 12.33, 12.34
    extrapleural 4.45
    gastrointestinal bleeding localization
        13.21
    intracranial 12.18
        calcification 12.30
    mediastinal 4.45
    mediastinal cyst, CT 4.53
    perinephric 8.1
    post-chest trauma 4.45
    prevertebral 6.10
    pulmonary 4.25, 4.27, 4.45
    rectosigmoid junction 6.43
    soft-tissue calcification 9.3
    spinal mass,
        extradural 2.22
        intradural 2.24
    splenic 6.5
    subdural, *see* Subdural haematoma
    surface enhancement of brain 12.31
Haemochromatosis **437**
    chondrocalcinosis 3.11
    density increase in CT liver 7.16
    hepatic calcification 7.6
    hepatomegaly 7.5
    intervertebral disc calcification 2.12
Haemodialysis related cysts 8.15
Haemoglobinopathies
    avascular necrosis 1.40
    coarse trabecular bone pattern 1.14
    Erlenmeyer flask deformity 1.47
    splenic imaging 13.17
Haemolytic anaemia
    skull vault,
        'hair-on-end' 12.14
        increased density 12.7
        thickening 12.5
    small/absent sinuses 11.11
    splenomegaly 7.18
Haemomediastinum: subclavian vein
    catheterization 5.20
Haemopericardium 4.45
Haemophilia **438**
    arthritis + osteoporosis 3.3
    arthritis + periosteal reaction 3.5
    avascular necrosis 1.40
    femoral intercondylar notch erosion 3.9
    premature closure of growth plate 1.3
    widespread air-space disease 4.15
Haemophilic pseudotumour 438
    lucent lesions, grossly expansile 1.23
Haemophilus influenzae: pneumatocoeles
    4.9
Haemopoiesis, extramedullary 4.51
Haemosiderosis
    density increase in CT liver 7.16
    idiopathic pulmonary 4.15
    pulmonary opacities 4.23

Haemothorax 4.37
    pleural calcification 4.42
    post-chest trauma 4.45
    rib fracture 4.45
    subclavian vein catheterization 5.20
    unilateral elevated hemidiaphragm 4.40
'Hair-on-end' 1.31, **12.14**
    haemangioma 437, 12.1
    meningioma 12.8
    sickle-cell anaemia 480
    thalassaemia 484
Hajdu–Cheney syndrome 1.54, 12.16
Hamartoma
    accelerated skeletal maturation 1.2
    benign: abdominal mass in neonate 6.5
    CT mediastinal mass containing fat
        4.52
    pulmonary nodule, solitary 4.25
    renal 8.12
    temporal lobe, calcification 12.26
Hand: trident + coarse trabecular pattern
    441
Hand–foot syndrome (sickle-cell dactylitis)
    480
    periosteal reaction 1.36
Hand–Schüller–Christian disease **439**,
    12.2
    vertebral collapse 2.3
Hashimoto's thyroiditis 13.9
Head
    in AIDS, in children 415
    injury: pulmonary oedema 4.17
    large in infancy **12.19**
Heart
    calcified thrombus 5.8
    complete block, fetal 14.13
    gross enlargement **5.1**
    hypoplastic left 5.17
    left border, bulge **5.7**
    multiple valvular disease 5.1
    small **5.2**
    valve calcification **5.9**
    see also entries beginning Cardiac
Heel pad thickness, increased **9.7**
Heller's operation 6.12
Hemidiaphragm
    bilateral elevated **4.41**
    unilateral elevated **4.40**
Hemihypertrophy: asymmetrical
    maturation of bone 1.4
Hemiplegia: unilateral elevated
    hemidiaphragm 4.40
Hemithorax
    bilateral hypertransradiant **4.6**
    increased density **4.8**
    opaque 4.4
    unilateral hypertransradiant **4.5**
Hemivertebra: scoliosis 2.1
Henoch-Schönlein purpura
    duodenal folds thickened 6.26
    small bowel thickened folds 6.30
Heparin: osteoporosis 1.29

Hepatic, entries beginning, *see* Liver
Hepatitis
  acute: colloid liver scan 13.15
  chronic active 13.17
  low density CT liver 7.17
  non visualization of gallbladder with
      HIDA 13.16
  serum 7.5
  splenomegaly 7.18
  ultrasound,
    generalized hyperechoic 7.9
    generalized hypoechoic 7.8
Hepatobiliary scintigraphy 13.16
Hepatoblastoma
  in child 6.6
  focal hyperdense CT lesion 7.14
  in neonate 6.5
Hepatocellular disease: non-visualization
    of gallbladder 13.16
Hepatoma 7.5
  calcification 7.6
  colloid liver scan 13.15
  CT lesions,
    focal hyperdense 7.14
    focal hypodense 7.13
  gallium uptake 13.7
  ultrasound,
    focal hyperechoic 7.10
    focal hypoechoic 7.11
Hepatomegaly 7.5
  gastric indentation 6.17
Hepatosplenomegaly
  in AIDS, in children 415
  bilateral elevated hemidiaphragms 4.41
Hereditary telangiectasia (Osler–Weber–
    Rendu syndrome) 6.9
Hernia, *see individual hernia*
Herpes oesophagitis 6.13
Hexadactyly 1.5
Hiatus hernia
  gastric dilatation 6.21
  haematemesis 6.9
  oesophageal stricture 6.14
  oesophageal ulceration 6.13
  pneumonia, slowly resolving/recurrent
      4.10
  posterior mediastinal masses 4.51
HIDA, non visualization of gallbladder
    13.16
Hilar adenopathy, in AIDS in children
    415
Hilar cyst: middle mediastinal mass 4.50
Hilar enlargement, *see* Lung
Hilar lymph nodes
  'eggshell' calcification **4.32**
  enlargement 4.11
Hippel–Lindau syndrome, *see* von
    Hippel–Lindau syndrome
Hirschsprung's disease
  intestinal obstruction in neonate 6.7
  megacolon 6.40
Histamine liberators 4.48

Histiocytosis X **439–440**
  expanded pituitary fossa 12.23
  'floating' teeth 11.15
  honeycomb lung 4.20
  lucent bone lesions with calcium/bone
      1.25
  mandibular lesion, cystic 11.14
  orbital hyperostosis 11.10
  orbital masses, CT 11.2
  rib lesion, focal 1.50
  ring shadows 4.47
  skull vault 12.4
    lucency 12.2
    lucency + sclerosis 12.3
  teeth, loss of lamina dura 11.16
  vertebral collapse 2.2, 2.3
  see also Eosinophilic granuloma
Histoplasmoma: solitary pulmonary
    nodule 4.25
Histoplasmosis
  adrenal calcification 7.22
  bilateral hilar enlargement 4.31
  hepatic calcification 7.6
  ileal lesions 6.35
  intracranial calcification 12.27
  lung cavities 4.27
  pneumonia + enlarged hilum 4.11
  pneumonia 4.15
  pulmonary calcification 4.29
  pulmonary nodules, multiple 4.26
  pulmonary opacities 4.23
  pulmonary upper zone fibrosis 4.33
  splenic calcification 7.19
  splenomegaly 7.18
  unilateral hilar enlargement 4.30
Hodgkin's disease 446
  lung cavities 4.27
  middle mediastinal mass 4.50
  thymic mass 4.54
  vertebral body, ivory 2.10
  see also Lymphoma
Holt–Oram syndrome
  cardiovascular involvement 5.19
  carpal fusion 1.56
Homocystinuria **440**
  arachnodactyly 1.53
  cardiovascular involvement 5.19
  osteoporosis 1.29
  scoliosis 2.1
Homogentisic acid 417
Homozygous achondroplasia 1.6
Honeycomb lung **4.20**, 4.37
Hookworm infestation: thickened
    duodenal folds 6.26
Human chorionic gonadotrophin (hCG)
    14.6, 14.22
Humerus, erosion of medial metaphysis
    1.48
Hunter's syndrome 441, 1.7
  cardiovascular involvement 5.19
Hurler's syndrome **440–441**, 1.7
  cardiovascular involvement 5.19

Hurler's syndrome (*cont.*)
  erosion of medial metaphysis 1.48
  vertebral body,
    beaks 2.15
    scalloping 2.16
Hyaline (articular) cartilage calcification
    421, 437, **3.11**
Hyaline membrane disease 4.46
Hydatid disease
  cardiac calcification 5.8
  cerebral 12.33
    CT 2.34
  CT lesions,
    focal hyperdense 7.14
    focal hypodense 7.13
  extradural spinal mass 2.22
  hepatic calcification 7.6
  hepatomegaly 7.5
  intracranial calcification 12.27
  lucent bone lesions 1.23
  lung cavities 4.27
  pulmonary nodules,
    multiple 4.26
    solitary 4.25
  rectosigmoid junction indentation 6.43
  renal calcification 8.2
  renal cysts 8.14
    CT 8.15
  right sided diaphragmatic humps 4.39
  skull vault 12.1
  splenic calcification 7.19
  vertebral body enlargement 2.7
Hydatidiform mole 14.4, 14.22
Hydranencephaly: large head 12.19
Hydrocalycosis 8.24
Hydrocephalus
  accelerated skeletal maturation 1.2
  basilar invagination 12.13
  benign external 12.19
  congenital and acquired 12.19
  cranial thinning 12.13
  craniostenosis 12.15
  J-shaped sella 12.24
  large head in infancy 12.19
  obstructive 12.18
  raised intracranial pressure 12.18
  raised serum alphafeto protein (AFP)
    14.10
  sutures widening 12.20
  vertebral body scalloping 2.16
Hydrometrocolpos
  abdominal mass in neonate 6.5
  ruptured 7.7
Hydronephrosis
  abdominal mass,
    in child 6.6
    in neonate 6.5
  bilateral: large smooth kidneys 8.10
  in child 6.6, **8.17**
  fetal 14.12, 14.13
  nephrogram 8.18
  raised AFP 14.10

  renal imaging 13.20
  renal induced hypertension 8.20
  renal mass 8.16
Hydroxy vitamin D therapy 9.5
Hyperaemia: premature closure of growth
    plate 1.3
Hypercalcaemia
  idiopathic, of infancy 1.8
  metastatic pulmonary calcifications 4.29
  renal calcification 8.2
  renal calculi 8.3
  soft-tissue calcification 9.5
Hypercalciuria: renal calcification 8.2
Hyperlipidaemia: avascular necrosis 1.40
Hypernephroma: gallium uptake 13.7
Hyperostosis
  benign, skull vault 12.8
  endosteal 12.6
  orbital **11.10**
Hyperoxaluria: renal calcification 8.2, 8.3
Hyperparathyroidism **441–442**, 471
  basal ganglia calcification 12.29
  bone scans 13.4
  brown tumours, *see* Brown tumours of
    hyperparathyroidism
  chondrocalcinosis 3.11
  clavicle, erosion/absence of outer end
    1.49
  distal phalangeal destruction 1.54
  'floating' teeth 11.15
  mandibular lesion, cystic 11.14
  osteopenia, generalized 1.28
  pancreatic calcification 7.20
  primary **441–442**
  pulmonary calcifications 4.29
  renal calcification 8.2
  renal calculi 8.3
  rib notching 1.52
  sacroiliitis, bilateral symmetrical 3.12
  secondary 9.2, 9.3, 9.5
  sella erosion and osteoporosis 12.25
  skull vault 12.1
    lucent lesions 12.4
  soft-tissue calcification 9.2, 9.3, 9.5
  symphysis pubis widening 3.14
  teeth, loss of lamina dura 11.16
Hyperphosphatasia: skull density increase
    12.6
Hypertension
  fetal growth retardation 14.14
  large aortic arch 5.10
  left ventricle enlargement 5.6
  malignant 12.25
  renal-induced **8.20**
Hyperthyroidism
  accelerated skeletal maturation 1.2
  anterior mediastinal mass 4.49
  craniostenosis 12.15
  left ventricle enlarged 5.6
  osteoporosis 1.29
  pulmonary arteries enlarged 5.15
Hypertrophic osteoarthropathy (HOA) **1.34**

periosteal reactions 1.33
Hyperuricaemia 435
    renal calculi 8.3
Hypervitaminosis A: generalized increased
        bone density 1.8
Hypervitaminosis D
    generalized increased bone density 1.8
    intracranial calcification 12.27
    renal calcification 8.2
    renal calculi 8.3
    soft-tissue calcification 9.5
    solitary dense metaphyseal band 1.43
Hypoalbuminaemia: ascites 6.4
Hypochondroplasia
    dwarfing skeletal dysplasia 1.5
    narrow spinal canal 2.19
Hypogammaglobulinaemia
    bronchiectasis 4.14
    pneumonia 4.10
    small bowel nodules 6.32
Hypoglycaemia: neonatal respiratory
        distress 4.46
Hypogonadism
    gynaecomastia 9.1
    osteoporosis 1.29
    retarded skeletal maturation 1.1
Hypoparathyroidism 443
    basal ganglia calcification 12.29
    intracranial calcification 12.27
Hypophosphataemia, X-linked 1.30
Hypophosphatasia 443–444, 1.6
    antenatal diagnosis 14.13
    cupping of metaphyses 1.46
    defective ossification of skull vault
        12.17
    dense vertical metaphyseal lines 1.44
    fraying of metaphyses 1.45
    osteomalacia/rickets 1.30
Hypopituitarism 12.22
    gynaecomastia 9.1
    retarded skeletal maturation 1.1
Hypoplastic left heart: neonatal
        pulmonary venous congestion
        5.17
Hypoproteinaemia
    duodenal folds thickened 6.26
    pulmonary oedema 4.17
    small bowel, thickened folds 6.30
Hypotension
    bilateral small smooth kidneys 8.8
    nephrographic pattern 8.18
Hypothalamus, masses: accelerated
        skeletal maturation 1.2
Hypothermia: neonatal respiratory distress
        4.46
Hypothyroidism
    congenital, *see* Cretinism
    expanded pituitary fossa 12.23
    retarded skeletal maturation 1.1
    thyroid imaging 13.9
Hypoxia: enlarged pulmonary arteries
        5.15

I–Cell disease 1.7
Idiopathic hypercalcaemia of infancy:
        bone density increase 1.8
Idiopathic interstitial fibrosis: honeycomb
        lung 4.20
Idiopathic pulmonary arterial hypertension
        5.1
Idiopathic pulmonary haemosiderosis
        4.15
Idiopathic sexual precocity: accelerated
        skeletal maturation 1.2
Ileocaecal valve 427
Ileum
    atresia 6.7
    carcinoids 6.35
    dilated **6.28**
    lymphoma 6.35
    metastases 6.35
    obstruction in neonate 6.7
    terminal, lesions **6.35**
Ill health, chronic: retarded skeletal
        maturation 1.1
Immune deficiency states
    bronchiectasis 4.14
    pneumonia 4.10
    see also Hypogammaglobulinaemia
Immune hydrops 14.9
Immunoglobulin deficiency, pneumonia
        4.10
Immunological incompetence: slowly
        resolving/recurrentpneumonia
        4.10
Immunosuppressives 13.6
    avascular necrosis 1.40
    slowly resolving/recurrent pneumonia
        4.10
Imperforate anus 6.5
    bladder fistula 8.29
    immaturity in neonate 6.7
    megacolon 6.40Incomplete mole
        (triploidy) 14.22
Indium (S111sIn) scans 13.6
Indomethacin: avascular necrosis 1.40
Infantile cortical hyperostosis (Caffey's
        disease) 1.8
    bone density increase 1.8
    bone sclerosis + periosteal reaction
        1.12
    periosteal reactions 1.31, 1.35
Infantile hypertrophic pyloric stenosis:
        gastric dilatation 6.21
Infantile polycystic disease 6.5, 8.14
    nephrogram 8.18
Infarcts: premature closure of growth
        plate 1.3
Infection
    localization **13.6**
    premature closure of growth plate 1.3
    see also individual infections
Infectious mononucleosis
    hepatomegaly 7.5
    splenomegaly 7.18

Infective colitis: infection localization 13.6
Inferior vena cava
    obstruction 5.14
    thrombosis,
        ascites 6.4
        protein-losing enteropathy 6.34
        renal vein thrombosis 8.21
Inflammatory bowel disease
    infection localization 13.6
    retarded skeletal maturation 1.1
    sacroiliitis, bilateral symmetrical 3.12
    see also Crohn's disease; Ulcerative
        colitis
Influenza: widespread air-space disease
    4.15
Infraclinoid aneurysm
    exophthalmos, unilateral 11.1
    superior orbital fissure enlargement 11.8
Inguinal hernia: intestinal obstruction in
    neonate 6.7
Innominate artery
    compression 4.2
    tortuous 4.49
Inorganic dust, pneumoconioses 4.21
Inspissated milk 6.7
Insulinoma 451, 7.21
Internal auditory meatus 12.10
Interpedicular distance, widened **2.20**
Interstitial emphysema, *see* Emphysema,
    interstitial
Interstitial fibrosis: gallium uptake 13.7
Interstitial ossification 4.29
Intervertebral disc
    calcification **2.12**
    spinal mass 2.22
Intervertebral joint disorders: spinal block
    2.21
Intervillous thrombosis 14.19
Intestinal duplication cyst 4.51
Intestinal infarction 6.1
    pneumoperitoneum 6.2
Intestinal obstruction
    abdominal mass in neonate 6.5
    closed-loop: gasless abdomen 6.3
    gasless abdomen 6.3
    in neonate **6.7**, 6.27
Intestine
    abnormalities of rotation **6.8**
    duplication 6.5
    malrotation 6.8, 6.27
    perforation: pneumoperitoneum 6.2
    see also Bowel; Colon; *entries beginning*
        Gastrointestinal
Intra-abdominal gas, extraluminal **6.1**
Intra-abdominal tumour: bilateral elevated
    hemidiaphragms 4.41
Intracerebral haematoma 12.18
Intracranial abscess 12.26
Intracranial calcification
    basal ganglia **12.29**
    curvilinear **12.30**
    multifocal **12.27**

parasella **12.28**
unifocal **12.26**
Intracranial injury, non-accidental 457
Intracranial masses: accelerated skeletal
    maturation 1.2
Intracranial pressure, decreased: skull
    vault thickening 12.5
Intracranial pressure, raised **12.18**
    brain isotope angiogram 13.11
    erosion of sella 12.25
    expanded pituitary fossa 12.23
    optic foramen enlarged 11.7
    optic nerve enlargement 11.3
    pulmonary oedema 4.17
    sutures widened 12.20
Intrahepatic duct, dilated 13.15
Intraorbital calcification **11.9**
Intrapleural infusion 5.20
Intrarenal artery, compression by 8.11,
    8.24
Intrasellar mass 12.23
Intraspinal mass
    pedicle erosion/destruction/absence 2.5
    scoliosis 2.1
    spinal block 2.21
    widened interpedicular distance 2.20
    see also Spinal mass
Intrathymic haemorrhage 4.49
Intrauterine growth retardation, *see*
    Growth retardation
Intrauterine infections 14.14
    thickened placenta 14.20
Intrauterine perforation: solitary
    radiolucent metaphysealband
    1.41
Intraventricular haemorrhage: non-
    accidental injury 457
Intussusception 13.21, 13.22
Invasive mole 14.22
Iodine scanning, whole body **13.8**
Iron-deficiency anaemia: 'hair-on-end'
    skull vault 12.14
Iron overload 437
    density increase in CT liver 7.16
Ischaemic colitis
    aphthous ulcers 6.42
    'thumbprinting' in colon 6.41
    toxic megacolon 6.39
Islet cell tumour, CT 7.21

Jaundice, obstructive
    colloid liver scan 13.15
    osteomalacia/rickets 1.30
Jejunal atresia 6.7
Jejunal dilatation **6.28**, 6.33
Jejunal diverticulosis: malabsorption 6.33
Jejunal malrotation and volvulus 6.7
Jejunal obstruction
    fetal 14.12
    in neonate 6.7

Jeune's thoracic dysplasia, *see* Asphyxiating thoracicdysplasia of Jeune
Joints **3.1–3.15**
   increased uptake on bone scans 13.1
Jugular foramen syndrome: skull base metastases 12.12
Jugular reflux 13.11
Juvenile chronic arthritis **444–445**
   arthritis mutilans 3.7
   arthritis + periosteal reaction 3.5
   atlanto-axial subluxation 2.11
   block vertebrae 2.9
   carpal fusion 1.56
   femoral intercondylar notch erosion 3.9
   intervertebral disc calcification 2.12
   monoarthritis 3.1
   periosteal reactions 1.35
   premature closure of growth plate 1.3
   protrusio acetabuli 3.13
Juvenile polyposis 6.36
   hypertrophic osteoarthropathy 1.34

Kala-azar
   hepatomegaly 7.5
   splenomegaly 7.18
Kaposi's sarcoma, in AIDS 412, 413
Kartagener's syndrome
   bronchiectasis 4.14
   cardiovascular involvement 5.19
   small/absent sinuses 11.11
Kerley B lines **4.19**
Kidney
   abscess 8.2, 8.11, 8.22
      CT lesions 8.13
      imaging 13.20
   absent 8.1, 8.5
   acute cortical necrosis 8.2, 8.10
   acute tubular necrosis 8.10, 8.18
   adenoma 8.12
   arterial occlusion 8.18
   bilateral large smooth **8.10**
   bilateral parenchymal disease 8.20
   bilateral small smooth **8.8**
   blood clot 8.23
   bowel overlying 8.6
   calcification **8.2**
   calculi 8.2, **8.3**, 8.23
   calyx,
      dilatation 8.11, **8.24**
      five or less 8.7
      non-visualization **8.22**
      radiolucent filling defect **8.23**
   carcinoma 8.12
      calcification 8.2
      imaging 13.20
      renal cysts 8.14
      squamous cell 8.12, 8.23
      transitional cell 8.12, 8.23
      see also Renal cell carcinoma; Renal tumours

compensatory hypertrophy 8.9
congenital absence 8.1, 8.5
congenital hypoplasia 8.7
cortical cysts 8.14
crossed fused ectopia 8.9
cystic hamartoma 8.15
cysts, *see* Renal cyst
dilated collecting system 8.7
disease: fetal growth retardation 14.14
displaced 8.1
dromedary hump 8.11
'drooping flower' appearance 8.11, 8.22, 8.30
duplex 8.6, 8.9, 8.30
   + hydronephrotic upper moiety 8.11
   non-visualization of renal calyx 8.22
ectopic 6.5, 8.1, 8.5, 8.16
   abdominal mass in neonate 6.5
extraparenchymal cysts 8.14
fetal lobulation 8.6
focal hypodense CT lesion **8.13**
focal/segmental cystic dysplasia 8.14
hamartoma 8.12, 8.15
hilar lip 8.11
infarction 8.6, 8.13
   unilateral small smooth kidney 8.7
infundibulum,
   obstructed 8.22
   wide 8.24
ischaemia, nephrographic pattern 8.18
leukaemic infiltration 8.10, 8.12
localized hypertrophy 8.11
lymphoma involvement 8.12
medullary calcification 8.2
medullary cystic disease 8.14
medullary cysts 8.14
medullary sponge 8.2, 8.10, 8.14
   nephrogram 8.18
megacalyces 8.24
metastases 8.12, 8.13, 13.20
multicystic 8.5, 8.9, 8.14
   abdominal mass in neonate 6.5
   CT 8.15
   in newborn and young 8.16
multicystic dysplastic 14.12, 14.13
   raised AFP 14.10
non-visualization during excretion urography **8.5**
obstructed 8.9
outline,
   localized bulge **8.11**
   loss on plain film **8.1**
papillary necrosis, *see* Renal papillary necrosis
papilloma 8.23
parapelvic cyst 8.14
pelvis, radiolucent filling defect **8.23**
polycalycosis 8.24
polycystic, *see* Polycystic disease
post-obstructive atrophy 8.7, 8.24
prominent septum of Bertin 8.11
pyelogenic (calyceal) cyst 8.14

Kidney (*cont.*)
  reflux nephropathy, *see* Reflux
    nephropathy
  reflux without obstruction 8.17
  small-volume collecting system 8.7
  spleen impression 8.6, 8.11
  squamous metaplasia (cholesteatoma)
    8.23
  stricture 8.24
  transplant, rejected 8.2, 13.6
  trauma: imaging 13.20
  unilateral large smooth **8.9**
  unilateral scarred 8.6
  unilateral small smooth 8.7
  see also entries beginning Renal
Klebsiella pneumoniae
  lobar pneumonia 4.12
  lung cavities 4.27
  lung consolidation + bulging of fissures
    4.13
  pneumatocoeles 4.9
Klinefelter's syndrome: gynaecomastia 9.1
Klippel–Feil syndrome
  basilar invagination 12.13
  block vertebrae 2.9
Klippel–Trenaunay–Weber syndrome 1.4
Kniest syndrome 1.5
  coronal cleft vertebral bodies 2.14
  narrow spinal canal 2.19
  platyspondyly 2.4
Kwashiorkor: pancreatic calcification 7.20

Lactase deficiency: malabsorption 6.33
Ladd, congenital fibrous bands 6.7
Laron dwarfism: retarded skeletal
    maturation 1.1
Laryngeal carcinoma
  infraglottic 4.3
  supraglottic 4.3
Laryngeal cyst 4.2
Laryngeal oedema: acute upper airway
    obstruction 4.1
Laryngeal papilloma 4.2
Laryngeal polyp 4.2
Laryngeal stenosis: bilateral
    hypertransradiant hemithoraces
    4.6
Laryngomalacia: chronic upper airway
    obstruction 4.2
Laryngo-tracheobronchitis: acute upper
    airway obstruction 4.1
Lead poisoning
  basal ganglia calcification 12.29
  generalized increased bone density 1.8
  intracranial calcification 12.27
  raised intracranial pressure 12.18
  solitary dense metaphyseal band 1.43
Left atrial appendage, enlarged 5.7
Left atrium
  enlarged 4.7, **5.5**
  myxoma 5.5, 5.16

Left heart failure: enlarged right ventricle
    5.4
Left-to-right shunt 5.17
  pulmonary arteries enlarged 5.15
  right ventricle enlarged 5.4
  small aortic arch 5.11
Left ventricle
  enlarged **5.6**
  hypoplastic, neonatal cyanosis 5.18
Left ventricular failure
  Kerley B lines 4.19
  left atrium enlarged 5.5
  pulmonary veins enlarged 5.16
Leg, length discrepancy 2.1
Legionnaire's disease: pneumatocoeles 4.9
Leiomyoma
  'bull's eye' lesions in stomach 6.22
  cystic 6.46
  dysphagia 6.10
  gastric 6.17
  gastrointestinal bleeding localization
    13.21
  oesophageal strictures 6.14
  oesophageal ulceration 6.13
  uterus enlargement 14.25
Leiomyosarcoma
  oesophageal strictures 6.15
  oesophageal ulceration 6.13
  retroperitoneal cystic mass 6.45
  small bowel strictures 6.29
Leontiasis ossea 434, 11.1, 12.7
  see also Fibrous dysplasia
Leprosy 455
  arthritis mutilans 3.7
  distal phalangeal destruction 1.54
  soft-tissue calcification 9.2
Leptomeningeal cyst 12.2
Leri–Weil disease (dyschondrosteosis):
    Madelung deformity 1.57
Letterer–Siwe disease **440**
Leukaemia
  acute myeloid, splenomegaly 7.18
  bilateral large smooth kidneys 8.10,
    8.12
  erosion of medial metaphysis 1.48
  exophthalmos, unilateral 11.1
  lucent bone lesions with calcium/bone
    1.25
  'moth-eaten' bone 1.25
  orbital masses, CT 11.2
  periosteal reaction 1.35
  photopenic area on bone scan 13.3
  skull vault 12.2
  solitary radiolucent metaphyseal band
    1.41
  splenomegaly 7.18
  sutures widened 12.20
  teeth, loss of lamina dura 11.16
  widespread air-space disease 4.15
Leydig cell tumours: gynaecomastia 9.1
Limestone workers: pulmonary opacities
    4.22

Linear pneumatosis intestinalis 6.1
Linitis plastica 6.17, **6.19**
Lipodystrophy: accelerated skeletal
    maturation 1.2
Lipoma
  breast 10.4, 10.7
  calcification 12.26
  cerebral, CT 12.33, 12.34
  of cord, spinal block 2.21
  of corpus callosum 12.30
  CT mediastinal mass containing fat
    4.52
  gastric 6.17
  parosteal 9.3
  spinal mass 2.23
Liposarcoma
  CT mediastinal mass containing fat
    4.52
  soft-tissue calcification 9.3
  soft-tissue ossification 9.6
Liquor volume **14.8**
Liver
  abscess 7.11, 7.13
    colloid liver scan 13.15
    right sided diaphragmatic humps 4.39
    unilateral elevated hemidiaphragm
      4.40
  adenoma 7.10
    colloid scans 13.15
    focal hyperdense CT lesion 7.14
    focal hypodense CT lesion 7.13
  amyloid infiltration 13.15
  bright **7.9**
  calcification **7.6**
    CT 7.14
    fetal/neonatal **7.7**
  CT, *see* Computerized tomography
  cyst 7.11, 7.13
    abdominal mass in neonate 6.5
    colloid liver scan 13.15
    fetal 14.12
    focal hypodense CT liver lesion 7.13
  disease: pulmonary oedema 4.17
  failure,
    osteomalacia/rickets 1.30
    pleural effusion 4.34
  fatty infiltration 13.15
    CT 7.13
    generalized low density CT 7.15
    hepatomegaly 7.5
    ultrasound 7.9, 7.10
  focal nodular hyperplasia,
    CT 7.13
    focal hyperdense CT lesion 7.14
    ultrasound 7.10
  granuloma 7.6
  haemorrhage 7.14
  herniated 4.51
  infarction 7.13
  ischaemic infarcts 7.7
  lymphoma 7.11, 7.17
  metastases 7.5

bone scans increased uptake 13.2
  calcification 7.6
  colloid liver scan 13.15
  focal hyperdense CT lesions 7.14
  focal hyperechoic ultrasound 7.10
  focal hypoechoic ultrasound 7.11
  right sided diaphragmatic humps 4.39
  necrosis: increased uptake on bone
    scans 13.2
  scans **13.15**
  tumours,
    calcification 7.6, 7.7
    colloid liver scan 13.15
    focal hyperdense CT lesions 7.14
    focal hypodense CT lesions 7.13
    generalized hypoechoic ultrasound 7.8
    generalized low density CT 7.15
  ultrasound, *see* Ultrasound, liver
Loa loa, soft-tissue calcification 9.2
Lobectomy
  unilateral hypertransradiant hemithorax
    4.5
  unilateral pulmonary oedema 4.18
Löffler's syndrome: widespread air-space
    disease 4.15
Long bones
  abnormal modelling 12.6
  overgrowth 12.6
Loose body, calcified **3.10**
Looser's zones 462
Lung
  abscess, *see* Pulmonary abscess
  agenesis 4.4
    increased density of hemithorax 4.8
    neonatal respiratory distress 4.46
  cavitation: infarction 4.27
  cavities **4.27**
  collapse 4.4
    bilateral elevated hemidiaphragms
      4.41
    increased density of hemithorax 4.8
    lobar pneumonia 4.12
    pneumonia + enlarged hilum 4.11
    unilateral elevated hemidiaphragm
      4.40
    ventilation perfusion mismatch 13.12
  consolidation 4.8
    + bulging of fissures **4.13**
    lobar pneumonia 4.12
    pneumonia + enlarged hilum 4.11
    right sided diaphragmatic humps 4.39
  contusion,
    localized air-space disease 4.16
    post-chest trauma 4.45
    unilateral pulmonary oedema 4.18
  cyst, traumatic 4.45
  cystic adenoma 14.9
  disease,
    diffuse: enlarged right ventricle 5.4
    drug-induced **4.48**
    gallium uptake 13.7
    restrictive: rib notching 1.52

Lung (*cont.*)
  fibrotic disease 4.41
  haematoma 4.25, 4.27, 4.45
  hamartoma 4.25
  hilar enlargement **4.30, 4.31**
    bilateral **4.31**
    drug-induced 4.48
    unilateral **4.30**
  honeycomb **4.20**, 4.37
  lobar enlargement 4.13
  overexpansion 4.6
  re-expansion: pulmonary oedema 4.17
  septal lines **4.19**
  sequestration,
    lung cavities 4.27
    solitary pulmonary nodule 4.25
  tear: pneumomediastinum 4.38
  tumours,
    pneumothorax 4.37
    see also Bronchial carcinoma;
      Pulmonary metastases
  unequal size/lucency/vascularity **4.4**
  upper zone fibrosis **4.33**
  see also entries beginning Pulmonary
Lye ingestion 6.10, 6.15
Lymphadenopathy
  in AIDS 413
    in children 415
  dysphagia 6.10
  hilar 4.11, 4.15
  intrathoracic 446
  mediastinal 4.15
  paratracheal 4.31
  vertebral bodies scalloping 2.17
Lymphangiectasia
  malabsorption 6.33
  protein-losing enteropathy 6.34
  pulmonary 14.9
  small bowel, thickened folds 6.30
Lymphangioma
  mediastinal cyst CT 4.53
  mesenteric cystic lesion, CT 6.46
  orbital masses, CT 11.2
  retroperitoneal cystic mass 6.45
Lymphangitis carcinomatosa
  bilateral hilar enlargement 4.31
  increased density of hemithorax 4.8
  Kerley B lines 4.19
Lymphatic insufficiency: periosteal
    reactions 1.33
Lymphatic obstruction
  ascites 6.4
  duodenal folds thickened 6.26
  protein-losing enteropathy 6.34
  small bowel, thickened folds 6.30
Lymph nodes
  enlargement: hilar enlargement 4.30,
    4.31
  hilar: egg-shell calcification 4.30, **4.32**
  intramammary 10.4, 10.5, 10.6, 10.8
  mediastinal,
    anterior mediastinal mass 4.49

  'eggshell' calcification 4 32
  middle mediastinal mass 4.50
Lymphocoele: retroperitoneal cystic mass
    6.45
Lymphogram: pulmonary opacities 4.22
Lymphogranuloma venereum: colonic
    strictures 6.37
Lymphoma 446–449
  adrenal mass, CT 7.23
  in AIDS 412, 413
  air-space disease,
    localized 4.16
    widespread 4.15
  ascites 6.4
  bone density increase 1.9
  bone scans 13.4
  bone sclerosis + periosteal reaction
    1.12
  brain 449
  'bull's eye' lesions in stomach 6.22
  central nervous system 449
  cobblestone duodenal cap 6.24
  colonic strictures 6.37
  colon and rectum in 448
  duodenal folds, thickened 6.26
  dysphagia 6.10
  'eggshell' calcification of lymph nodes
    446, 4.32
  exophthalmos, unilateral 11.1
  gallium uptake 13.7
  gastric 447, 6.17
  gastric folds, thick 6.18
  gastrointestinal tract 446–448
  hepatomegaly 7.5
  hilar enlargement,
    bilateral 4.31
    unilateral 4.30
  hypertrophic osteoarthropathy 1.34
  ileal lesions 6.35
  intrathoracic lymphadenopathy 446
  ivory vertebral body 2.10
  kidneys, bilateral large smooth 8.10,
    8.12
  linitis plastica 6.19
  liver,
    focal hypoechoic ultrasound 7.11
    low density 7.17
  lucent bone lesions with calcium/bone
    1.25
  lucent medullary lesions, ill-defined 1.21
  maxillary antrum, opaque 11.12
  metaphyseal band, solitary radiolucent
    1.41
  nasopharyngeal mass 11.17
  oesophageal strictures 6.15
  oesophageal ulceration 6.13
  opacity with air bronchogram 4.28
  optic nerve enlargement 11.3
  orbital masses, CT 11.2
  ovarian mass 14.27
  parathyroid imaging 13.10
  pleural effusion 4.36

prevertebral soft-tissue mass 11.18
protein-losing enteropathy 6.34
pulmonary, in AIDS 412
pulmonary disease 446
pulmonary opacities 4.23, 4.28
renal lesions, focal hypodense CT 8.13
retroperitoneal lymphadenopathy 448
rib lesion + soft-tissue mass 4.44
sclerotic bone lesions,
    multiple 1.11
    solitary 1.10
skeleton in 448
small bowel,
    dilatation 447, 6.28
    multiple nodules 6.32
    strictures 447, 6.29
    thickened folds 6.31
splenic imaging 13.17
splenomegaly 7.18
superior orbital fissure enlargement 11.8
surface enhancement of brain 12.31
sutures, widened 12.20
'thumbprinting' in colon 6.41
thymic mass 4.54
vertebra, solitary collapsed 2.2
Lymphosarcoma: opacity with air
    bronchogram 4.28

McCune–Albright syndrome 434
    accelerated skeletal maturation 1.2
McGregor's line 12.13
Macleod's syndrome
    unilateral hypertransradiant hemithorax
        4.5
    unilateral pulmonary oedema 4.18
Macrocysts, fetal 14.13
Macroglossia, dysphagia 6.11
Madelung deformity 1.57
Maffucci's syndrome 432
Malabsorption 6.33
Malaria
    hepatomegaly 7.5
    splenomegaly 7.18
Malformation syndromes: retarded
        skeletal maturation 1.1
Mallory-Weiss syndrome 6.12
    haematemesis 6.9
Malnutrition
    retarded skeletal maturation 1.1
    small heart 5.2
Mammography 10.1–10.13
    benign conditions mimicking
        malignancy 10.3
    benign lesions with typical appearances
        10.4
    benign vs. malignant 10.1, 10.2
    calcification 10.2
        disappearance 10.9
    'comet-tail' appearance 10.4
    large well-defined opacity 10.7
    microcalcification 10.2, 10.3

mixed density well-defined single
        opacity 10.8
    oedematous breast 10.10
    radiation risk 10.13
    soft-tissue opacity,
        multiple well-defined 10.6
        single well-defined 10.5
Mandible
    cystic adamantinoma 11.14
    cystic lesion 11.14
    metastases 11.14
Mannosidosis 1.7
Marble workers: pulmonary opacities 4.22
Marfan's syndrome 449
    aortic aneurysm 5.10
    arachnodactyly 1.53
    cardiovascular involvement 5.19
    protrusio acetabuli 3.13
    rib notching 1.52
    scoliosis 2.1
    vertebral body scalloping 2.16
Maroteaux–Lamy syndrome 1.7
Marshall syndrome: accelerated skeletal
        maturation 1.2
Mastectomy: unilateral hypertransradiant
        hemithorax 4.5
Mastocytosis
    bone density increase 1.9
    duodenal folds, thickened 6.26
    malabsorption 6.33
    osteoporosis 1.29
    small bowel,
        multiple nodules 6.32
        thickened folds 6.31
Mastoiditis 12.4
Maternal deprivation: retarded skeletal
        maturation 1.1
Maxillary antrum
    carcinoma 11.12, 11.13
    cysts 11.12, 11.13
    leontiasis ossea of 11.1
    mass 11.13
    opaque 11.12
    polyp 11.13
Measles: bronchiectasis 4.14
Meatal stenosis 8.30
Meckel's diverticulum 13.21, 13.22
    gastrointestinal bleeding 13.21, 13.22
Meconium aspiration syndrome 4.46
Meconium ileus 6.7
Meconium peritonitis 7.7
Meconium plug syndrome 6.7
Mediastinal abscess 4.53
Mediastinal cysts 4.53
Mediastinal displacement 4.8
Mediastinal emphysema, *see* Emphysema
Mediastinal fibrosis
    pulmonary veins enlargement 5.16
    superior vena cava, enlarged 5.13
Mediastinal haematoma 4.45
Mediastinal infusion 5.20
Mediastinal lipomatosis 4.52

Mediastinal lymphadenopathy, in AIDS, in
    children 415
Mediastinal lymph nodes, *see* Lymph
    nodes
Mediastinal mass
    anterior **4.49**
    CT, containing fat **4.52**
    middle **4.50**
    posterior **4.51**
    superior vena cava, enlarged 5.13
    unilateral hilar enlargement 4.30
Mediastinal shift 4.8
    neonatal respiratory distress 4.46
Mediastinal tumours
    anterior 4.32
    bronchial stenosis/occlusion 4.7
    dysphagia 6.10
    oesophageal strictures 6.14
    pulmonary oedema 4.17
Mediastinum, post-chest trauma 4.45
Medullary sponge kidney, *see* Kidney
Medulloblastoma 12.32
    CT 12.32, 12.33
    spinal metastases 2.23
Megacalyces 8.24
Megacolon
    adult **6.39**
    child **6.40**
    non-toxic **6.39**
    toxic **6.39**
        gas in wall of colon 6.38
        pneumoperitoneum 6.2
Megalencephaly 12.19
Meig's syndrome
    ascites 6.4
    pleural effusion 4.34, 4.35
Melanoma
    bone metastases 1.16
    'bull's eye' lesions in stomach 6.22
    oesophageal ulceration 6.13
    optic nerve enlargement 11.3
    splenic imaging 13.17
Melnick–Needles syndrome
    (osteodysplasty) 1.8, 12.6, 12.17
Melorheostosis: bone sclerosis +
    periosteal reaction 1.12
Mendelson's syndrome: pulmonary
    oedema 4.17
Ménétrier's disease 6.18
    protein-losing enteropathy 6.34
    stomach abnormality + thickened small
        bowel folds 6.31
Meningeal disease, disseminated 12.31
Meningeal neoplasms: surface
    enhancement of brain 12.31
Meningioma
    brain isotope angiogram 13.11
    CT 12.33, 12.34
    exophthalmos, unilateral 11.1
    expanded pituitary fossa 12.23
    intracranial calcification 12.26
    optic nerve enlargement 11.3

orbital, *see* Orbital meningioma
    parasellar calcification 12.28
    periosteal reactions 1.31
    petrous bone destruction 12.10
    sella erosion and osteoporosis 12.25
    skull base, increased density 12.9
    skull vault,
        'hair-on-end' 12.14
        increased density 12.8
    spinal mass 2.23
    superior orbital fissure enlargement
        11.8
Meningitis
    in AIDS 415
    tuberculous,
        calcification 12.26
        parasellar calcification 12.28
        surface enhancement of brain 12.31
Meningocoele
    anterior sacral 6.44
        scalloping 2.18
    anterior thoracic 4.51
    CT mediastinal cyst 4.53
    retroperitoneal cystic mass 6.45
    skull vault lucency + sclerosis 12.3
Menkes kinky hair syndrome 12.16
Menke's syndrome, non-accidental injury
    vs. 1.37
Mesenteric cyst 14.12
    abdominal mass in neonate 6.5
    CT **6.46**
Mesenteric infarction
    gas in bowel wall 6.1
    gasless abdomen 6.3
    gas in portal veins 7.4
Mesenteric lymphadenopathy, in AIDS 413
Mesoblastic nephroma 6.5
Mesodermal diseases: scoliosis 2.1
Mesomelic dysplasia 14.13
Mesothelial cyst 6.46
Mesothelioma 420
    cystic 6.46
    hypertrophic osteoarthropathy 1.34
    increased density of hemithorax 4.8
    local benign 4.43
    pleural effusion 4.36
    pleural masses, local 4.43
    rib lesion + soft-tissue mass 4.44
Metacarpal(s), short 1.55
Meta iodo benzyl guanidine (MIBG)
    13.18
Metaphyseal band
    alternating radiolucent/dense 1.42
    solitary dense **1.43**
    solitary radiolucent **1.41**
Metaphyseal chondrodysplasia 1.5
    cupping of metaphyses 1.46
    osteomalacia/rickets 1.30
Metaphyseal dysplasia, *see* Pyle's disease
Metaphyseal fractures 456
    solitary radiolucent metaphyseal band
        1.41

Metaphyseal lines, dense vertical **1.44**
Metaphyses
  cupping **1.46**
  fraying **1.45**
  medial of proximal humerus, erosion
    1.48
Metastases
  bone scans 13.4, 13.5
    increased uptake 13.1
  bone sclerosis with periosteal reaction
    1.12
  brain isotope angiogram 13.11
  parathyroid imaging 13.10
  sclerotic bone lesions 1.10, 1.11
  skeletal **1.16**
  whole body iodine scanning **13.8**
  see also individual anatomical regions,
    tumours
Metatarsal(s), short **1.55**
Metatropic dwarfism, *see* Dwarfism
Mica, pneumoconiosis 4.21
Microcephaly 12.15
Microglioma 449
  CT 12.33, 12.34
Micrognathia 4.46
  chronic upper airway obstruction 4.2
Mikity–Wilson syndrome (pulmonary
    dysmaturity) 4.46
  ring shadows 4.47
Milk–alkali syndrome
  renal calcification 8.2
  renal calculi 8.3
  soft-tissue calcification 9.5
Mitral valve
  calcification 5.9
  disease,
    gross cardiac enlargement 5.1
    right ventricle enlarged 5.4
  incompetence,
    left atrium enlarged 5.5
    left ventricle enlarged 5.6
  prolapse: myocardial perfusion imaging
    13.13
  stenosis,
    Kerley B lines 4.19
    left atrium enlarged 5.5
    pulmonary calcifications 4.29
    pulmonary veins enlarged 5.16
Moniliasis
  dysphagia 6.10
  oesophageal ulceration 6.13
Monoarthritis **3.1**
Monroe, foramen of, stenosis 12.19
Morgagni hernia
  anterior mediastinal mass 4.49
  CT mediastinal mass containing fat
    4.52
  right sided diaphragmatic humps 4.39
Morquio's syndrome **450**, 1.7
  atlanto-axial subluxation 2.11
  cardiovascular involvement 5.19
  irregular/stippled epiphyses 1.39

platyspondyly 2.4
vertebral body,
  beaks 2.15
  scalloping 2.16
'Moth-eaten bone' 1.25
Moulage sign 6.33
Mucocoele: unilateral exophthalmos 11.1
Mucocutaneous candidiasis 6.13
Mucolipidoses: dysostosis multiplex 1.7
Mucopolysaccharidoses
  dysostosis multiplex 1.7
  J-shaped sella 12.24
  osteoporosis 1.29
  see also individual diseases
Mucus plug, bronchial occlusion 4.7
Multicentric reticulohistiocytosis 1.54
Multicystic kidney, *see* Kidney
Multiple Endocrine Neoplasia (MEN)
    syndromes 441, **450–451**, 7.23
Multiple epiphyseal dysplasia 1.5, 1.39
Multiple myeloma **451–452**
  bone lesions,
    ill-defined lucent medullary 1.21
    lucent with calcium/bone 1.25
    lucent medullary 452, 1.20
    multiple sclerotic 1.11
    subarticular lucent 1.24
  bone scans 13.5
    photopenic area 13.3
  clavicle, erosion/absence of outer end
    1.49
  distal phalangeal destruction 1.54
  excessive callus formation 1.15
  'floating' teeth 11.15
  kidneys, bilateral large smooth 8.10
  nephrogram 8.18
  pedicle erosion/destruction/absence 2.5
  pulmonary calcifications 4.29
  rib lesion, focal 1.50
  rib lesion + soft-tissue mass 4.44
  sacral scalloping 2.18
  skull vault 12.1, 12.4
  solitary collapsed vertebra 2.2
  teeth, loss of lamina dura 11.16
Muscular dystrophy: scoliosis 2.1
Mushroom workers' lung 433, 4.21, 4.31
Myasthenia gravis
  dysphagia 6.10
  thymic tumours 4.45, 4.49
Mycobacterial infection, in AIDS 412
Mycobacterium tuberculosis: lung
  consolidation + bulging
  offissures 4.13
Mycoplasma infection
  pleural effusion 4.36
  pneumonia + enlarged hilum 4.11
  unilateral hilar enlargement 4.30
Myelocoele: antenatal diagnosis 14.13
Myelofibrosis
  bone scans 13.4
  hepatomegaly 7.5
  splenomegaly 7.18

Myeloma
    brain isotope angiogram 13.11
    peak age incidence 1.18
    site of origin 1.17
    see also Multiple myeloma
Myelomeningocoele 455, 12.18
    antenatal diagnosis 14.13
    distal phalangeal destruction 1.54
    scoliosis 2.1
    widened interpedicular distance 2.20
Myelosclerosis
    bone density increase 1.9
    skull vault density 12.7
Myocardial calcification 5.8
Myocardial infarction
    bone scans, increased uptake 13.2
    calcified 5.8
    gated blood pool imaging 13.14
    infection localization 13.6
    myocardial perfusion imaging 13.13
Myocardial ischaemia: enlarged left
        ventricle 5.6
Myocardial mass: bulge on left heart
        border 5.7
Myocardial perforation: subclavian vein
        catheterization 5.20
Myocardial perfusion imaging 13.13
Myocarditis
    calcification after 5.8
    gallium uptake 13.7
    infection localization 13.6
    left ventricle enlargement 5.6
    myocardial perfusion imaging 13.13
Myositis ossificans 9.6
    increased uptake on bone scans 13.2
    soft-tissue calcification 9.3
Myositis ossificans progressiva, congenital
        9.4, 9.6
Myxoedema: heel pad thickness increase
        9.7
Myxoma
    cardiac calcification 5.8
    left atrial 5.5, 5.16
    right atrial 5.3

Nasal angiofibroma: chronic upper airway
        obstruction 4.2
Naso-gastric aspiration: gasless abdomen
        6.3
Naso-gastric intubation
    dysphagia 6.10
    oesophageal strictures 6.14
Nasopharyngeal carcinoma 11.17
    hypertrophic osteoarthropathy 1.34
    petrous bone destruction 12.10
    pneumocephalus 12.21
Nasopharynx
    abscess 11.17
    mass in 11.17
    neoplasms 11.17
Near-drowning 4.17

Neck 11.1–11.18
Necrotizing enterocolitis
    gas in portal veins 7.4
    gas in stomach wall 6.23
    gas in wall of colon 6.38
    megacolon after 6.40
    pneumoperitoneum 6.2
Negative predictive value 15(404-5)
Nelson's syndrome 12.23
Neonatal abdominal mass 6.5
Neonatal cyanosis 5.18
Neonatal dysphagia 6.11
Neonatal dysplasia, lethal 1.6
Neonatal intestinal obstruction 6.7
Neonatal liver calcification 7.7
Neonatal pulmonary venous congestion
        5.17
Neonatal renal masses 8.16
Neonatal respiratory distress 4.46
Neonatal rickets 1.30
Neonatal stress 6.5
Nephrectomy 8.1
    partial 8.22
Nephritis
    acute focal bacterial 8.13
    acute interstitial 8.10
    radiation 8.7
Nephroblastomatosis 8.12, 8.16
Nephrocalcinosis 8.2
Nephrographic patterns 8.18
Nephroma
    mesoblastic 6.5, 8.12, 8.16
    multilocular cystic 8.12
Nephropathy
    analgesic 8.20
    reflux, *see* Reflux nephropathy
    urate 436, 8.10
Nephrosis, congenital: fetal hydrops 14.9
Nephrotic syndrome
    ascites 6.4
    duodenal folds thickened 6.26
    pleural effusion 4.34, 4.35
    renal vein thrombosis 8.21
Nerve injury: subclavian vein
        catheterization 5.20
Nerve root trauma 4.45
Neural tube defects: antenatal diagnosis
        14.13
Neuraminidase deficiency 1.7
Neurenteric cyst: posterior mediastinal
        masses 4.51
Neuroblastoma
    abdominal mass in neonate 6.5
    adrenal calcification 7.22
    adrenal masses, CT 7.23
    in children 6.6
    exophthalmos, unilateral 11.1
    metastases 1.48
        bone 1.16
        focal rib lesion 1.50
        'hair-on-end' skull vault 12.14
    MIBG imaging 13.18

orbital masses, CT 11.2
prevertebral soft-tissue mass 11.18
skull vault 12.2
sutures, widened 12.20
Neuroectodermal diseases: scoliosis 2.1
Neuro-enteric cyst 6.10
CT mediastinal cyst 4.53
Neurofibroma
'bull's' eye' lesions in stomach 6.22
CT mediastinal mass containing fat
4.52
enlarged optic foramen 11.7
gastric 6.17
interosseous 454
intraorbital calcification 11.9
rib lesion + soft-tissue mass 4.44
skull vault 12.1, 12.8
spinal mass 2.23
Neurofibromatosis 453–454
'bare' orbit 11.6
'bull's eye' lesions in stomach 6.22
exophthalmos, unilateral 11.1
honeycomb lung 4.20
J-shaped sella 12.24
large head 12.19
mediastinal cyst, CT 4.53
optic foramen, enlarged 11.7
orbit, enlarged 11.5
petrous bone destruction 12.10
posterior mediastinal masses 4.51
pseudoarthrosis 1.38
renal induced hypertension 8.20
rib notching 1.51, 1.52
ring shadows 4.47
scoliosis 2.1
soft-tissue calcification 9.2
superior orbital fissure enlargement 11.8
vertebral body scalloping 2.16
Neurogenic tumours: posterior mediastinal
mass 4.51
Neuromuscular disease
osteoporosis 1.29
vertebral bodies, beaks 2.15
Neuropathic arthropathy 455
arthritis + bone density preservation
3.4
arthritis mutilans 3.7
calcified loose body 2.22
excessive callus formation 1.15
Neuropathic disease: distal phalangeal
destruction 1.54
Neutropenia, drug-induced 4.48
Niemann–Pick disease
Erlenmeyer flask deformity 1.47
erosion of medial metaphysis 1.48
hepatomegaly 7.5
Nipples: increased uptake on bone scans
13.2
Nissen fundoplication 6.17
Nocardiosis
lung cavities 4.27
rib lesion + soft-tissue mass 4.44

Nodular lymphoid hyperplasia 6.24, 6.36
duodenal 6.24
liver, *see* Liver
multiple nodules in small bowel 6.32
Non-accidental injury 456–458
excessive callus formation 1.15
periosteal reaction 1.36
skeletal lesions vs. 1.37
solitary radiolucent metaphyseal band
1.41
Non-Hodgkin's lymphoma 446, 447
CT renal lesions 8.13
small bowel strictures 6.29
thick gastric folds 6.18
see also Lymphoma
Non-ossifying fibroma (fibrous cortical
defect) 458, 1.17
lucent medullary lesion + eccentric
expansion 1.22
osteomalacia/rickets 1.30
peak age incidence 1.18
site of origin 1.17
Noonan's syndrome: cardiovascular
involvement 5.19
Nuclear medicine 13.1–13.22

Oat cell carcinoma 7.23
Obesity
bilateral elevated hemidiaphragms 4.41
in children 1.2
CT mediastinal mass containing fat
4.52
generalized low density liver CT 7.15
heel pad thickness increase 9.7
Obstetric ultrasonography 14.1
Obstructive airways disease
right ventricle enlarged 5.4
ventilation perfusion mismatch 13.12
see also Upper airway obstruction
Occipital condyle syndrome: skull base
metastases 12.12
Occipital fracture, depressed 456
Occiput, anomalies 12.13
Ochronosis, *see* Alkaptonuria
Ocular tumours: optic nerve enlargement
11.3
Odontoid process, congenital absence/
hypoplasia 2.11
Oedema
acute upper airway obstruction 4.1
air-space disease 4.16
peripheral: heel pad thickness increase
9.7
widespread air-space disease 4.15
see also Pulmonary oedema
Oesophagitis 6.13
in AIDS, in children 415
reflux 6.13, 6.16
Oesophagoscopy, diverticula after 6.12
Oesophagus
atresia 4.2, 6.3

Oesophagus atresia (*cont.*)
 dysphagia 6.11
 carcinoma,
  chronic upper airway obstruction 4.3
  oesophageal ulceration 6.13
  strictures 6.14, 6.15
 caustic ingestion 6.13
 cyst, CT mediastinal cyst 4.53
 dilated 4.51
 diverticula **6.12**
 erosions 6.13
 fundoplication 6.15
 leiomyoma 6.10, 6.14, 6.13
 leiomyosarcoma 6.15, 6.13
 lymphoma 6.10, 6.15, 6.13
 monilial infection 6.10, 6.13
 perforation, pneumomediastinum 4.38
 reflux stricture, dysphagia 6.10
 rupture 4.45
  pleural effusion 4.36
 stasis 6.13
 strictures 6.10
  intramural diverticula 6.12
  irregular **6.15**
  peptic **6.14**
  smooth **6.14**
 tertiary contractions **6.16**
 tumours,
  dysphagia 6.10
  haematemesis 6.9
  tertiary contractions 6.16
 ulceration **6.13**
 varices,
  bleeding localization 13.21
  cobblestone duodenal cap 6.24
  haematemesis 6.9
  thick gastric folds 6.18
 vascular rings, dysphagia 6.11
Oligaemia
 congenital heart disease 4.6
 neonatal cyanosis 5.18
Oligodendroglioma: intracranial
  calcification 12.26
Oligohydramnios: abnormal liquor volume
  14.8
Oligosaccharidoses: dysostosis multiplex
  1.7
Ollier's disease 432
Omphalocoele 14.11
 antenatal diagnosis 14.13
 raised AFP 14.10
Oncocytoma: CT lesions 8.13
Ophthalmic artery aneurysm 11.7
Opportunistic infections
 in AIDS 412, 414, 415
 drug-induced 4.48
Optic chiasm glioma
 accelerated skeletal maturation 1.2
 J-shaped sella 12.24
 parasellar calcification 12.28
Optic enuritis 11.3
Optic foramen, enlarged **11.7**

Optic nerve enlargement **11.3**
Optic nerve glioma 11.3, **11.4**
 CT orbital mass 11.2
 enlarged optic foramen 11.7
 exophthalmos, unilateral 11.1
 oribal meningioma vs. **11.4**
Orbit
 'bare' 11.1, 11.5, **11.6**
 calcification **11.9**
 enlarged **11.5**
 hyperostosis **11.10**
Orbital blow-out fracture 11.13
Orbital haemangioma 11.8, 11.9
Orbital lesions, unilateral exophthalmos
  11.1
Orbital masses, in children, CT **11.2**
Orbital meningioma **11.4**
 'bare' orbit 11.6
 exophthalmos, unilateral 11.1
 hyperostosis 11.10
 intraorbital calcification 11.9
 optic foramen enlargement 11.7
 optic nerve glioma vs. **11.4**
 superior orbital fissure enlargement 11.8
Orbital metastases 11.1, 11.6, 11.7
 hyperostosis 11.10
Orbital pseudotumour 11.1, 11.2
 optic foramen enlarged 11.7
 optic nerve enlargement 11.3
Orbital syndrome: skull base metastases
  12.12
Osler-Weber-Rendu syndrome (hereditary
  telangiectasia) 6.9
Ossification
 cranial 12.13
 defective,
  skull vault **12.17**
  wide sutures 12.20
 paravertebral 2.13
 pulmonary **4.29**
 soft-tissue **9.4**, 9.6
Osteitis condensans ilii 3.12
Osteitis pubis
 fusion/bridging symphysis pubis 3.15
 widening of symphysis pubis 3.14
Osteoarthritis
 arthritis + bone density preservation
  3.4
 distal phalangeal destruction 1.54
 fusion/bridging symphysis pubis 3.15
 monoarthritis 3.1
 protrusio acetabuli 3.13
 sacroiliitis, bilateral asymmetrical 3.12
 subarticular lucent bone lesions 1.24
Osteoblastic metastases
 bone density increase 1.9
 vertebral pedicle, dense 2.6
 see also Bone metastases
Osteoblastoma 459
 bone sclerosis + periosteal reaction
  1.12
 extradural spinal mass 2.22

lucent bone lesions with calcium/bone
1.25
osteomalacia/rickets 1.30
peak age incidence 459, 1.18
scoliosis 2.1
site of origin 1.17
solitary bone lesions + lucent centre
1.13
solitary sclerotic bone lesion 1.10
vertebral pedicle, dense 2.6
Osteochondral fracture: calcified loose
body 2.22
Osteochondritides: avascular necrosis 1.40
Osteochondritis dissecans: calcified loose
body 2.22
Osteochondroma **459**
focal rib lesion 1.50
peak age incidence 459, 1.18
site of origin 1.17
Osteochondromatosis, synovial 9.5
Osteodysplasty (Melnick–Needles
syndrome) 12.6, 12.17
bone density increase 1.8
Osteodystrophy: bone scans 13.4
Osteodystrophy, renal, *see* Renal
osteodystrophy
Osteogenesis imperfecta **460–461**, 1.6
antenatal diagnosis 14.13
basilar invagination 12.13
cardiovascular involvement 5.19
excessive callus formation 1.15
neonatal respiratory distress 4.46
non-accidental injury vs. 1.37
osteoporosis 1.29
platyspondyly 2.4
pseudoarthrosis 1.38
rib notching 1.52
skull vault, defective ossification 12.17
types 460
Osteogenesis imperfecta tarda: vertebral
body scalloping 2.16
Osteogenic sarcoma **461**
bone sclerosis + periosteal reaction
1.12
ill-defined lucent medullary lesions 1.21
lucent bone lesions with calcium/bone
1.25
peak age incidence 461, 1.18
periosteal reactions 1.31
site of origin 1.17
Osteoid neoplasms: lucent bone lesions
with calcium/bone 1.25
Osteoid osteoma **462**
bone sclerosis + periosteal reaction
1.12
distal phalangeal destruction 1.54
lucent bone lesions with calcium/bone
1.25
peak age incidence 462, 1.18
scoliosis 2.1
site of origin 1.17
solitary bone lesions with lucent centre

1.13
vertebral pedicle, dense 2.6
Osteolysis, post-traumatic 1.49
Osteolytic metastases 3.14
Osteoma
of calvarium 12.26
exophthalmos, unilateral 11.1
ivory 12.8
peak age incidence 1.18
pneumocephalus 12.21
sclerotic bone lesions,
multiple 1.11
solitary 1.10
skull vault 12.8
Osteomalacia **462**, **1.30**
basilar invagination 12.13
coarse trabecular pattern 1.14
osteopenia 1.28
periosteal reaction 1.36
protrusio acetabuli 3.13
sella erosion and osteoporosis 12.25
teeth, loss of lamina dura 11.16
Osteomyelitis
bone scans 13.4
bone sclerosis + periosteal reaction
1.12
distal phalangeal destruction 1.54
extradural spinal mass 2.22
lucent bone lesions with calcium/bone
1.25
lucent medullary lesions, ill-defined 1.21
non-accidental injury vs. 1.37
orbital hyperostosis 11.10
periosteal reaction 1.36
rib lesion, focal 1.50
skull vault lucent lesions 12.4
+ sclerosis 12.3
symphysis pubis widening 3.14
tuberculous 12.1
Osteonecrosis **480**
subarticular lucent bone lesions 1.24
Osteopathia striata (Voorhoeve's disease)
1.11
dense vertical metaphyseal lines 1.44
Osteopenia **452**
asymmetrical maturation of bone 1.4
generalized **1.28**
regional **1.27**
Osteopetrosis **463–464**
antenatal diagnosis 14.13
Erlenmeyer flask deformity 1.47
generalized bone density increase 1.8
metaphyseal bands,
radiolucent/dense 1.42
solitary dense 1.43
orbital hyperostosis 11.10
skull density increase 12.6
skull vault density increase 12.7
Osteophyte 2.22
detached 3.10
Osteopoikilosis: multiple sclerotic bone
lesions 1.11

Osteoporosis 1.28, **1.29**
    arthritis with **3.3**
    bone scans 13.5
    coarse trabecular pattern 1.14
    disuse induced 1.29
    iatrogenic 1.29
    periosteal reaction 1.36
    protrusio acetabuli 3.13
    regional migratory 1.27
    sella **12.25**
    sella erosion and osteoporosis 12.25
    teeth, loss of lamina dura 11.16
    transient, of hip 1.27
    vertebral collapse 2.2, 2.3
Osteoporosis circumscripta 464
    lucent bone lesions 1.25
    skull vault 12.1
Osteosarcoma
    calcified pulmonary metastasis 4.29
    'hair-on-end' skull vault 12.14
    parosteal 9.3, 9.6
Osteosclerosis 12.7
Otitis media, chronic 12.11
    in AIDS 415
    skull base density increase 12.9
Ovarian hypogonadism 1.29
Ovary
    abscess 14.27
    adenocarcinoma 14.27
    cyst 14.12
        abdominal mass in a child 6.6
        abdominal mass in neonate 6.5
    cystic teratoma 14.27
    fibroma 6.4, 14.27
    masses **14.27**
    metastases 14.27
    normal ultrasound **14.26**
    polycystic 14.24, 14.27
    simple cystic structures 14.26, 14.27
    teratoma 14.27
        in child 6.6
    tumours,
        ascites 6.4
        bone metastases 1.16
Overhydration: neonatal pulmonary
        venous congestion 5.17
Ovulation 14.26
Ovum, blighted (anembryonic pregnancy)
        14.4, **14.5**
Oxycephaly 12.15

Pachydermoperiostosis 12.16
    periosteal reactions 1.33
Paget's disease **464–465**
    active (osteolytic) 464
    basilar invagination 12.13
    bone density increase 1.9
    bone scans 13.4
        increased uptake 13.1
    brain isotope angiogram 13.11
    coarse trabecular pattern 1.14

    complications 465
    inactive (osteosclerotic) 464
    left ventricle enlarged 5.6
    orbital hyperostosis 11.10
    protrusio acetabuli 3.13
    pulmonary arteries, enlarged 5.15
    rib lesion, focal 1.50
    sclerotic bone lesions,
        multiple 1.11
        solitary 1.10
    sinuses small/absent 11.11
    skull base, density increase 12.9
    skull vault, density increase 12.7, 12.8
    spinal mass, extradural 2.22
    teeth, loss of lamina dura 11.16
    vertebral body,
        enlargement 2.7
        ivory 2.10
        squaring 2.8
Pain, congenital insensitivity 455, 1.37,
        1.54
Pancreas
    abscess, CT 7.21
    adenocarcinoma, CT 7.21
    annular,
        dilated duodenum 6.27
        gasless abdomen 6.3
        intestinal obstruction in neonate 6.7
    calcification **7.20**
    carcinoma 6.45
        calcification 7.20
        gastrocolic fistula 6.20
        linitis plastica 6.19
        malabsorption 6.33
    cyst, fetal 14.12
    cystadenoma 6.45, 7.20
    dysfunction: malabsorption 6.33
    mass 7.23
        CT **7.21**
    metastases, CT 7.21
    pseudocyst 6.45, 6.46
        calcification 7.20
        CT mediastinal cyst 4.53
        gastric indentation 6.17
    'rest' 6.17
    'bull's eye' lesions in stomach 6.22
    tumour: gastric indentation 6.17
Pancreatectomy: malabsorption 6.33
Pancreatitis
    alcoholic 7.20
    avascular necrosis 1.40
    biliary: non visualization of gallbladder
        13.16
    duodenal folds thickened 6.26
    focal: CT 7.21
    gasless abdomen 6.3
    gastric folds thickened 6.18
    gastrocolic fistula 6.20
    hereditary, calcification 7.20
    infection localization 13.6
    malabsorption 6.33
    pleural effusion 4.34, 4.35

retroperitoneal fibrosis 8.26
splenic imaging 13.17
unilateral elevated hemidiaphragm 4.40
Panhypopituitarism: retarded skeletal
 maturation 1.1
Papilloma
 breast 10.5, 10.6
 cerebral, CT 12.34
 choroid plexus 12.26, 12.32, 12.33
 CT 12.33
Paraaortic cystic nodes 6.45
Paraduodenal hernia 6.8
Paragonimiasis: intracranial calcification
 12.27
Paralysis
 asymmetrical maturation of bone 1.4
 excessive callus formation 1.15
Paralytic ileus 6.21
 duodenum dilated 6.27
 intestinal obstruction in neonate 6.7
 megacolon 6.39, 6.40
 small bowel dilatation 6.28
Paranasal sinus, carcinoma 11.1
Paraoesophageal cyst: middle mediastinal
 mass 4.50
Paraplegia
 non-accidental injury vs. 1.37
 sacroiliitis, bilateral symmetrical 3.12
 soft-tissue ossification 9.6
Paraquat poisoning 4.17
Parasellar calcification 12.28
Parasellar chordoma 11.8, 12.28
Parasellar mass 12.23, 12.25
Parasellar metastases 12.25
Parasellar and middle fossa syndrome:
 skull base metastases 12.12
Parathyroid adenoma, imaging 13.10
Parathyroid carcinoma 13.10
Parathyroid hyperplasia 13.10
Parathyroid imaging 13.10
Paratracheal cyst 4.53
 middle mediastinal mass 4.50
Paravertebral abscess 4.51
Paravertebral masses 4.51
Paravertebral ossification 2.13
Park's lines 1.42
Parosteal lipoma 9.3
Parosteal osteosarcoma 9.3, 9.6
 peak age incidence 1.18
Patent ductus arteriosus (PDA) 5.17
 large aortic arch 5.10
 left atrium enlarged 5.5
 left ventricle enlarged 5.6
Pelkan spurs 479
Pellegrini–Stieda syndrome: soft-tissue
 calcification 9.2
Pelvicalyceal system, gas in 8.4
Pelvic lipomatosis 6.44, 8.26
Pelvic tumours
 benign: pleural effusion 4.35
 rectosigmoid junction indentation 6.43
 sacral scalloping 2.18

Pelviureteric junction obstruction 8.17
 abdominal mass in neonate 6.5
Pemphigus
 dysphagia 6.10
 oesophageal strictures 6.14
'Pepper pot skull' 12.1
Peptic ulcer
 gas in stomach wall 6.23
 gastritis 6.18
 gastrocolic fistula 6.20
 haematemesis 6.9
 pharyngeal/oesophageal diverticula 6.12
 pneumoperitoneum 6.2
Periarthritis, calcific 9.5
Periarticular soft-tissue calcification 9.5
Pericardial calcification 5.8
Pericardial cyst
 anterior mediastinal mass 4.49
 bulge on left heart border 5.7
 CT mediastinal cyst 4.53
 diaphragmatic hump 4.39
Pericardial effusion
 azygos vein enlarged 5.14
 in fetus 14.9
 gross cardiac enlargement 5.1
Pericardial fat pad 4.39
 anterior mediastinal mass 4.49
Pericardial sac defect 5.7
Pericarditis, constrictive
 ascites 6.4
 azygos vein enlarged 5.14
 duodenal folds, thickened 6.26
 gallium uptake 13.7
 hepatomegaly 7.5
 protein-losing enteropathy 6.34
 pulmonary vein enlargement 5.16
 small heart 5.2
 superior vena cava enlargement 5.13
Pericolic abscess: colonic strictures 6.37
Perihilar pneumonia 4.30
Perinephric abscess: loss of renal outline
 8.1
Perinephric cyst 8.14
Perinephric fat 8.1
Perinephric haematoma: loss of renal
 outline 8.1
Periodontal cyst 11.14
Periodontal disease: 'floating' teeth 11.15
Periosteal reactions 1.31
 arthritis with 3.5
 bilaterally asymmetrical 1.36
 bilaterally symmetrical,
  in adults 1.33
  in children 1.35
 bone sclerosis with 1.12
 Codman triangle (single lamina/
  lamellated) 1.31
 continuous with destroyed cortex 1.31
 divergent spiculated ('sunray') 1.31
 parallel spiculated ('hair-on-end') 1.31
 solitary/localized 1.32
 types 1.31

Peritoneal dialysis: pneumoperitoneum 6.2
Peritoneal metastases
 ascites 6.4
 rectosigmoid junction indentation 6.43
Peritonitis
 ascites 6.4
 plastic 7.7
Pertechnetate 13.22
 free 13.2
Perthes' disease 1.39
 avascular necrosis 1.40
Pertussis
 bronchiectasis 4.14
 unilateral hilar enlargement 4.30
Petrositis, apical 12.10
Petrous bone, *see* Temporal bone, petrous part
Peutz-Jeghers' syndrome 6.17
 colonic polyps 6.36
 small bowel nodules 6.32
Peyer's patches, hypertrophy 6.32
Pfeiffer's syndrome 12.15
Phaeochromocytoma 7.23
 adrenal calcification 7.22
 bone metastases 1.16
 gallium uptake 13.7
 MIBG imaging 13.18
Phalangeal destruction, distal **1.54**
Phalangeal sclerosis, diffuse terminal **3.8**
Pharyngeal diverticula **6.12**
Pharyngeal pouch 11.18
 dysphagia 6.10
 pneumonia, slowly resolving/recurrent 4.10
Pharyngocoele, lateral 6.12
Phenobarbitone: osteomalacia/rickets 1.30
Phenylbutazone: avascular necrosis 1.40
Phenytoin
 distal phalangeal destruction 1.54
 osteomalacia/rickets 1.30
 skull vault density increase 12.7
Phimosis 8.30
Phleboliths 7.6, 7.19, 9.3
 intraorbital calcification 11.9
Phrenic nerve palsy: unilateral elevated hemidiaphragm 4.40
Pierre Robin syndrome
 chronic upper airway obstruction 4.2
 dysphagia 6.11
Pigeon breeders' lung 4.21
Pigmented villonodular synovitis
 arthritis + bone density preservation 3.4
 arthritis + preserved/widened joint space 3.6
 monoarthritis 3.1
 subarticular lucent bone lesions 1.24
Pineal displacement 12.18
Pinealoma
 calcification 12.26
 CT 12.33, 12.34
 spinal metastases 2.23

Pituitary adenoma 12.23
 CT 12.33, 12.34
 intracranial calcification 12.26
 parasellar calcification 12.28
 sella erosion and osteoporosis 12.25
Pituitary fossa
 expanded **12.23**
 small **12.22**
Pituitary tumours 12.23
Placenta
 abnormal/cystic 14.11
 abnormalities **14.18**
 development **14.15**
 grading **14.16**
 thickened **14.20**
 thin **14.21**
 in twin pregnancies **14.17**
Placental abruption 14.19
Placental haemorrhage **14.19**
Placental insufficiency: fetal growth retardation 14.14
Placental maturation impairment: fetal growth retardation 14.14
Placenta praevia 14.18
 classification and associations 14.18
Plagiocephaly 12.15
Plague pneumonia 4.13
Plasmacytoma **451**
 'hair-on-end' skull vault 12.14
 lucent bone lesions 1.23
 nasopharyngeal mass 11.17
 rib lesion, focal 1.50
 solitary collapsed vertebra 2.2
Platybasia 12.13
Platyspondyly, in childhood **2.4**
Pleonaemia 5.18
Pleural calcification **4.42**
Pleural disease
 hemidiaphragm, unilateral elevated 4.40
 pulmonary oedema, unilateral 4.18
Pleural effusion **4.34**
 aortic aneurysm 5.10
 extrathoracic disease causing **4.35**
 in fetus 14.9
 fibrin balls 4.43
 hemithorax, increased density 4.8
 local pleural masses 4.43
 malignant, bone scans 13.2
 neonatal respiratory distress 4.46
 normal chest X-ray **4.36**
 right sided diaphragmatic humps 4.39
 ventilation perfusion mismatch 13.12
Pleural fibroma 4.43
 hypertrophic osteoarthropathy 1.34
Pleural masses **4.43**
Pleural metastases 4.43
Pleurisy: unilateral elevated hemidiaphragm 4.40
Pleuro-pericardial cyst 4.39, 4.49
Pleuroperitoneal canal, persistence 4.51
Pleuroperitoneal fistula 6.2
Plombage 4.43

Plummer–Vinson syndrome: oesophageal strictures 6.15
Plummer–Vinson web, dysphagia 6.10
Pneumatocoeles **4.9**
   ring shadows 4.47
Pneumatosis, cystic 6.23
Pneumatosis coli 6.1, 6.41
   gas in wall of colon 6.38
   pneumoperitoneum 6.2
Pneumatosis intestinalis, linear 6.1
Pneumocephalus **12.21**
Pneumoconioses **4.21**
   'eggshell' calcification of lymph nodes 4.32
   honeycomb lung 4.20
   Kerley B lines 4.19
   pulmonary opacities 4.23
Pneumocystis carinii
   in AIDS 412
      in children 414
   widespread air-space disease 4.15
Pneumomediastinum **4.38**, 6.2
   bronchial/tracheal injury 4.45
Pneumonia
   in AIDS 412, 414
   aspiration, *see* Aspiration pneumonia
   enlarged hilum **4.11**
   Friedländer's 4.13
   hemithorax increased density 4.8
   lobar **4.12**
   localized air-space disease 4.16
   multifocal, pulmonary opacities 4.23
   neonatal respiratory distress 4.46
   opacity with air bronchogram 4.28
   perihilar 4.30
   plague 4.13
   pneumothorax 4.37
   primary **4.11**
   pulmonary nodule, solitary 4.25
   resolving by fibrosis 4.10
   secondary 4.11
   slowly resolving/recurrent **4.10**
   staphylococcal 4.13
   ventilation perfusion mismatch 13.12
   viral 4.11, 4.15
   widespread air-space disease 4.15
Pneumonitis
   aspiration 4.45
   chemical 4.21
   diffuse, drug-induced 4.48
   drug-induced 4.48
   radiation 4.8, 4.28
Pneumoperitoneum 4.37, 6.1, **6.2**
   bilateral elevated hemidiaphragms 4.41
Pneumothorax **4.37**
   pneumoperitoneum 6.2
   post-chest trauma 4.45
   rib fracture 4.45
   spontaneous 4.37
   subclavian vein catheterization 5.20
   unilateral hypertransradiant hemithorax 4.5

Poisoning
   bone density increase 1.8, 1.9
   pulmonary oedema 4.17
   solitary dense metaphyseal band 1.43
Poland's syndrome: unilateral hypertransradiant hemithorax

Poliomyelitis
   rib notching 1.52
   scoliosis 2.1
   unilateral hypertransradiant hemithorax 4.5
Polyarteritis nodosa
   aphthous ulcers 6.42
   bilateral large smooth kidneys 8.10
   pulmonary arteries enlarged 5.1
   renal induced hypertension 8.20 **sp 8.20
   right ventricle enlarged 5.4
   ventilation perfusion mismatch 13.12
Polyarthritides **3.2**
Polycalycosis 8.24
Polycystic disease 8.14
   adult **467**, 8.14
      hypertension 8.20
      unilateral large smooth kidney 8.9
   autosomal dominant, antenatal diagnosis 14.13
   autosomal recessive, antenatal diagnosis 14.13
   bilateral large smooth kidneys 8.10
   of childhood **466**, 8.14, 8.18
   CT 8.15
   hepatomegaly 7.5
   infantile **466**, 8.14, 8.18
      renal mass 8.16
   neonatal respiratory distress 4.46
   nephrography 8.18
   of newborn **466**, 8.14, 8.18
      abdominal mass 6.5
      renal mass 8.16
Polycystic ovary syndrome 14.24, 14.27
Polycythaemia: craniostenosis 12.15
Polycythaemia rubra vera
   avascular necrosis 1.40
   hepatomegaly 7.5
   splenic imaging 13.17
Polydactyly: short rib 14.13
Polyhydramnios 14.8
Polyposis
   juvenile 1.34
   small bowel nodules 6.32
Polyposis coli, familial 6.17, 6.36
Polyps
   adenomatous 6.17
      gastric carcinoma 6.17
   antro-choanal 4.2, 11.17
   colonic **6.36**
   gastric 6.17
   hamartomatous 6.17
   hyperplastic 6.17
Polyvinyl chloride tank cleaners 1.54

Porencephalic cyst 12.33
  CT 12.34
Porphyria: distal phalangeal destruction
  1.54
Portal hypertension
  enlarged azygos vein 5.14
  splenomegaly 7.18
Portal vein
  gas in 6.1, **7.4**
  preduodenal: intestinal obstruction 6.7
  thromboemboli 7.7
  thrombosis, low density CT liver 7.17
Positive predictive value **15**(404)
Post-cricoid carcinoma 11.18
Posterior cranial fossa
  elevation of floor 12.13
  neoplasms **12.32**
Post-pericarditis: calcification 5.8
Post-pneumonectomy: increased density of
  hemithorax 4.8
Post-radiation myelopathy: spinal mass
  2.24
Post-traumatic osteolysis: clavicle outer
  end, erosion/absence 1.49
Potassium tablets, enteric coated 6.29
Pott's procedure 4.18
Pouch of Douglas, fluid in 14.6
Preduodenal portal vein: intestinal
  obstruction 6.7
Pregnancy
  anembryonic (blighted ovum) 14.4, **14.5**
  avascular necrosis 1.40
  azygos vein enlarged 5.14
  bilateral elevated hemidiaphragms 4.41
  ectopic, *see* Ectopic pregnancy
  endometrial thickening, *see* Endometrial
    thickening
  first trimester, indications for
    ultrasound **14.3**
  generalized low density liver CT 7.15
  intrauterine, absent + positive
    pregnancy test **14.7**
  liquor volume **14.8**
  molar 14.22
  normal, ultrasound features **14.2**
  symphysis pubis widening 3.14
  test, positive + absent intrauterine
    pregnancy **14.7**
  twin, *see* Twin pregnancies
Premature rupture of membranes 14.8
Prenatal infections: irregular/stippled
  epiphyses 1.39
Presbyoesophagus 6.16
Prevertebral abscess: dysphagia 6.10
Prevertebral haematoma 6.10
Prevertebral soft-tissue mass, cervical
  region **11.18**
Primitive neuroectodermal tumours
  (PNET): spinal metastases 2.23
Progeria
  osteoporosis 1.29
  rib notching 1.52

Progressive massive fibrosis (PMF) 424,
  481–482, 4.26
  lung cavities 4.27
  opacity with air bronchogram 4.28
  pulmonary upper zone fibrosis 4.33
Progressive systemic sclerosis, *see*
  Scleroderma
Prolactinoma 12.23
  CT 12.33, 12.34
Proptosis 11.1, 11.3
Prostaglandin EU1u therapy 1.37
Prostate carcinoma: dilated ureter 8.25
Prostate tumour metastases 1.50
  bone 1.16
  skull base 12.12
  spinal 2.2
Prostheses, infected 13.6
Protein deficiency: osteoporosis 1.29
Protein-losing enteropathy **6.34**
  duodenal folds thickened 6.26
  small bowel thickened folds 6.30
Protrusio acetabuli **3.13**
'Prune-belly' syndrome 8.30
  abdominal mass in neonate 6.5
Pseudoachondroplasia
  cupping of metaphyses 1.46
  dwarfing skeletal dysplasia 1.5
  vertebral bodies, beaks 2.15
Pseudoarthrosis **1.38**
Pseudobulbar palsy: dysphagia 6.10
Pseudogout 421
Pseudohypoparathyroidism **467**
  accelerated skeletal maturation 1.2
  basal ganglia calcification 12.29
  intracranial calcification 12.27
  narrow spinal canal 2.19
  osteoporosis 1.29
  short metacarpals 1.55
Pseudolymphoma: thick gastric folds 6.18
Pseudomembranous colitis
  'thumbprinting' in colon 6.41
  toxic megacolon 6.39
Pseudo-obstruction, of intestine 6.39
Pseudopolydystrophy of Maroteaux 1.7
Pseudopseudohypoparathyroidism **467**
  basal ganglia calcification 12.29
  intracranial calcification 12.27
  narrow spinal canal 2.19
  osteoporosis 1.29
  short metacarpals 1.55
Pseudoxanthoma elasticum: haematemesis
  6.9
Psoriatic arthropathy **468**
  arthritis + bone density preservation
    3.4
  arthritis + periosteal reaction 3.5
  arthritis + preserved/widened joint
    space 3.6
  arthritis mutilans 3.7
  atlanto-axial subluxation 2.11
  distal phalangeal destruction 1.54
  femoral intercondylar notch erosion 3.9

paravertebral ossification 2.13
periosteal reaction 1.36
sacroiliitis 3.12
vertebral body squaring 2.8
Pulmonary, for additional entries, *see*
   Lung
Pulmonary abscess 4.27
   consolidation + bulging of fissures 4.13
   hypertrophic osteoarthropathy 1.34
   pneumonia, slowly resolving/recurrent
      4.10
   pulmonary nodules, multiple 4.26
Pulmonary adenoma: pulmonary nodules,
   solitary 4.25
Pulmonary agenesis, *see* Lung
Pulmonary arterial hypertension
   bilateral hypertransradiant hemithoraces
      4.6
   hilar enlargement 4.30
      bilateral 4.31
   idiopathic 5.1
   right ventricle enlargement 5.4
   valve calcification 5.9
Pulmonary arteriovenous malformation
   pulmonary nodule 4.25, 4.26
   rib notching 1.51
Pulmonary artery
   aberrant left 6.10, 6.11
   aneurysm 4.30
   calcification 4.32
   congenital absence/hypoplasia 4.18
   enlarged 5.15
   left, anomalous origin 4.7
   post-stenotic dilatation 4.30
   stenosis, bilateral hypertransradiant
      hemithoraces 4.6
   systemic artery shunts 4.18
   unilateral hilar enlargement 4.30
Pulmonary atresia
   neonatal cyanosis 5.18
   right-sided aortic arch 5.12
   + ventricular septal defect 5.18
Pulmonary bullae 4.5
Pulmonary calcification/ossification 4.29
Pulmonary capillary wall permeability
      4.17, 4.48
Pulmonary dysmaturity, *see*
      Mikity–Wilson syndrome
Pulmonary embolic disease 469–470
   see also Pulmonary embolism;
      Pulmonary infarction
Pulmonary embolism
   acute minor 469–470
   acute/subacute massive 469
   chronic 470
   drug-induced 4.48
   hemithorax,
      bilateral hypertransradiant 4.6
      unilateral hypertransradiant 4.5
   hilar enlargement, unilateral 4.30
   pleural effusion 4.36
   right ventricle enlarged 5.4

ventilation perfusion mismatch 13.12
Pulmonary eosinophila, drug-induced
   4.48
Pulmonary fibrosis
   drug-induced 4.48
   pneumoconioses 4.21
   right ventricle enlarged 5.4
   upper zone 4.33
Pulmonary haematoma
   chest trauma 4.45
   lung cavities 4.27
   solitary pulmonary nodule 4.25
Pulmonary haemorrhage
   drug-induced 4.48
   neonatal respiratory distress 4.46
   pulmonary opacities 4.23
   widespread air-space disease 4.15
Pulmonary hypoplasia: increased density
   of hemithorax 4.8
Pulmonary infarction 469
   localized air-space disease 4.16
   lung cavities 4.27
   pleural effusion 4.34
   pulmonary nodule, solitary 4.25
   unilateral elevated hemidiaphragm 4.40
   see also Pulmonary embolic disease
Pulmonary lymphangiectasia: fetal
   hydrops 14.9
Pulmonary lymphoid hyperplasia: in AIDS
   in children 414
Pulmonary metastases
   bone 1.16
   calcified 4.29
   hypertrophic osteoarthropathy 1.34
   lung cavities 4.27
   pleural effusion 4.36
   pulmonary nodules,
      multiple 4.26
      solitary 4.25
   rib lesion + soft-tissue mass 4.44
   solitary calcifying/ossifying 4.29
Pulmonary nodule
   multiple 4.26
   solitary 4.25
      calcification within 4.29
Pulmonary oedema 4.17
   drug-induced 4.48
   increased density of hemithorax 4.8
   localized air-space disease 4.16
   post-chest trauma 4.45
   pulmonary opacities 4.23
   unilateral 4.18
   widespread air-space disease 4.15
Pulmonary oligaemia: rib notching 1.51
Pulmonary opacities
   air bronchogram 4.28
   multiple 4.23, 4.24
   multiple pin-point 4.22
Pulmonary ossification 4.29
Pulmonary ostodystrophy: bone scans
   13.4
Pulmonary sequestration 4.25, 4.27

Pulmonary stenosis 5.9
  neonatal cyanosis 5.18
  right ventricle enlargement 5.4
Pulmonary valve
  calcification 5.9
  stenosis 5.9
Pulmonary vascular resistance 5.17
Pulmonary veins, enlarged **5.16**
Pulmonary venous congestion, neonatal
  5.17
Pulmonary venous hypertension
  interstitial ossification 4.29
  Kerley B lines 4.19
  pulmonary arteries enlarged 5.15
  pulmonary calcifications, multiple 4.29
Purgative abuse 6.39
Pus, localization 13.6
Pycnodysostosis
  bone density increase 1.8
  clavicle, erosion/absence of outer end
    1.49
  increased skull density 12.6
  skull vault,
    defective ossification 12.17
    increased density 12.7
Pyelonephritis 8.5
  acute 8.9
    nephrogram 8.18
  chronic, hypertension 8.20
  xanthogranulomatous, *see*
    Xanthogranulomatous
    pyelonephritis
Pyeloureteritis cystica 8.24
Pyle's disease (metaphyseal dysplasia) 1.8,
    12.6
  skull vault increased density 12.7
Pyloric stenosis
  hypertrophic, gasless abdomen 6.3
  infantile hypertrophic: gastric dilatation
    6.21
Pyocele: opaque maxillary antrum 11.12
Pyogenic abscess
  cerebral, CT 12.34
  focal hypodense CT liver lesion 7.13
Pyogenic arthritis, *see* Arthritis, pyogenic
Pyogenic spondylitis: vertebral collapse
    2.3
Pyonephrosis 8.5, 8.9
Pyrophosphate arthropathy 421
Pyruvate kinase deficiency: 'hair-on-end'
    skull vault 12.14

Radiation
  ascites 6.4
  solitary dense metaphyseal band 1.43
Radiation enteritis 6.30
  ileal lesions 6.35
  small bowel strictures 6.29
Radiation nephritis: unilateral small
    smooth kidney 8.7

Radiation osteitis: rib lesion + soft-tissue
    mass 4.44
Radiation pneumonitis
  increased density of hemithorax 4.8
  opacity with air bronchogram 4.28
Radiotherapy, conditions due to
  avascular necrosis 1.40
  bladder fistula 8.29
  bone scans, photopenic area 13.3
  colonic strictures 6.37
  duodenal folds, thickened 6.26
  dysphagia 6.10, 6.15
  'eggshell' calcification of lymph nodes
    4.32
  increased density of hemithorax 4.8
  linitis plastica 6.19
  localized air-space disease 4.16
  malabsorption 6.33
  mammographic changes 10.9, 10.10
  oesophageal strictures 6.15
  oesophageal ulceration 6.13
  orbital hyperostosis 11.10
  protein-losing enteropathy 6.34
  pulmonary calcifications 4.29
  pulmonary oedema 4.17
  pulmonary upper zone fibrosis 4.33
  renal induced hypertension 8.20
  retrorectal space widening 6.44
  scoliosis 2.1
  skull vault lucent lesions 12.4
  small bowel,
    dilatation 6.28
    thickened folds 6.30
  small pituitary fossa 12.22
  spinal mass 2.24
  ventilation perfusion mismatch 13.12
Raynaud's disease: distal phalangeal
    destruction 1.54
Receiver operating characteristic (ROC)
    curves **15**(405)
Rectal prolapse 6.43
Rectosigmoid junction
  abscess 6.43
  anterior indentation **6.43**
  haematoma 6.43
  tumours 6.43
Rectum
  carcinoma: retrorectal space widening
    6.44
  metastases 6.44
  polyps 6.36
  tumours: bone metastases 1.16
Reduplication cyst 14.12
Reflex sympathetic dystrophy syndrome,
    see Sudeck's atrophy
Reflux nephropathy 8.6
  pseudotumour 8.11
  unilateral scarred kidney 8.6
Reflux oesophagitis 6.13
  tertiary oesophageal contractions 6.16
Reiter's syndrome 470–471
  arthritis + bone density preservation
    3.4

arthritis + osteoporosis 3.3
arthritis + periosteal reaction 3.5
arthritis mutilans 3.7
paravertebral ossification 2.13
periosteal reaction 1.36
sacroiliitis, bilateral asymmetrical 3.12
vertebral body squaring 2.8
Reliability 15(404)
Renal, for additional entries beginning, *see*
    Kidney
Renal agenesis 14.8
    raised serum AFP 14.10
Renal anomalies, fetal 14.11, 14.12
    antenatal diagnosis 14.13
    raised serum AFP 14.10
Renal artery
    aneurysm 8.20
        renal calcification 8.2
    arteriosclerosis 8.20
    arteriovenous fistula 8.20
    fibromuscular dysplasia 8.20
    occlusion 8.5
    stenosis 8.20
        unilateral small smooth kidney 8.7
    thrombosis/embolism 8.20
Renal carcinoma, *see* Kidney, carcinoma;
        Renal cell carcinoma; Renal
        tumours
Renal cell carcinoma 8.11, **8.12**
    bone metastases 1.16
    CT lesions,
        focal hyperdense liver 7.14
        focal hypodense 8.13
    cystic 8.14, 8.15
    non-visualization of renal calyx 8.22
    pulmonary metastases 4.25
    renal induced hypertension 8.20
    renal vein thrombosis 8.21
Renal cyst 466, 8.11, **8.14**
    in children 466, 6.6
    CT **8.15**
    haemodialysis related 8.15
    imaging 13.20
    multiple 8.11
    radiolucent filling defect 8.23
Renal dysplasia 8.9, 8.14
    unilateral scarred kidney 8.6
Renal failure
    acute-on-chronic 8.18
    chronic: pulmonary calcifications 4.29
    expanded pituitary fossa 12.23
    intracranial calcification 12.27
    nephrographic pattern 8.18
    oedematous breast 10.10
    pulmonary oedema 4.17
    retarded skeletal maturation 1.1
    soft-tissue calcification 9.5
Renal imaging: cortical defects **13.20**
Renal mass: in newborn and young **8.16**
Renal metastases 8.12, 8.13
    imaging 13.20
Renal osteodystrophy **471**
    bone density increase 1.9

bone scans 13.4
callus formation, excessive 1.15
increased bone density 1.8
osteomalacia/rickets 1.30
rib lesion + soft-tissue mass 4.44
skull vault,
    increased density 12.7
    thickening 12.5
sutures widened 12.20
Renal papillary necrosis 8.2, 8.10, 8.14,
        8.19
    acute 8.10
        nephrogram 8.18
    bilateral small smooth kidneys 8.8
Renal sinus lipomatosis 8.23
Renal tubular acidosis 463
    calcification 8.2
    osteomalacia/rickets 1.30
Renal tubular disease: osteomalacia/rickets
        1.30
Renal tubular necrosis, acute 8.18.8.10
Renal tumours 8.5, 8.11, **8.12**
    focal hypodense CT lesions **8.13**
    hypertension 8.20
    rib metastases 1.50
    spinal metastases 2.2
    see also Kidney, carcinoma; Renal cell
        carcinoma
Renal vein occlusion 8.5
Renal vein thrombosis 8.7, **8.21**
    abdominal mass in neonate 6.5
    hypertension 8.20
    large smooth kidney,
        bilateral 8.10
        unilateral 8.9
    nephrographic pattern 8.18
    in newborn and young 8.16
Respiratory distress
    adult 4.17, 4.45
    neonatal **4.46**
Respiratory papillomatosis: chronic upper
        airway obstruction 4.2
Respiratory tract **4.1–4.54**
Reticuloses
    middle mediastinal mass 4.50
    posterior mediastinal masses 4.51
Reticulum cell sarcoma
    ill-defined lucent medullary lesions 1.21
    lucent bone lesions with calcium/bone
        1.25
    peak age incidence 1.18
    site of origin 1.17
Retinoblastoma
    enlarged optic foramen 11.7
    intraorbital calcification 11.9
    optic nerve enlargement 11.3
Retroperitoneal cystic mass **6.45**
Retroperitoneal cystic tumour 6.45
Retroperitoneal fibrosis **8.26**
    dilated ureter 8.25
    protein-losing enteropathy 6.34
    small bowel, thickened folds 6.30
Retroperitoneal gas 6.1

Retroperitoneal lymphadenopathy
in AIDS 413
in children 415
in lymphoma 448
Retroperitoneal mass
in children 6.6
in neonate 6.5
Retroperitoneal tumours 8.26
gastric indentation 6.17
Retropharyngeal abscess
acute upper airway obstruction 4.1
atlanto-axial subluxation 2.11
Retropharyngeal haemorrhage: acute
upper airway obstruction 4.1
Retroplacental haemorrhage 14.19
Retrorectal space, widening **6.44**
Retrosternal goitre 4.49
'Reversed bat's wing' sign 4.15
Rhabdomyosarcoma
bladder filling defect 8.27
nasopharyngeal mass 11.17
orbital masses, CT 11.2
petrous bone destruction 12.11
unilateral exophthalmos 11.1
Rhesus incompatibility 14.9
thickened placenta 14.20
Rheumatic fever: cardiac calcification 5.8
Rheumatic heart disease: valve
calcification 5.9
Rheumatoid arthritis **472–473**
arthritis + osteoporosis 3.3
arthritis + periosteal reaction 3.5
arthritis mutilans 3.7
atlanto-axial subluxation 2.11
avascular necrosis 1.40
block vertebrae 2.9
carpal fusion 1.56
clavicle, erosion/absence of outer end
1.49
complications **473**
femoral intercondylar notch erosion 3.9
gas in wall of colon 6.38
monoarthritis 3.1
pleural effusion 4.36
protrusio acetabuli 3.13
rib notching 1.52
sacroiliitis, bilateral asymmetrical 3.12
splenomegaly 7.18
subarticular lucent bone lesions 1.24
terminal phalangeal sclerosis, diffuse 3.8
vertebral body squaring 2.8
Rheumatoid lung, honeycomb lung 4.20
Rheumatoid nodules
lung cavities 4.27
pulmonary 4.26
Rib
dysplastic 2.1
focal lesion (solitary/multiple) **1.50**
fractures 4.37, 4.44
bone scans 13.4
chest radiograph 4.45
healed 1.50

non-accidental injury 456
unilateral elevated hemidiaphragm
4.40
lesion + adjacent soft-tissue mass **4.44**
notching,
inferior surface **1.51**
superior surface **1.52**
resection 4.8
'Ribbon ribs' 1.51
Rickets **474**, **1.30**
basilar invagination 12.13
craniostenosis 12.15
metaphyseal bands, radiolucent/dense
1.42
metaphyses,
cupping 1.46
fraying 1.45
neonatal 1.30
non-accidental injury vs. 1.37
periosteal reaction 1.35
protrusio acetabuli 3.13
renal osteodystrophy 471
retarded skeletal maturation 1.1
sutures widened 12.20
vitamin D dependent 1.30
Rickettsial infections: splenomegaly 7.18
Riedel's lobe 7.5
Riedel's thyroiditis 13.9
Right atrium
enlarged **5.3**
myxoma 5.3
Right heart obstruction 4.6
Right-to-left shunts 4.6
Right ventricle
enlarged **5.4**
failure: enlarged right atrium 5.3
'Rind' sign 434
Ring shadows in child **4.47**
Rokitansky–Aschoff sinuses 7.2
Rubella
cardiovascular involvement 5.19
congenital 1.44, 14.9
dense vertical metaphyseal lines 1.44
fetal hydrops 14.9
intracranial calcification 12.27
renal induced hypertension 8.20
'Rugger jersey' spine 463
Russell–Silver dwarfism: asymmetrical
maturation of bone 1.4

Sacral agenesis 6.7
Sacral meningocoele, anterior 2.18, 6.44
Sacral tumours: retrorectal space widening
6.44
Sacrococcageal teratoma: fetal hydrops
14.9
Sacroiliitis **3.12**
bilateral asymmetrical **3.12**
bilateral symmetrical **3.12**
Sacrum, anterior scalloping **2.18**
Saethre–Chotzen syndrome 12.15

Salmonella infections: toxic megacolon 6.39
Sanfilippo's syndrome 1.7
Sarcoid granuloma: bronchial stenosis/ occlusion 4.7
Sarcoidosis 475–477
  bone 476–477
  'eggshell' calcification of lymph nodes 475, 4.32
  gallium uptake 13.7
  hepatic/gastrointestinal 476
  hilar enlargement,
    bilateral 4.31
    unilateral 4.30
  honeycomb lung 4.20
  intrathoracic 475
  joint 476
  Kerley B lines 4.19
  low density CT liver 7.17
  lung cavities 4.27
  middle mediastinal mass 4.50
  myocardial perfusion imaging 13.13
  neurologic 476
  ocular 476
  parathyroid imaging 13.10
  phalangeal destruction, distal 1.54
  pulmonary opacities 475, 4.23
  pulmonary upper zone fibrosis 4.33
  renal calcification 8.2
  renal calculi 8.3
  skin 475
  skull vault 12.1
    lucent lesions 12.4
  soft-tissue calcification 9.5
  splenomegaly 7.18
  surface enhancement of brain 12.31
  terminal phalangeal sclerosis, diffuse 3.8
  widespread air-space disease 4.15
Scaphocephaly 12.15
Schatzki ring 6.10
Scheie's syndrome 1.7
Scheuermann's disease: vertebral collapse 2.3
Schistosomiasis
  bilateral hypertransradiant hemithoraces 4.6
  bladder calcification 8.28
  bladder filling defect 8.27
  colonic polyps 6.36
  colonic strictures 6.37
  dilated ureter 8.25
  periportal hyperechoic ultrasound 7.12
  pulmonary arteries enlarged 5.1
  seminal vesicle/vas deferens calcification 8.31
  'thumbprinting' in colon 6.41
Schmincke's tumour: hypertrophic osteoarthropathy 1.34
Schmorl's nodes 2.3
Scleroderma 478
  arthritis + osteoporosis 3.3
  avascular necrosis 1.40

distal phalangeal destruction 1.54
duodenal folds, decreased/absent 6.25
duodenum, dilated 6.27
dysphagia 6.10
gallium uptake 13.7
gas in wall of colon 6.38
honeycomb lung 4.20
malabsorption 6.33
oesophageal strictures 6.14
pneumonia, slowly resolving/recurrent 4.10
renal induced hypertension 8.20
rib notching 1.52
small bowel dilatation 6.28
soft-tissue calcification 9.3, 9.5
teeth, loss of lamina dura 11.16
terminal phalangeal sclerosis, diffuse 3.8
Sclerosing adenosis 10.3
Sclerosing osteomyelitis of Garré 1.10
Sclerosteosis 1.8, 12.6
Scoliosis 2.1
  congenital 2.1
  hemidiaphragm, unilateral elevated 4.40
  idiopathic 2.1
  loss of renal outline 8.1
  painful 2.1
  unilateral hypertransradiant hemithorax 4.5
Scorpion venom: distal phalangeal destruction 1.54
Scurvy 479
  cupping of metaphyses 1.46
  metaphyseal band, solitary radiolucent 1.41
  non-accidental injury vs. 1.37
  osteoporosis 1.29
  periosteal reaction 1.35
Sebaceous cyst
  breast 10.5, 10.7
  calcified 12.26
  skull vault 12.8
Sella
  empty 12.23
  erosion 12.25
  J-shaped 12.24
  osteoporosis 12.25
  see also entries beginning Parasellar
Seminal vesicles, calcification 8.31
Seminoma
  anterior mediastinal mass 4.49
  pulmonary metastases 4.25
Sensitivity 15(404)
Septal (Kerley B) lines 4.19
Sexual precocity: accelerated skeletal maturation 1.2
Shock lung, see Adult respiratory distress syndrome
Short rib polydactyly syndromes 1.6, 14.13
'Shoulder sign' 6.21
Sickle-cell anaemia 480
  avascular necrosis 1.40

Sickle-cell anaemia (*cont.*)
  bilateral large smooth kidneys 8.10
  'hair-on-end' skull vault 480, 12.14
  premature closure of growth plate 1.3
  renal papillary necrosis 8.19
  short metacarpal/metatarsal 1.55
  splenic calcification 7.19
  vertebral collapse 2.3
Sickle-cell dactylitis (Hand–foot syndrome)
    480, 1.36
Siderosis 4.21
  pulmonary opacities 4.23
Silicoproteinosis 481
Silicosis 481–482, 4.21
  complicated 481–482
    see also Progressive massive fibrosis
      (PMF)
  complications 482
  'eggshell' calcification of lymph nodes
    4.32
  hilar enlargement, bilateral 4.31
  pleural calcification 4.42
  pulmonary calcifications, multiple 4.29
  pulmonary opacities 4.22, 4.23
  simple 481
Simple bone cyst, *see* Bone cyst
Sinus, small/absent 11.11
Sinusitis 11.13
  in AIDS 415
  brain isotope angiogram 13.11
  chronic: pneumonia 4.10
  in cystic fibrosis 430
  infection localization 13.6
Sinus venosus defect 5.14
Sipple's syndrome 451
Sjögren's syndrome: rib notching 1.52
Skeletal dysplasia 1.5
  antenatal diagnosis 14.13
  bone density increase, generalized 1.8
  fetal hydrops 14.9
  see also Bone dysplasia
Skeletal injuries, non-accidental 456–457
Skeletal maturation
  generalized accelerated 1.2
  retarded 1.1
Skeletal metastases, *see* Bone metastases
Skin disorders
  dysphagia 6.10
  oesophageal strictures 6.14
Skin tumours: bone metastases 1.16
Skull 12.1–12.20
  fractures: non-accidental injury 456
  increased density, bone dysplasia +
    12.6
Skull base
  increased density 12.9
  metastases 12.9, 12.12
  primary neoplasms 12.12
Skull vault
  defective ossification 12.17
  density increase,
    generalized 12.7

  localized 12.8
  depressed fracture 12.8
  generalized thickening in children 12.5
  'hair-on-end', *see* 'Hair-on-end'
  lucency,
    adult 12.1
    child 12.2
    multiple lesions 12.4
    + surrounding sclerosis 12.3
  metastases 12.1, 12.2, 12.4, 12.7, 12.8
  neoplasms 12.8
  non-homogeneous sclerosis 12.5
Sly's syndrome 1.7
Small bowel, *see* Bowel, small
Small left colon syndrome 6.7
Snake venom
  distal phalangeal destruction 1.54
  pulmonary oedema 4.17
Soft tissues 9.1–9.7
  bone scans, increased uptake 13.2
  conglomerate calcification 9.3
  linear/curvilinear calcification 9.2
  opacity, mammography 10.5
  ossification 9.6
  periarticular calcification 9.5
  prevertebral mass in cervical region
    11.18
  'sheets' of calcification/ossification 9.4
  tumours,
    increased uptake on bone scans 13.2
    skull vault density increase 12.8
Solitary sclerotic bone lesions 1.10
Soto's syndrome (cerebral gigantism)
  accelerated skeletal maturation 1.2
  large head 12.19
Space-occupying lesion
  raised intracranial pressure 12.18
  wide sutures 12.20
Specificity 15(404)
Sphenoid carcinoma 11.7, 11.17
Sphenoid dysplasia 11.6, 12.24
Sphenoid mucocoele 11.7
Sphenoid wing, metastases 11.8
Spherocytosis, hereditary: 'hair-on-end'
  skull vault 12.14
Sphincter of Oddi, incompetence 7.3
Spina bifida
  antenatal diagnosis 14.13
  megacolon 6.40
  photopenic area on bone scan 13.3
  raised serum AFP 14.10
Spinal abscess: extradural spinal mass
  2.22
Spinal block 2.21
Spinal canal
  narrow 2.19
  tumour: vertebral body scalloping 2.16
Spinal cord
  contusion 2.24
  trauma 4.45
Spinal mass
  extradural 2.22

intradural,
    extramedullary **2.23**
    intramedullary **2.24**
    see also Intraspinal mass
Spinal metastases, solitary 2.2
Spinal muscular atrophy: scoliosis
    2.1
Spine **2.1–2.24**
    bony outgrowths **2.13**
    dwarfing skeletal dysplasia 1.5
    fracture 2.3, 4.45
    infection,
        ivory vertebral body 2.10
        scoliosis 2.1
        spinal block 2.21
        vertebral collapse 2.2, 2.3
    operative fusion 2.12
    wedge fractures 2.3
Spleen
    accessory 7.23
    amyloid infiltration 13.17
    cyst 7.19
    imaging **13.17**
    vascular occlusion 13.17
Splenectomy 13.17
Splenic abscess: unilateral elevated
    hemidiaphragm 4.40
Splenic artery atherosclerosis 7.19
Splenic calcification **7.19**
Splenic flexure
    gaseous distension 4.40
    ischaemia 6.37
Splenic haematoma, in neonate 6.5
Splenic lobulation 7.23
Splenomegaly **7.18**
    gastric indentation 6.17
Splenunculus 13.17
Spondylitis
    vertebral collapse 2.3
    see also Tuberculosis, spondylitis
Spondyloarthritis 428
Spondyloepiphyseal dysplasia: dwarfing
    skeletal dysplasia 1.5
Spondyloepiphyseal dysplasia congenita
    14.13
    platyspondyly 2.4
Spondyloepiphyseal dysplasia tarda:
    platyspondyly 2.4
Spondylometaphyseal dysplasia: dwarfing
    skeletal dysplasia 1.5
Spondylosis
    intervertebral disc calcification 2.12
    vertebral pedicle, dense 2.6
Spondylo–epiphyseal dysplasia: atlanto-
    axial subluxation 2.11
Sprengel's shoulder 2.9
Spring water cyst 4.39, 4.49
Sprue: protein-losing enteropathy 6.34
Squamous cell carcinoma
    bladder 8.28
    bone metastases 1.16
    kidney 8.12, 8.23

'Stacked coin' appearance 6.26, 6.30
Stagnant loop syndrome 6.33
Stannosis 4.21
    pulmonary opacities 4.22, 4.23
Staphylococcus aureus
    lobar pneumonia 4.12
    lung cavities 4.27
    monoarthritis 3.1
    pneumatocoeles 4.9
    pulmonary nodules, multiple 4.26
Statistics **15**(404)
Sternal fracture 4.45
Sternal metastases 4.49
Sternal tumours 4.49
Steroid therapy 455
    avascular necrosis 1.40
    CT mediastinal mass containing fat
        4.52
    excessive callus formation 1.15
    gas in the wall of the colon 6.38
    infection localization 13.6
    osteoporosis 1.29
    pneumonia, slowly resolving/recurrent
        4.10
    retarded skeletal maturation 1.1
Stomach
    abnormality + thickened small bowel
        folds 6.31
    'bull's eye' (target) lesions 6.17, **6.22**
    carcinoma 6.17, 6.18
        gastrocolic fistula 6.20
        haematemesis 6.9
        linitis plastica 6.19
        protein-losing enteropathy 6.34
        thick gastric folds 6.18
    corrosive injury 6.19
    dilatation **6.21**
        acute, gas in portal veins 7.4
    erosions, haematemesis 6.9
    fibrosis 6.21
    filling defects **6.17**
    gaseous distension 4.40
    gas in wall **6.23**
    heterotopic mucosa 6.24
    leiomyoma 447, 6.17, 6.22
    lipoma 6.17
    lymphoma 6.17, 6.18, 6.22
        linitis plastica 6.19
    masses **6.17**
    metastases 6.17
        gastrocolic fistula 6.20
        linitis plastica 6.19
        submucosal 6.17, 6.22
    mucosa, ectopic 13.22
    neurofibroma 6.17, 6.22
    obstruction 6.21
        at cardia 6.16
    polyps 6.17
    pseudolymphoma 6.18
    radiotherapy injury 6.19
    thick folds **6.18**
    tumours **6.17**

Stomach tumours *(cont.)*
  bone metastases 1.16
    gastric dilatation 6.21
    submucosal 6.17
  ulcer, *see* Peptic ulcer
  see also entries beginning Gastric,
    Gastrointestinal
Storage diseases
  large head 12.19
  see also individual storage diseases
Streptococcus pneumoniae
  lobar pneumonia 4.12
  lung consolidation + bulging of fissures
    4.13
  pneumatocoeles 4.9
Streptococcus pyogenes 4.12
Stress response: claw osteophytes 2.13
'String sign' 6.21
Strongyloides
  duodenal folds,
    decreased/absent 6.25
    thickened 6.26
  malabsorption 6.33
  non-dilated small bowel, thickened folds
    6.31
Sturge–Weber syndrome 12.26
Subamniotic haemorrhage 14.19
Subarachnoid haemorrhage 12.18
Subchorionic haemorrhage 14.19
Subclavian artery
  aberrant right 6.10, 6.11
  puncture 5.20
Subclavian obstruction: rib notching 1.51
Subclavian vein catheterization,
  complications 5.20
Subdural haematoma 12.19
  brain isotope angiogram 13.11
  calcification 12.26
  non-accidental injury 457
Subglottic haemangioma 4.2
Subphrenic abscess
  colloid liver scan 13.15
  hemidiaphragm,
    bilateral elevated 4.41
    unilateral elevated 4.40
  pleural effusion 4.34, 4.35
  right sided diaphragmatic humps 4.39
Subphrenic inflammatory disease 4.40
Subpleural haematoma 4.44
Subpulmonary effusion 4.40, 4.41
Subungual exostosis: distal phalangeal
  destruction 1.54
Sudeck's atrophy (reflex sympathetic
  dystrophy syndrome) 1.27
Sunray spiculation 7.6, 12.20
Superior mesenteric artery (SMA) 6.8
Superior mesenteric artery (SMA)
  syndrome: dilated duodenum
    6.27
Superior mesenteric vein (SMV) 6.8
Superior orbital fissure, enlargement 11.7,
    11.8

Superior sagittal sinus thrombosis 12.18
Superior vena cava
  enlarged **5.13**
    obstruction 5.14
    rib notching 1.51
Super scan 13.1
Supraglottic carcinoma of larynx 4.3
Supraspinatus tendinitis 9.2
Symphalangism, carpal fusion 1.56
Symphysis pubis
  fusion/bridging **3.15**
  widening **3.14**
Syndesmophytes 2.13
Synovial osteochondromatosis 9.5
  calcified loose body 2.22
Synovioma: soft-tissue calcification 9.5
Synovitis
  enteropathic 428
  pigmented villonodular, *see* Pigmented
    villonodular synovitis
Syphilis
  aortic valve calcification 5.9
  bone sclerosis + periosteal reaction
    1.12
  congenital,
    non-accidental injury vs. 1.37
    periosteal reaction 1.35
    solitary radiolucent metaphyseal band
      1.41
  fetal hydrops 14.9
  optic nerve enlargement 11.3
  periosteal reactions 1.31
  renal induced hypertension 8.20
  seminal vesicle/vas deferens calcification
    8.31
  skull vault 12.1
Syringomyelia 455
  distal phalangeal destruction 1.54
  intradural spinal mass 2.24
  vertebral body scalloping 2.16
Systemic lupus erythematosus **483**
  arthritis + osteoporosis 3.3
  atlanto-axial subluxation 2.11
  avascular necrosis 1.40
  bilateral large smooth kidneys 8.10
  drug-induced lung disease 4.48
  gallium uptake 13.7
  pleural effusion 4.36
  renal induced hypertension 8.20
  rib notching 1.52
  splenomegaly 7.18
  terminal phalangeal sclerosis, diffuse 3.8
  ventilation perfusion mismatch 13.12

Tabes dorsalis 455
Tachycardia, fetal 14.13
Tachypnoea of newborn, transient 4.46
Takayasu's disease: renal induced
    hypertension 8.20
Talc
  pleural calcification 4.42
  pneumoconiosis 4.21

Tamponade: subclavian vein
    catheterization 5.20
Tapeworm: thickened duodenal folds 6.26
Teeth
  'floating' 439, **11.15**, 12.2
  loss of lamina dura **11.16**
Telangiectasia: gastrointestinal bleeding
    localization 13.21
Temporal bone, petrous part
  destruction,
    apex **12.10**
    middle ear **12.11**
  metastases 12.10
Temporomandibular joint, articular fossa,
    destruction 12.11
Tendinitis
  calcific 13.2
  soft-tissue calcification 9.2
  supraspinatus 9.2
Teratodermoid: CT mediastinal cyst 4.53
Teratoma
  abdominal mass,
    in child 6.6
    in neonate 6.5
  anterior mediastinal mass 4.49
  cerebral, calcified 12.26
  CT mediastinal cyst 4.53
  CT mesenteric cystic lesion 6.46
  intracranial, calcification 12.30
  ovarian 6.6, 14.27
  prevertebral soft-tissue mass 11.18
  sacrococcygeal 6.40, 6.44
  of testis: gynaecomastia 9.1
Testicular feminization: gynaecomastia 9.1
Testicular hypogonadism 1.29
Testicular teratoma 6.45, 9.1
Testis
  teratoma: gynaecomastia 9.1
  tumours: bone metastases 1.16
Tetradermoid 4.52
Thalassaemia 484
  craniostenosis 12.15
  fetal hydrops 14.9
  'hair-on-end' skull vault 12.14
Thallium imaging 13.13
Thanatophoric dwarfism, *see* Dwarfism
Theca–lutein cysts 14.22
Thermal injuries
  distal phalangeal destruction 1.54
  premature closure of growth plate 1.3
Thoracentesis 4.17
  pulmonary oedema 4.18
Thoracic cage, abnormal 4.46
Thoracic duct obstruction: pleural effusion
    4.34
Thoracic dysplasia, asphyxiating, *see*
    Asphyxiating thoracicdysplasia of
    Jeune
Thoracic mass: fetal hydrops 14.9
Thoracolumbar junction: abscess 2.22
Thoracotomy: unilateral elevated
    hemidiaphragm 4.40

Thorotrast 7.6, 7.19
Thromboangiitis obliterans 8.20
Thromboembolism
  pulmonary arteries enlarged 5.15
  unilateral pulmonary oedema 4.18
  see also individual thromboembolic
    disease
Thymic cyst, CT mediastinal cyst 4.53
Thymic hyperplasia 4.54
Thymic mass, CT **4.54**
Thymic tumours 4.49
Thymolipoma 4.54
  CT mediastinal mass containing fat
Thymoma 4.54
Thymus
  anterior mediastinal mass 4.49
  enlargement 4.49
Thyroid acropachy: periosteal reaction
    1.33
Thyroid Binding Globulin 13.8
Thyroid gland
  abscess 13.9
  adenoma, imaging 13.9
  carcinoma 13.9
    chronic upper airway obstruction 4.3
  ectopic 13.9
  ectopic hormone production 13.9
  imaging, photopenic (cold) areas **13.9**
  nodules 13.10
  tumours,
    bone metastases 1.16
    spinal metastases 2.2
Thyroiditis 13.9
Thyrotoxicosis: enlarged pulmonary
    arteries 5.15
Tolosa Hunt syndrome 12.12
Tonsils, grossly enlarged: upper airway
    obstruction 4.2
TORCH complex 7.7
Torulosis
  intracranial calcification 12.27
  pulmonary opacities 4.23
  surface enhancement of brain 12.31
Total anomalous pulmonary venous
    drainage (TAPVD)
  neonatal cyanosis 5.18
  neonatal pulmonary venous congestion
    5.17
  pulmonary veins enlarged 5.16
  right atrium enlarged 5.3
  superior vena cava enlarged 5.13
'Tower-shaped' skull 12.15
Toxic megacolon, *see* Megacolon
Toxoplasmosis
  in AIDS 413
  basal ganglia calcification 12.29
  fetal hydrops 14.9
  intracranial calcification 12.27
  optic nerve enlargement 11.3
Trachea
  intubation: upper airway obstruction
    4.2, 4.3

Trachea (*cont.*)
  laceration/fracture 4.45
  malignancy: upper airway obstruction 4.3
  perforation: pneumomediastinum 4.38
  stenosis: bilateral hypertransradiant hemithoraces 4.6
Tracheomalacia: upper airway obstruction 4.2
Tracheo-oesophageal fistula 4.2
  'H'-type 4.10
Traction diverticulum 6.12
Traction spurs 2.13
Transfusion reaction: pulmonary oedema 4.17
Transient tachypnoea of newborn 4.46
Transitional cell carcinoma
  bladder 8.27, 8.28
  bone metastases 1.16
  renal 8.12, 8.23
    CT lesions 8.13
Transplant, renal: rejection 8.2, 13.6
Transposition of great arteries
  neonatal cyanosis 5.18
  right-sided aortic arch 5.12
  small aortic arch 5.11
Trapezium–trapezoid fusion 1.56
Trauma
  chest, *see* Chest, trauma
  cupping of metaphyses 1.46
  non-accidental injury vs. 1.37
  premature closure of growth plate 1.3
Tricuspid atresia 5.3
  left atrium enlarged 5.5
  neonatal cyanosis 5.18
  right-sided aortic arch 5.12
Tricuspid incompetence
  right atrium enlarged 5.3
  superior vena cava enlarged 5.13
Tricuspid regurgitation, isolated, calcification 5.9
Tricuspid stenosis
  enlarged right atrium 5.3
  hepatomegaly 7.5
Tricuspid valve calcification 5.9
Trigonocephaly 12.15
Triphyllocephaly 12.15
Triploidy 14.22
  fetal hydrops 14.9
  thickened placenta 14.20
Triquetral–lunate fusion 1.56
Trisomies: fetal hydrops 14.9
Trisomy 13
  cardiovascular involvement 5.19
  osteoporosis 1.29
  renal cysts 8.14
Trisomy 18
  cardiovascular involvement 5.19
  irregular/stippled epiphyses 1.39
  osteoporosis 1.29
  renal cysts 8.14
  retarded skeletal maturation 1.1

Trisomy 21, *see* Down's syndrome
Trophoblastic tumour, metastatic 4.6
Tropical sprue 6.33
  dilated small bowel 6.28
  protein-losing enteropathy 6.34
Tropical ulcer: periosteal reactions 1.31
Truncus arteriosus
  neonatal cyanosis 5.18
  right-sided aortic arch 5.12
Trypanosomiasis: hepatomegaly 7.5
Tuberculoma
  calcification 12.26
  CT 12.33, 12.34
  intracranial calcification 12.27
  pulmonary nodules, solitary 4.25
Tuberculosis
  adrenal calcification 7.22
  arthritis,
    femoral intercondylar notch erosion 3.9
    monoarthritis 3.1
  ascites 6.4
  bladder calcification 8.28
  colonic strictures 6.37
  dilated ureter 8.25
  gastrocolic fistula 6.20
  granuloma, focal hyperdense CT lesion 7.14
  hepatic calcification 7.6
  ileal lesions 6.35
  kidney,
    calcification 8.2
    cysts 8.14
    non-visualization of calyx 8.22
    non-visualization during excretion urography 8.5
    unilateral scarred 8.6
  linitis plastica 6.19
  lung cavities 4.27
  miliary: pulmonary opacities 4.23
  optic nerve enlargement 11.3
  osteitis: rib lesion + soft-tissue mass 4.44
  pedicle erosion/destruction/absence 2.5
  periosteal reactions 1.31
  petrous bone destruction 12.11
  pneumonia 4.15
    slowly resolving/recurrent 4.10
  primary,
    bilateral hilar enlargement 4.31
    hilar lymph-node enlargement 4.11
    lobar pneumonia 4.12
    pleural effusion 4.36
    pneumonia + enlarged hilum 4.11
    unilateral hilar enlargement 4.30
  pulmonary,
    pneumonia 4.10
    upper zone fibrosis 4.33
  pulmonary calcification 4.29
    multiple 4.29
  renal induced hypertension 8.20
  seminal vesicle/vas deferens calcification 8.31

skull vault 12.1
small bowel, thickened folds 6.31
soft-tissue calcification 9.3
spinal mass, extradural 2.22
splenic calcification 7.19
splenomegaly 7.18
spondylitis,
    vertebral bodies scalloping 2.17
    vertebral collapse 2.3
subarticular lucent bone lesions 1.24
ventilation perfusion mismatch 13.12
vertebrae, block 2.9
widespread air-space disease 4.15
Tuberous sclerosis 484–485, 12.27
    basal ganglia calcification 12.29
    cardiovascular involvement 5.19
    honeycomb lung 4.20
    intracranial calcification 12.27
    multiple sclerotic bone lesions 1.11
    renal cysts 8.14
Tubulovillous adenoma 6.36
Tumoral calcinosis 9.5
Turcot's syndrome: colonic polyps 6.36
Turner's syndrome 486
    cardiovascular involvement 5.19
    carpal fusion 1.56
    fetal hydrops 14.9
    Madelung deformity 1.57
    osteoporosis 1.29
    retarded skeletal maturation 1.1
    short metacarpals 1.55
Turricephaly 12.15
Twin pregnancies
    fetal hydrops 14.9
    placenta and membranes in 14.17
    raised serum AFP 14.10
Tylosis: oesophageal strictures 6.10,
    6.15
Typhoid
    small bowel nodules 6.32
    splenomegaly 7.18
Typhus, splenomegaly 7.18

Ulcerative colitis 487
    colonic polyps 6.36
    colonic strictures 6.37
    complications 487
    hypertrophic osteoarthropathy 1.34
    ileal lesions 6.35
    infection localization 13.6
    protein-losing enteropathy 6.34
    retrorectal space widening 6.44
    sacroiliitis, bilateral symmetrical 3.12
    'thumbprinting' in colon 487, 6.41
    toxic megacolon 487, 6.39
Ultrasound
    breast disease 10.11
    liver,
        focal hyperechoic 7.10
        focal hypoechoic 7.11
        generalized hyperechoic 7.9

        generalized hypoechoic 7.8
        periportal hyperechoic 7.12
    obstetric and gynaecological 14.1–

        in first trimester 14.3
        measurements for dating 14.1
        normal pregnancy 14.2
Umbilical artery, single + structural
    anomaly 14.11
Umbilical vein catheterization: gas in
    portal veins 7.4
Upper airway obstruction
    acute 4.1
    chronic,
        in adults 4.3
        in child 4.2
    neonatal respiratory distress 4.46
    see also Obstructive airways disease
Urachus, patent 8.29
Uraemia: cardiac calcification 5.8
Urate nephropathy 436, 8.10
Ureter
    calculus 8.25
    dilated 8.25
    gas in 8.4
    medially placed 8.26
    megaureter 8.25
    obstruction 8.25, 8.26
        nephrogram 8.18
    retrocaval 8.25, 8.26
    stricture 8.25
Ureteric artery collaterals 8.23
Ureteric diversion 8.4
Ureterocoele 8.25, 8.27
    ectopic 6.5, 8.30
Ureterovesical obstruction: hydronephrosis
    in child 8.17
Urethra
    foreign body, calculus 8.30
    stricture 8.30
Urethral diverticulum, anterior 8.30
Urethral valves, posterior 8.30
    abdominal mass in neonate 6.5
Urinary tract 8.1–8.29
    gas in 6.1, 8.4
    infection,
        dilated ureter 8.25
        hydronephrosis in child 8.17
        seminal vesicle/vas deferens
            calcification 8.31
    obstruction 8.14
Urine, extravasation 8.26
Urogenital anomalies: symphysis pubis
    widening 3.14
Urolithiasis 436
Uropathy, chronic obstructive 8.5
Uterus
    carcinoma: bone metastases 1.16
    enlarged 14.25
    normal ultrasound 14.23
    sarcoma 14.25
Uveoparotid fever 477

Vaginal stenosis 6.5
Vagotomy
  paralytic ileus after 6.21
  small bowel dilatation after 6.28
van Buchem's disease 12.6
Varicella: multiple pulmonary
  calcifications 4.29
Vascular insufficiency: periosteal reactions
  1.33
Vascular occlusion: premature closure of
  growth plate 1.3
Vasculitis
  pulmonary arteries enlarged 5.1
  right ventricle enlarged 5.4
  small bowel thickened folds 6.30
  splenic imaging 13.17
  ventilation perfusion mismatch 13.12
Vas deferens, calcification 8.31
Vasoconstriction, peripheral arterial 5.15
Venous insufficiency: periosteal reactions
  1.33
Venous obstruction
  duodenal folds thickened 6.26
  oedematous breast 10.10
  protein-losing enteropathy 6.34
  small bowel thickened folds 6.30
Venous pressure, raised 7.5
Ventilation, artificial: pneumomediastinum
  4.38
Ventilation perfusion mismatch 470,
  13.12
Ventricle
  single: neonatal cyanosis 5.18
  see also Left ventricle; Right ventricle
Ventricular aneurysm 5.7
Ventricular septal defect (VSD)
  left atrium enlarged 5.5
  left ventricle enlarged 5.6
  neonatal cyanosis 5.18
  right-sided aortic arch 5.12
  right ventricle enlarged 5.4
Vertebrae
  anterior body beaks **2.15**
  anterior scalloping of body **2.17**
  block **2.9**
    scoliosis 2.1
  body enlarged **2.7**
  bony outgrowths of spine **2.13**
  butterfly: scoliosis 2.1
  collapsed,
    multiple **2.3**
    solitary **2.2**
  coronal cleft bodies **2.14**
  intervertebral disc calcification **2.12**
  ivory body **2.10**
  operative fusion 2.9
  pedicle,
    congenital absence 2.5
    erosion/destruction/absence **2.5**
    solitary dense **2.6**
  'picture frame' body 2.22

posterior element absent/hypoplastic 2.6
posterior scalloping of body **2.16**
squaring of body/bodies **2.8**
wedge: scoliosis 2.1
widened interpedicular distance **2.20**
Vertebra plana 2.4
Vertebrobasilar aneurysm 12.12
Vesico-intestinal fistula 8.4
Vesico-ureteric reflux 8.17, 8.25
Villous adenoma of intestine 6.34, 6.36
VIPoma 451
Viral infection
  bilateral hilar enlargement 4.31
  hepatomegaly 7.5
  oesophageal ulceration 6.13
  pleural effusion 4.36
  pnemonia 4.15
  pneumonia + enlarged hilum 4.11
  see also individual infections
Vitamin C deficiency, *see* Scurvy
Vitamin D deficiency: osteomalacia/rickets
  1.30
Vocal cord paralysis: upper airway
  obstruction 4.3
Volvulus
  fetal hydrops 14.9
  gasless abdomen 6.3
  gastric dilatation 6.21
  in neonate 6.7
Vomiting: gasless abdomen 6.3
von Hippel–Lindau syndrome
  CT renal cysts 8.15
  focal hypodense CT liver lesion 7.13
  retroperitoneal cystic mass 6.45
Von Recklinghausen's disease 453
  see also Neurofibromatosis
Voorhoeve's disease (osteopathia striata)
  1.11

Waldenström's macroglobulinaemia 6.32
Warfarin embryopathy: irregular/stippled
  epiphyses 1.39
'Water lily' sign 4.25, 4.26
Waterston shunt 4.18
Weaver syndrome: accelerated skeletal
  maturation 1.2
Wegener's granulomatosis
  bilateral large smooth kidneys 8.10
  lung cavities 4.27
  maxillary antrum 11.12, 11.13
  pulmonary nodules multiple 4.26
Werner's syndrome 451
  soft-tissue calcification 9.2
Whipple's disease
  duodenal folds thickened 6.26
  hypertrophic osteoarthropathy 1.34
  malabsorption 6.33
  protein-losing enteropathy 6.34
  sacroiliitis, bilateral symmetrical 3.12
  small bowel,
    multiple nodules 6.32

thickened folds 6.31
Williams–Campbell syndrome:
  bronchiectasis 4.14
Wilms' tumour 8.12
  abdominal mass 6.5, 6.6
  bone metastases 1.16
  non-visualization of renal calyx 8.22
  renal bulge 8.11
  renal imaging 13.20
  renal induced hypertension 8.20
Wilson's disease: chondrocalcinosis 3.11
Wimberger's sign 479
Wolman's disease: adrenal calcification
  7.22
Wormian bones 424, 12.7, **12.16**
Wrists, chronic stress in 1.45

Xanthogranulomatous pyelonephritis 8.5
  CT renal lesions 8.13
  hypertension 8.20

renal calcification 8.2
Xeromammography 10.13
X-linked hypophosphataemia:
  osteomalacia/rickets 1.30

Yersinia enterocolitis
  aphthous ulcers 6.42
  ileal lesions 6.35
  small bowel nodules 6.32
Yersinia pestis: lung consolidation +
  bulging of fissures 4.13

Zenker's diverticulum 6.12
Zollinger–Ellison syndrome 451
  duodenal folds thickened 6.26
  gastric folds thickened 6.18
  non-dilated small bowel, thickened folds
  6.31
  small bowel dilatation 6.28

Notes

Notes

Notes